PHYSIOTHERAPY IN
MUSCULOSKELETAL CONDITIONS

PHYSIOTHERAPY IN
MUSCULOSKELETAL CONDITIONS

Shweta Aggarwal

PEEPEE
PUBLISHERS AND DISTRIBUTORS (P) LTD.

Physiotherapy in Musculoskeletal Conditions

Published by
Pawaninder P. Vij and Anupam Vij
Peepee Publishers and Distributors (P) Ltd.
Head Office: 160, Shakti Vihar, Pitam Pura
Delhi-110034 (India)

Correspondence Address: **7/31, First Floor, Ansari Road**
Daryaganj, New Delhi-110002 (India)
Ph: 65195868, 23246245, 9811156083
e-mail: peepee160@yahoo.co.in
e-mail: peepee160@rediffmail.com
e-mail: peepee160@gmail.com
www.peepeepub.com

First Edition : 2015

ISBN: 978-81-8445-170-2

This book is dedicated to my mother,
who I know will always be my strength and
supports me from
wherever she is.

Preface

Physiotherapy is an integral part of rehabilitation of patients with musculoskeletal disorders in order to restore the full functions at the earliest and re-integrate the patient to daily routine.

As a Musculoskeletal Physiotherapist, I have tried to line out the basic clinical conditions dealt in clinical practice with relevant signs and symptoms, diagnostic criteria and orthopaedic management. The physiotherapeutic intervention has been explained in a detailed manner related to both conservative and surgical management of the conditions. Many of the treatment facts and schedules are based on the latest studies and research guidelines. Musculoskeletal physiotherapy is a vast subject and I have tried to cover the majority of topics, although I know there are still important topics that are left out which will be covered in next edition if given a chance.

The book will hopefully provide a good amount of knowledge and guidance to the students of physiotherapy and practising physiotherapists.

Any criticism and suggestion to improve the value of the book will be most welcome and highly appreciated. I have made all possible attempts to keep the mistakes to minimum but if you find any mistakes or need any clarification you can mail me at shweta.isic@gmail.com.

Shweta Aggarwal

Preface

Acknowledgements

This book is a result of constant encouragement from my husband and mother-in-law who always wants to see me at the highest peaks in my life shining as a star.

I cannot forget to mention my mentor Ms. Shallu Sharma whose continuous guidance and encouragement throughout my postgraduation and after has build up the confidence and a better Physiotherapist in me.

Special thanks to Mr. C.S. Ram who encouraged me to initiate this work under his guidance and to the publishing team for making this book a reality.

Long list of thanks to family and friends for their constant encouragement and appreciation.

Contents

UNIT ONE

FRACTURES AND DISLOCATIONS

CHAPTER 1

INTRODUCTION TO FRACTURES

DEFINITION OF FRACTURE

Fracture is defined as a break in the continuity of the bone which may either be complete, incomplete or a crack.

CLASSIFICATION OF FRACTURES

Fractures are classified clinically on the basis of the causative factors. They are categorized into following categories:
- Traumatic fractures.
- Fatigue fractures.
- Pathological fractures.
- Greenstick fractures.

Traumatic Fractures

A normal healthy bone can withstand a great amount of pressure, so a tremendous amount of force with greater momentum is required to produce a break in the bone. These are the most common type of fracture seen in day-to-day life. The fracture is caused by trauma to the bone previously free from the disease. The traumatic force could either be:
- Direct violence.
- Indirect violence.

The fractures caused by trauma are further classified on the basis of displacement and relationship with external environment.

On the Basis of Displacement

- *Displaced fractures*: The fractured fragments are displaced from their anatomical position either due to gravity, muscle pull or fracturing force.
- *Undisplaced fractures:* The fractured fragments are not displaced from their anatomical positions.

On the Basis Of Relationship with External Environment (Fig. 1.1)

- *Closed fractures:* This type of fracture is also known as simple fracture. The fractured fragments have no communication with the external environment. There is no obvious external injury at the fractured site i.e. overlying soft tissue and skin are intact.
- *Open fractures:* This type of fracture is also known as compound fracture. In this type of fracture the fractured fragments communicate with the external environment. The overlying skin and soft tissue are injured and the fractured fragments are visible. These types of fractures are prone to infections.

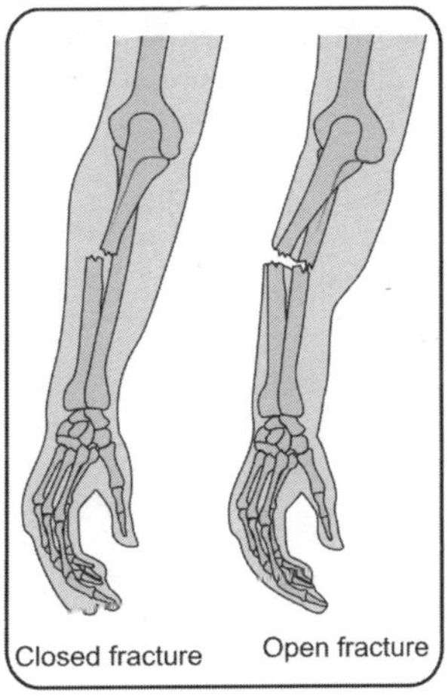

Fig. 1.1: Closed and open fractures

Fatigue Fractures

This type of fracture is also known as stress fracture. There is no obvious injury known for the required fracture. The fracture is caused by repeated stresses over a bone which may be minor in nature but present for a longer period of time.

The fatigue fractures are common in the bones of lower limb especially is metatarsals followed by fibula and the tibia. The fracture is characterized by pain, which is gradual in nature. The pain is aggravated by activity and is relived by rest. There is marked local tenderness over the affected bone. Fatigue fractures are commonly encountered by the dancers and the soldiers.

Pathological Fractures

As the name suggests, this type of fracture occurs in the bone which have an underlying pathological disorder. The bone is already weakened due to the disease that may be generalized or localized to a particular bone. The underlying bone often breaks down either by a minor trauma or spontaneously.

There are many causative factors for the pathological fractures ranging from inflammatory, neoplastic to hereditary. But the most common cause is osteoporosis. So the pathological fractures are often encountered in old aged patients whose bones are weakened by the osteoporosis. The most common sites of pathological fracture are vertebral bodies especially of thoracic and lumbar vertebrae, neck of femur and distal end of radius.

Greenstick Fractures (Fig. 1.2)

Greenstick fracture is a common name given to the fractures which are encountered in children especially below the age of 10 years. The bones of children are more resilient and springy, i.e., it could be easily bended. Any angulation force applied to the younger children can produce a break in the bone at the one end of the cortex and only a bend at the other end thus predisposing to an incomplete fracture.

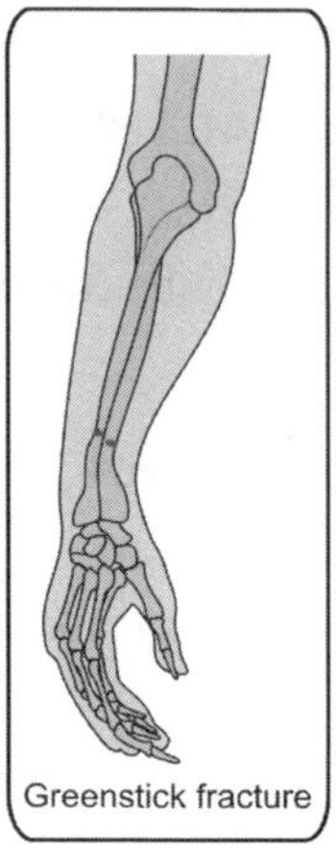

Fig. 1.2: Greenstick fractures

PATTERNS OF FRACTURES (Fig. 1.3)

The patterns of the fractures are described by the position of the fracture-line which is primarily determined by the nature of the causative force. The various patterns of the fractures are summarized in Table 1.1.

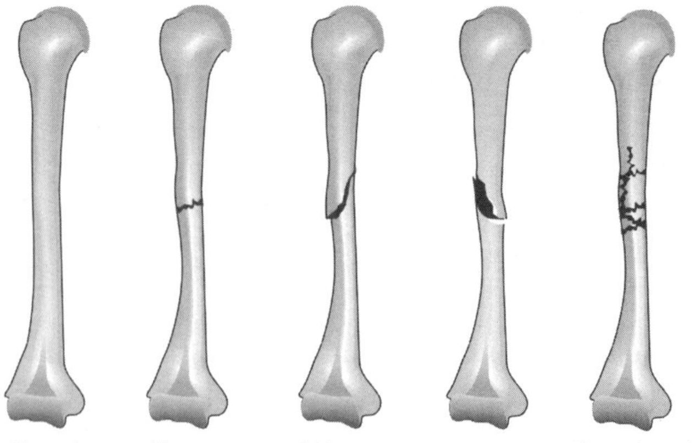

Fig. 1.3: Patterns of fractures

Table 1.1

Pattern of fracture	*Nature of fracture line*	*Causative force*
Transverse fracture	The fracture line is perpendicular to long axis of bone.	Bending force
Oblique fracture	Oblique	Bending force along the long axis of the bone.
Spiral fracture	Spirally running fracture line in more than one plane.	Twisting force
Comminuted fracture	There is no significant fracture line. The bone is crushed into many fragments.	Crushing or compression force.
Segmental fracture	Presence of two fracture lines in the same bone.	

CLINICAL EXAMINATION

The clinical examination of a patient with an injury, suspected to be a fracture begins as soon as he/she enters into the room. The following must be noticed carefully:

- State of ambulation of the patient.
- Any evident external injury.
- Age of the patient.

Before starting with the clinical examination and making a diagnosis following must be asked and notified as they could provide a general view regarding the injury.

- *Age of the patient:* There are different fractures which occur in a particular age-group as for example Colle's fracture is common in elderly people.
- *Mechanism of the injury:* It is important to know that how the patient has sustained the injury, it could give a fairly good idea about the expected fracture or dislocation. The mechanism could either be a fall, road traffic accident, or violence. Every mechanism is associated with a certain type of injury. As for example slipping in the bathroom leads to fracture of femoral neck.
- *External injury:* The patient must be asked and observed about any external injury because the treatment protocol may change completely in case of external injury and its severity.

CLINICAL FEATURES OF A FRACTURE

- *Pain:* The patient presents with immense pain at the fracture site which he/she experiences soon after the injury and which might be increasing as the time elapses.
- *Oedema:* As the patient experiences a fracture, the swelling do persist at the fractured site. The pressure of swelling at the site of injury could sometimes be misleading as the swelling can be present not only due to oedema but it could be due to haematoma, passive oedema etc. Sometimes a large amount of swelling could be present in absence of fracture as in case of soft tissue injuries and minimal swelling could be there in case of severe injuries like fracture neck of femur.
- *Deformity:* In case of displaced fracture, there is obvious deformity present at the fractured site. The deformity could alone be a characteristic feature of a certain fracture as Dinner fork deformity is characteristic of Colle's fracture. If severe oedema is there at the fractured site, the deformity may be unnoticed.
- *Signs of inflammation:* The signs of inflammation, i.e., pain, swelling, redness and warmth are obvious at the fractured site. Pain and swelling are already discussed. Redness is obvious just at looking at the area. As the

affected area is touched, it is sensed to be warmer than the rest of the limb. The local temperature of the area increases because of increased circulation to the injured area.

- *Ambulation:* This is of special importance in lower-limb fractures. The patient is unable to bear weight on the affected limb and would be ambulating using a walking aid or an assistive device (e.g., wheel chair).
- *Tenderness:* Tenderness means eliciting the pain by a minor pressure. As soon as the fracture occurs, tenderness could be elicited at the fracture site.
- *Muscle spasm:* The muscles proximal and distal to the fractured segments undergo a protective spasm. Because of this protected spasm it is difficult and painful for the patient to move the joints adjacent to the fractured segment.
- *Abnormal movement and crepitus:* In any part of the human body the movement is only possible at the joint, but in case of fracture there occurs movement between the fractured segments which is quite abnormal. The movement occurring at the fractured site produces grating between the bone ends thus producing a sound known as crepitus.

RADIOLOGICAL EXAMINATION

Radiological examination or imaging forms an important aspect of diagnosis of a fracture. It is important so that we can have a better view of the following:

- Fracture site.
- Extent of fracture.
- Displacement of fractured fragment.
- Deformity.
- Any associated injury.

Following techniques could be used:

- Plain radiograph (X-ray).
- Radioisotope scanning.
- Computed topography (CT).
- Magnetic resonance imaging (MRI).

HEALING OF FRACTURES

The healing of a fractured bone starts as soon as the fracture occurs through a series of various stages that follows each other until the bone is properly consolidated. The various stages of bone healing are as follows:

- Stage of haematoma.
- Stage of granulation tissue.
- Stage of callus.
- Stage of remodelling.
- Stage of modelling.

Stage of Haematoma

This is the initial stage in the process of fracture healing. As the bone fractures, the blood vessels also gets torned and results in the seepage of the blood in between the fractured fragments and around it. This stage usually lasts for about a week.

Stage of Granulation Tissue

This is the stage of proliferation of tissue both subperiosteal and endosteal. The proliferation of cells begins with the precursor cells, which lay down as intercellular matrix. The granulation tissue thus formed gives a soft anchorage to the healing bone but there is no structural rigidity at this stage. The haematoma formed earlier in the process of healing is pushed aside by the proliferating tissue and is subsequently reabsorbed. The stage lasts for about 2-3 weeks.

Stage of Callus

This is the stage which could be observed on a radiograph as a first sign of bone healing. In this stage the precursor cells gives rise to osteoblasts. The osteoblasts lay down an intercellular matrix of collagen and polysaccharide impregnated with calcium salts. There occurs formation of an immature bone or the callus. The texture of the bone at this stage is 'woven' in nature. This stage lasts from 4-12 weeks. This provides the healing bone with good strength along with the anchorage of the fractured fragments.

Stage of Remodelling

In this stage of fracture healing the callus formed earlier is transformed into a lamellar structure which is more mature in nature. The transformation occurs by the combined activity of osteoblasts and osteoclasts. This stage is of very long duration which lasts for a year or two.

Stage of Modelling

This stage of modelling is characterized by further strengthening of the fractured bone which occurs continuously for many years. As the patient resumes activities and the bone is loaded with stress and weight bearing, the process of modelling is initiated.

CLINICAL TESTS OF FRACTURE UNION

The radiological evidence is satisfactory diagnosis of fracture union. But the clinical diagnosis is also important preceding the radiological diagnosis. Following are the clinical signs of fracture union:

- Absence of mobility between the fractured fragments.
- Absence of tenderness.
- No or minimal pain on movement.

CHAPTER 2

FRACTURES OF UPPER EXTREMITY

FRACTURES OF CLAVICLE

The fracture of clavicle (Fig. 2.1) is a common injury amongst all age groups ranging from young to elderly.

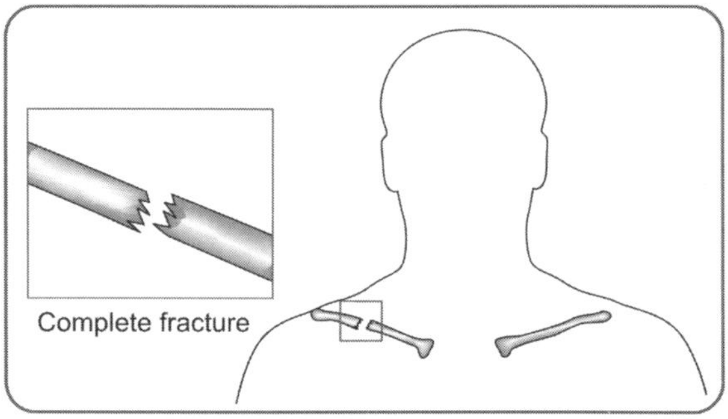

Fig. 2.1: Fracture of clavicle

Mechanism of Injury

- Fall on the shoulder.
- Fall on outstretched hand.

Most Common Site of Fracture

- Junction of middle and outer thirds of clavicle.
- Near the outer end of the clavicle.

Type of Fracture

The fracture that occurs in the clavicle is usually a displaced fracture.

Displacement (Fig. 2.2)

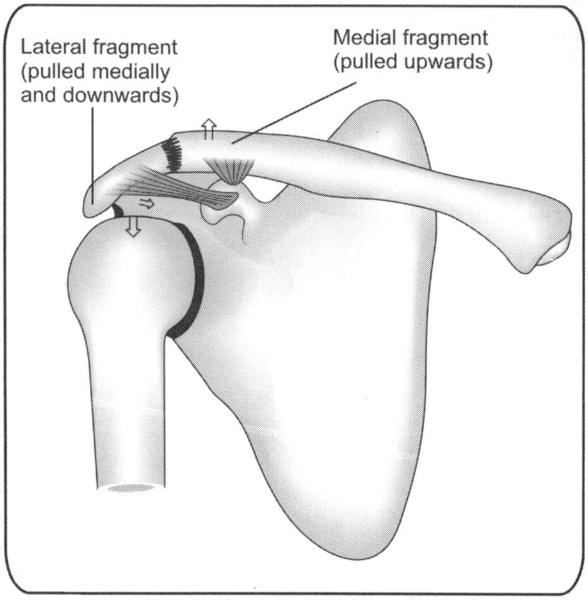

Fig. 2.2: Displaced clavicle fracture

- The lateral fragment is displaced medially and downwards due to:
  - Gravitational pull.
  - Pull by pectoralis major muscle.
  - Weight of the limb.
- The medial fragment is displaced upwards due to the pull of sternocleidomastoid (SCM) muscle attached to it.

Clinical Features

- Positive history of trauma.
- Pain.
- Swelling.

- Crepitus.
- Loss of normal contour of the bone which could be palpated as it is a subcutaneous bone.

Radiological Examination (Fig. 2.3)

The radiographic examination of the affected bone could confirm the presence of the fracture.

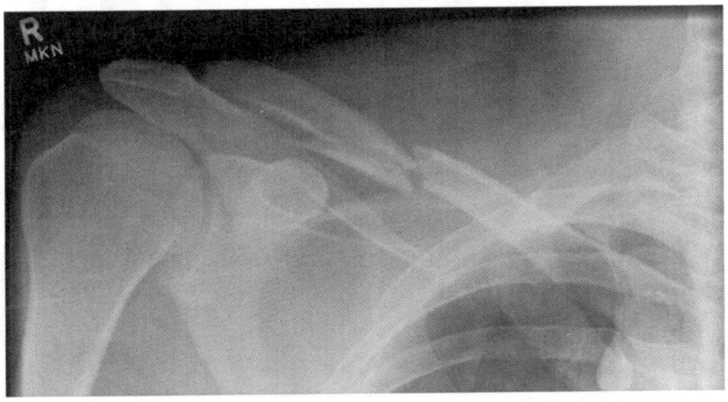

Fig. 2.3: Radiograph of fracture clavicle

Treatment

Conservative Treatment:

The fracture of the clavicle unites readily even if the fragments are widely displaced. Therefore reduction of the fractured segments is not required.

The part has to be immobilized for a short duration of time so that the pain and inflammation subsides and proper healing can occur. Following ways of immobilization can be used (Fig. 2.4):

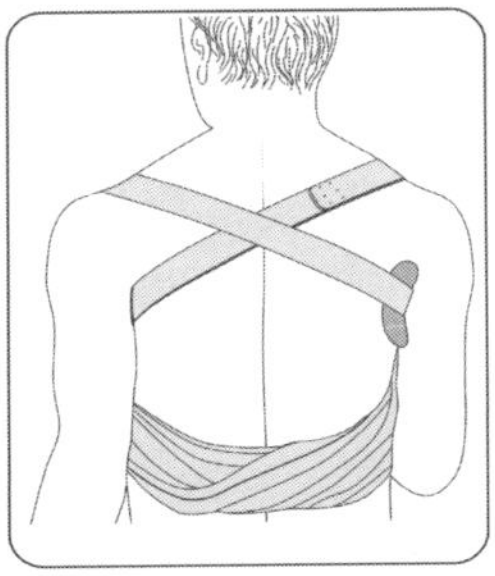

Figure of 8 bandage

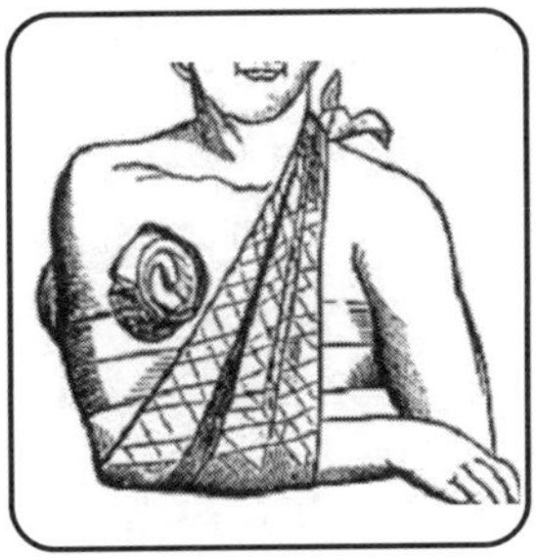

Triangular sling

Fig. 2.4: Immobilization techniques

- A triangular sling fully supporting the elbow and forearm to avoid gravitational force exerting any pull in the shoulder girdle and shoulder joint complex.
- The shoulders are braced up and holded in a figure of 8 bandage. The bandage is tied over a pad of cotton wool in each axilla and crossed between the scapula so as to brace the shoulders. The affected limb is then supported in a triangular sling.The bandage needs to be changed or tightened up after few days as it usually gets loosened.

Surgical Treatment:

Surgical treatment is rarely required in cases of fractures of clavicle. Some of the conditions requiring surgical intervention are as follows:

- Non-healing fracture.
- Severe neurovascular complications.
- Cosmetic appearance.

In cases treated with surgical intervention, the fractured fragments may be fixed up using a plate, stainless steel nail or pin.

Physiotherapy Management

Aim of Treatment:

- Regaining full range of motion at the shoulder complex.

During Immobilization:

Check for the following during the period of immobilization which is usually three weeks.

- Alignment of fractured bone ends.
- Proper positioning of scapula within figure of 8 bandage.
- Proper sling support.
- Neurovascular status of the affected limb.

Exercise Regime During Immobilization:

- Full range resistive movements to the elbow, forearm, wrist and hand.
- Isometrics to the shoulder.

During Mobilization:

- Start with small range relaxed movements.
- Codman's pendular exercises.
- Relaxed passive movements with patient in supine lying.

- Active shoulder exercises.
- Isometerics are advised at the terminal range of movements.
- Stretching to the shoulder in order to attain flexibility and to loosen the tightened structures.
- Resistive exercises in order to strengthen the shoulder muscles must be initiated using weight cuffs or dumbbells.

Day 0 – Week 1:

- Shoulder is stabilized in adduction and internal rotation with elbow in 90 degree of flexion.
- No range of motion to the shoulder.
- No strengthening exercises to the shoulder.

Week 2 – Week 4:

- Initiate gentle pendulum exercises to the shoulder as pain permits.
- No strengthening exercises to the shoulder.
- Initiate isometric exercises to the deltoid.

Week 4 – Week 6:

- At the end of week 6, gentle active range of motion to the shoulder is allowed.
- Limit abduction to 80°.
- Pendulum exercises to the shoulder with gravity eliminated.
- Initiate isometric exercises to the rotator cuff muscle along with deltoid.

Week 6 – Week 8:

- Active to active-assistive range of motion exercise to the shoulder in all planes.
- Initiate resistive exercises to the shoulder girdle muscles.
- Gradual weight bearing on the affected extremity is permitted.

Week 8 – Week 12:

- Active, active-assistive range of motion exercise to the shoulder.
- Encourage abduction.
- Isometric and isotonic resisted exercises to the shoulder girdle muscles.
- Full weight bearing on the affected extremity is allowed.

Home Exercise Regime

- Codman's pendular exercises.
- Ladder wall exercises.
- Assisted shoulder movements.
- Wand exercises.
- Functional use of the affected limb.

If the patient complains of pain at any stage the following pain relieving measures can be used:
- Hot packs.
- Short wave diathermy.
- Interferential therapy.
- TENS.

Complications

- Injury to subclavian vessels or brachial plexus.
- Malunion.
- Nonunion.
- Stiff shoulder.

FRACTURES OF SCAPULA

Fractures of the scapula is a rare injury and not so important because patients do well without any special treatment.

Mechanism of Injury

- Direct blow on the posterior aspect of thorax.
- Fall on the shoulder.

Displacement

Fractured fragments are usually undisplaced because they are held in position by muscles and fascia surrounding the scapula.

Sites of Fracture (Fig. 2.5)

Scapula may get fractured at different sites depending upon the mechanism of injury:
- Fracture of body of scapula.
- Fracture neck of scapula.
- Fracture of acromion process.
- Fracture of coracoid process.

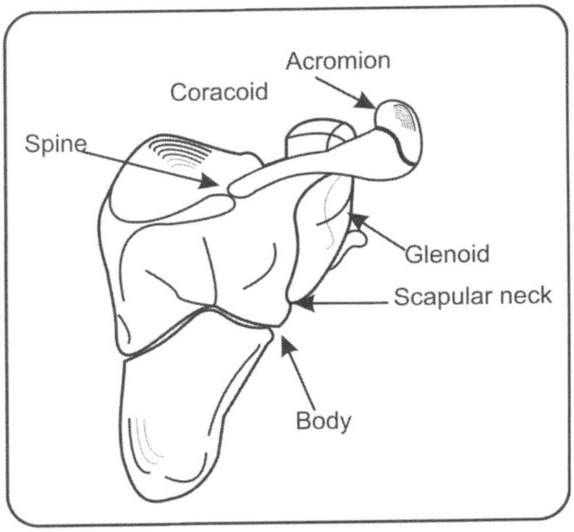

Fig. 2.5: Sites of scapula fracture

Clinical Features

- Severe pain.
- Extensive extravasation of blood into tissues.
- Widespread ecchymosis.

Treatment

A triangular sling for the period of two weeks is usually sufficient supporting the scapula and the shoulder. Surgical treatment is usually not necessary.

Physiotherapy Management

AIM:

To regain active full range movements of shoulder complex.

During Immobilization:

First two weeks: Treatment is based on the same outlines as for the clavicle fracture. The isometerics to the shoulder joint are initiated at an early stage.

During Mobilization:

Mobilization of the joints of shoulder girdle is easy as the period of immobilization is shorter and no stiffness thus develops in the joints.

- Proper pain relieving adjunct should be used as pain is a common feature of this type of fracture.
- Scapular muscle stabilization should be taught to the patient.
- Mobilization of all the components of shoulder girdle should be gradually progressed.
- Strengthening exercises by using:
  - Proprioceptive neuromuscular facilitation.
  - Dumbells.
  - Self-resistive exercises.

Prognosis

Prognosis of the fractured scapula is good. Full range, fairly strong movements of the shoulder complex should be obtained by 4-6 weeks.

FRACTURE OF GREATER TUBEROSITY OF HUMERUS

Fracture of greater tuberosity of humerus can occur in adult of any age group but is common amongst the elderly population.

Mechanism of Injury

- Fall on the shoulder.
- Direct trauma on the lateral aspect of the shoulder.
- Fall on outstretched hand.

Displacement (Fig. 2.6)

- The fracture could be undisplaced but comminuted.

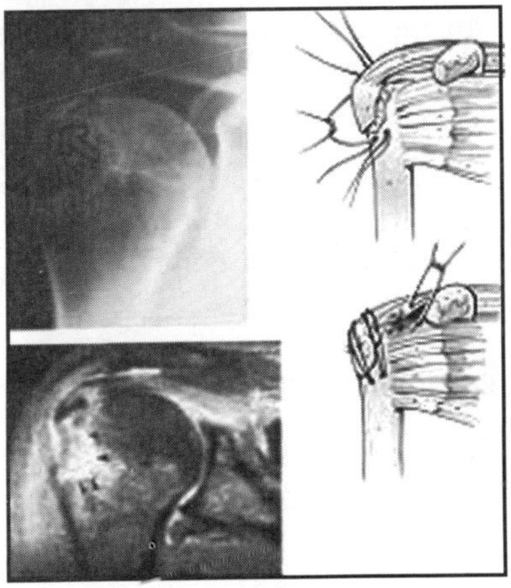

Fig. 2.6: Fracture of greater tuberosity of humerus

- The displacement of the fractured fragment results from the avulsion of the fractured segment by the strong contraction of the supraspinatus muscle.

Treatment

The treatment can either be purely conservative or surgical depending upon the type of the fracture.

Conservative Treatment

It is advised in case of undisplaced fracture. In this the healing takes place by use of sling for about two weeks. If conservative mode is followed in cases of displaced fracture reduction is brought about by bringing the arm into abduction and maintaining it there.

Surgical Treatment

It is advised in case of displaced fracture. It is quite cumbersome to maintain the limb in abduction following conservative management, therefore open reduction and internal fixation with a help of nail or screw is advised.

Physiotherapy Management

It aims at achieving the full range of motion of shoulder complex. The treatment runs on the same lines as for fracture clavicle or scapula. Following are some of the special considerations:

- Adhesion formation is quite common, therefore friction massage and ultrasonic is advised over the area of tenderness.
- Terminal arc movement is specially emphasized:
  - Abduction-Elevation
  - Flexion-Elevation

Functional recovery is gained by 6-8 weeks following injury.

FRACTURE OF NECK OF HUMERUS

The surgical neck of the humerus is most commonly fractured.

Aetiology

It is usually seen in elderly women. The cause may be regarded as osteoporosis.

Mechanism of Injury

- Fall on the shoulder.
- Fall on the outstretched hand.

Type of Fracture

The fracture type varies over a wider range:

- Impacted fracture.
- Severely displaced fracture.

Impacted Fracture (Fig. 2.7):

The fractured fragments are so impacted over each other that they are often missed on the radiographic evaluation. The whole part could be moved as one piece. The limb could be handled and moved passively through reasonable range of motion without causing much pain and discomfort.

Displaced or Unimpacted Fracture (Fig. 2.7):

The unimpacted displaced fractures are further categorized as adducted or abducted fracture depending upon position of distal fractured fragment.

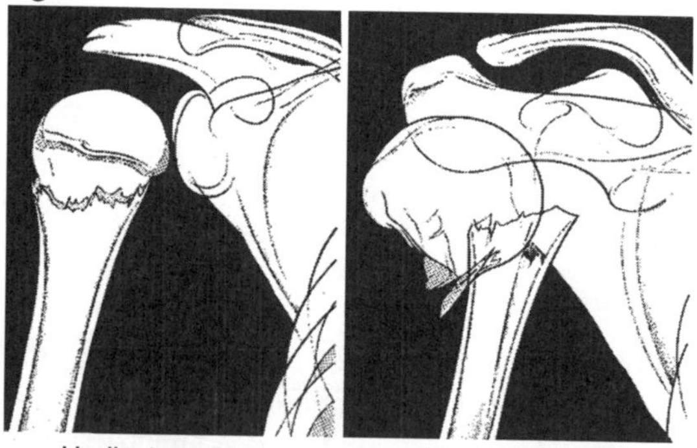

Fig. 2.7:

Adducted Unimpacted Fracture (Fig. 2.8):

In this type of fracture, the proximal fracture segment is abducted by the pull of supraspinatus

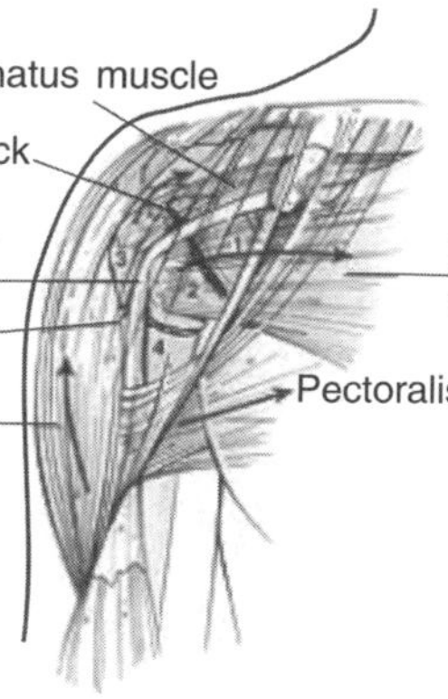

Fig. 2.8 : Adducted unimpacted fracture

while distal fragment is adducted by the pull of pectoralis major.

Abducted Unimpacted Fracture: The proximal fragment is at its own position but the lower fragment is abducted by the pull of deltoid muscle.

Clinical Diagnosis

Impacted fractures are often missed on radiographic evaluation; the patient may also be using the limb functionally. But complain of shoulder pain especially in elderly women with history of fall or trauma should be diagnosis carefully. External bruises are generally present.

Radiological Diagnosis (Fig. 2.9)

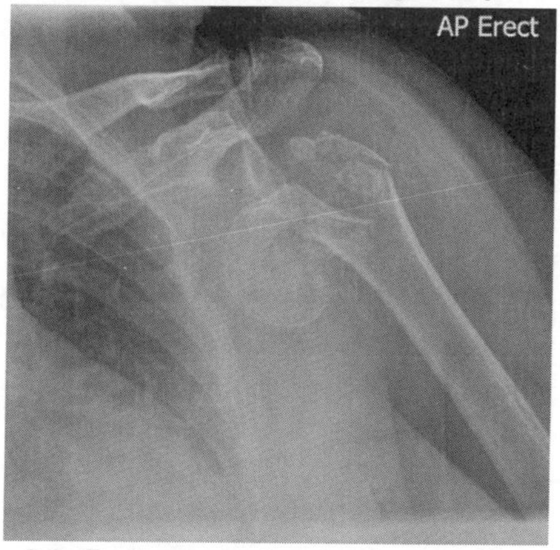

Fig. 2.9: Radiograph showing fractured neck of humerus

The following radiological views of the shoulder are undertaken:

- Anteroposterior view.
- Axial view.

Treatment

The treatment of fracture neck of humerus will depend upon the:

- Age of patient.
- Requirement of shoulder mobility.
- Type of fracture.

Impacted Fracture:

In cases of impacted fracture of neck of humerus, shoulder is immobilized with the help of triangular sling aided with arm-chest bandage.

Unimpacted Fracture:

In case of elderly person: In elderly patient encountered with unimpacted fracture of neck of humerus, the limb is immobilized in the triangular sling with no movement allowed at the shoulder joint.

In young person: In case of younger patients either of the following approaches could be used:

- Closed reduction and stabilization of fracture by multiple k-wires passed percutaneously under image intensifier control.
- Open reduction and internal fixation is indicated in severely displaced fracture.

Physiotherapy Management

As the fracture is commonly seen in elderly the basic aim of therapist is to regain full active range of motion of shoulder girdle so as to avoid stiff and painful shoulder.

During Immobilization:

- Pain relieving modalities can be used to relieve pain. The sling could be removed intermittently to use the modality. Following adjuncts can be used:
  - Cryotherapy.

- TENS.
- Diapulse.
- Ultrasonic therapy.

- Self resisted full range elbow, forearm, wrist and hand movements to be encouraged.
- Isometrics to the deltoid should be emphasized.
- Relaxed pendular movements in small range with arm in sling can be started as early as 1 week.

During Mobilization:

- In order to relieve pain and induce relaxation to the joint deep heating thermotherapy adjuncts can be used like:
  - Hot packs.
  - Short wave diathermy.
  - Ultrasonic.
- Range of motion exercises
  - Relaxed passive movements are essential. It should be progressed gradually to abduction and rotations.
  - Rhythmic pendular movements are initiated in small range. The movement should be initiated with flexion-extension swing and then progressed to abduction-adduction ranges.
  - Auto-assisted exercises using the contralateral limb should be taught to the patient.
  - Active shoulder mobilization should begin as the shoulder becomes pain free.
- Strengthening exercises
  - Active assisted movements should be practised within the available range.
  - As the active range of motion is achieved, resistive exercises should be started.
  - Good functional results could be achieved by 6-8 weeks.

Rehabilitation Following Proximal Humerus Fracture

Day 0 to Week 1:

- No shoulder and elbow range of motion exercise is allowed.
- No strengthening exercise to the shoulder and elbow are permitted.

Week 2 to Week 4:

- Patients treated conservatively can initiate pendulum exercises. Active to active-assisted exercise for range of motion are permitted.
- Avoid internal/external rotation of the shoulder.
- Initiate isometric exercises for shoulder musculature in patients treated conservatively.
- No strengthening exercises for the patient treated with surgical intervention.

Week 4 to Week 6:

- In patients treated conservatively regain full range of motion at elbow. Regain shoulder flexion/abduction upto 100°-110° with limited internal/external rotation. Continue pendulum exercises against gravity.
- Continue passive assisted range of motion exercises at shoulder in patients treated surgically.
- Isometric and isotonic exercises to the elbow musculature.
- Avoid exercise to the deltoid in patients treated surgically.
- Involved extremity can be used for dressing and self-care in patients treated conservatively and they can begin to bear weight on the affected extremity at the end of week 6.
- Patients treated surgically still need assistance and cannot bear weight on affected extremity.

Week 6 to Week 8:

- Active, active-assisted and passive range of motion exercises to shoulder and elbow in all planes as tolerated by the patient.
- Continue with isometric and isotonic strengthening exercises to elbow.
- Isometric exercises to the shoulder musculature must be continued.
- Initiate progressive resistive exercises for patients treated conservatively.
- Weight bearing on the involved extremity is permitted as tolerated by the patient.

Week 8 to Week 12:

- Active and passive range of motion to shoulder and elbow in all planes.
- Resisted exercises to the shoulder musculature with gradual increase in weight.
- Isokinetic exercises using appropriate equipment to improve strength and endurance.
- Initiate swimming.
- Sports such as golf and tennis can be resumed.
- Avoid contact sports till 6 months.

FRACTURE OF THE SHAFT OF HUMERUS

This fracture usually occurs in the middle third of humeral shaft and never includes articular or metaphyseal regions proximally or distally. This fracture can occur in patients of any age group.

Mechanism of Injury

There are many mechanisms which could lead to fracture of shaft of humerus like:

- Direct blow to the arm.
- Any twisting or bending force.
- Fall on the outstretched hand.
- Penetrating injury.

Classification

The fracture should be classified according to the anatomical position of fracture line on the humerus as the displacement or angulations of fractured segments is greatly affected by the position due to varying muscle pull at every different location. The fracture could be majorly classified as follows:

- *Fractures above pectoris major insertion:* The proximal humerus is abducted and externally rotated, secondary to the pull of rotator cuff muscles.
- *Fractures below the pectoralis major insertion and above the deltoid:* The proximal fragment is adducted and distal fragment is displaced proximally and laterally.
- *Fracture below the deltoid insertion:* The proximal fragment is abducted under the influence of deltoid muscle.

The fracture of the shaft of humerus could follow any pattern: Transverse, oblique, spiral, comminuted or segmental and could be either open or closed (Fig. 2.10).

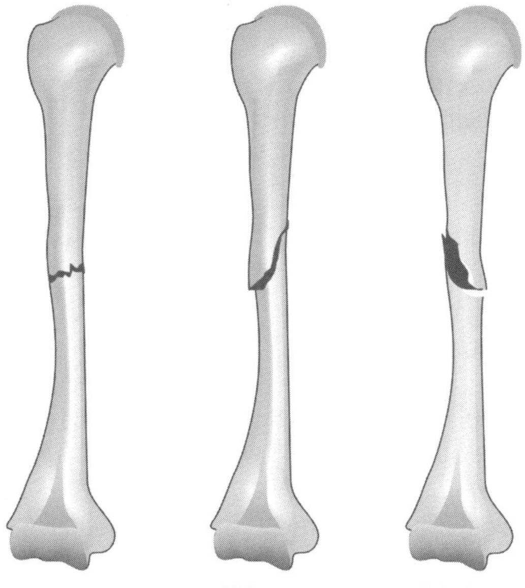

Fig. 2.10: Fracture patterns

Diagnosis

Diagnosis in cases of fracture of humeral shaft is not difficult as the patient present with classical signs and symptoms.

Radiographic Evaluation (Fig. 2.11)

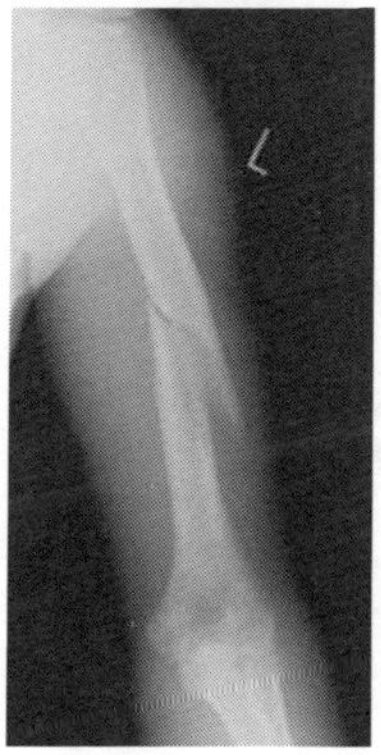

Fig. 2.11: Radiograph showing fracture shaft of humerus

Radiographs are taken to know the exact site and type of fracture. Radiographs of the whole arm including the elbow are to be taken.

Management

While dealing with the fracture in an acute case the main aim of orthopaedic treatment is alignment and stability of the fracture site. The orthopaedician could either follow the path of conservative treatment or surgical intervention.

Conservative Methods

If the displacement of the fragment is more than expected, fracture is reduced by traction and mobilization and is then stabilized by any of the following methods:

- *U-Slab:* This plaster slab extends from base of neck to lateral aspect of the arm and then to the medial aspect of arm by passing under the elbow. The slab is supported with a triangular sling.
- *Hanging cast (Fig. 2.12):* The plaster cast extends from proximal part of arm till the wrist with elbow at the position of 90° flexion. In this case the cast and the weight of the limb provide necessary traction.
- *Chest arm bandage:* This is usually used in young children below 5 years of age.
- *Coaptation splint.*
- *Functional bracing (Fig. 2.13).*

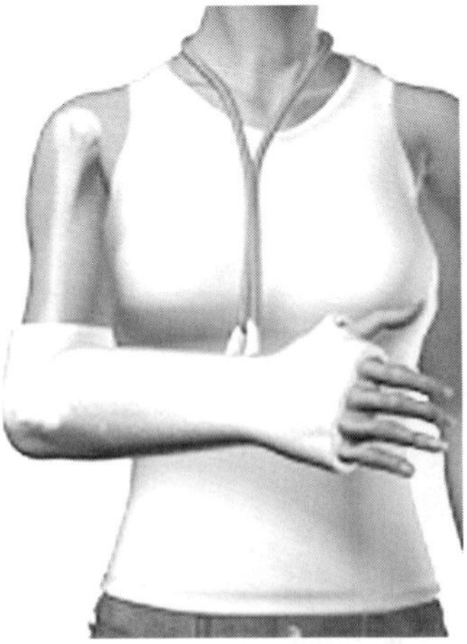

Fig. 2.12: Hanging cast

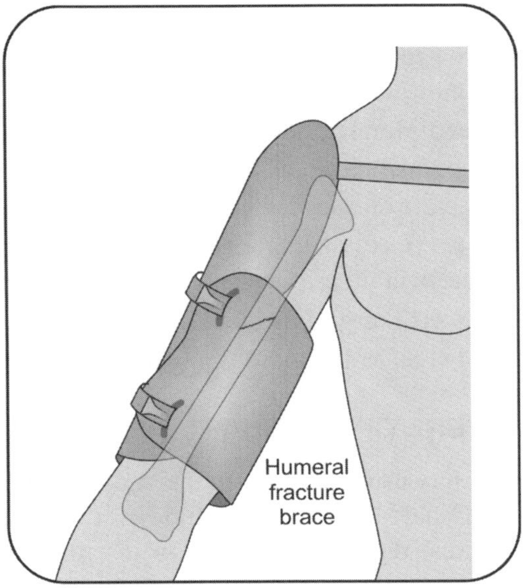

Fig. 2.13: Humeral fracture brace

Surgical Methods

Surgical intervention is considered if it is not possible to reduce the fracture by closed manipulation or in case of open fracture. The fracture could be treated by either:

- Open reduction and internal fixation.
- External fixation (Fig. 2.14)

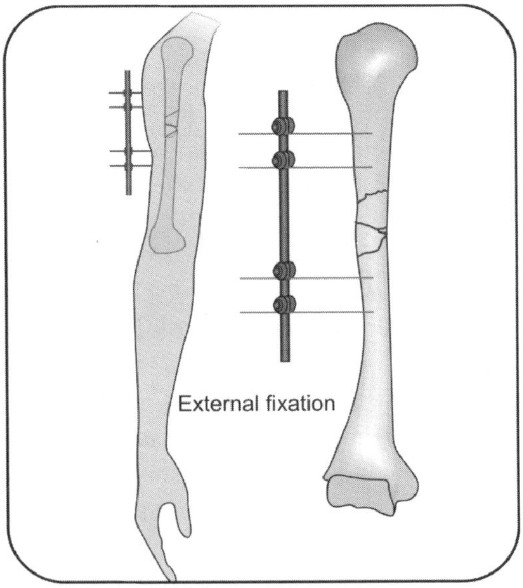

Fig. 2.14: External fixation

Open reduction and internal fixation:

- Intra medullary nail/rod (Fig. 2.15).
- Plate fixation (Fig. 2.16).

External fixation: It is used for open or closed fractures with severe soft tissue trauma or thermal injury, fractures with extensive comminution, floating elbow fracture or segmental humerus fractures.

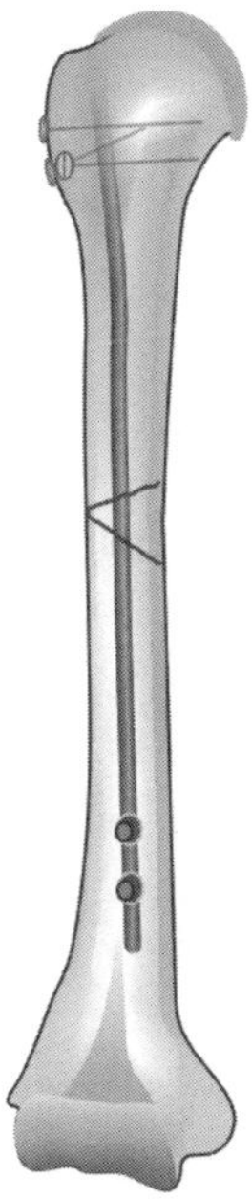

Fig. 2.15: Intramedullary (IM) rod in humeral fracture

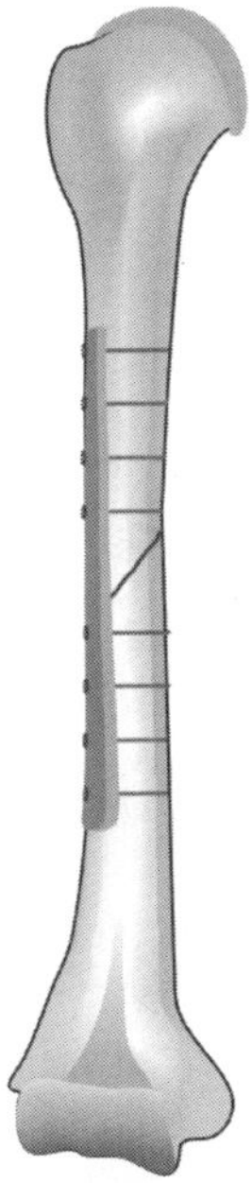

Fig. 2.16: Plate and screw fixation

Physiotherapy Management

AIMS of Treatment

- To restore full range of motion at shoulder and elbow joint in all planes.
- To improve the strength of the muscles affected by the fracture: Pectoralis major, deltoid, biceps, triceps.
- To improve and restore the function of involved extremity in self-care and personal hygiene.

Physiotherapy Intervention

Day of injury to one week:

- In cases treated by conservative means, no movement is allowed either at shoulder or elbow.
- In cases treated by surgical means, active and active assistive range of motion at shoulder and elbow is allowed. Pendulum exercises are incorporated.
- In every case, active range of motion is allowed at wrist and digits in order to reduce oedema and stiffness.
- Weight bearing on the affected extremity is not allowed.
- No strengthening exercises are initiated.

Second to fourth week:

- Active and active assistive exercises are prescribed to the shoulder and elbow.
- Isotonic exercises are given to the forearm muscles.
- Wrist musculature strengthening by ball squeezing exercise.
- In cases treated by internal fixation, minimal weight bearing is allowed on the affected extremity.
- Shoulder abduction is not allowed beyond 60 degree of range.

Four to six weeks:

- Weight bearing is allowed on affected extremity but it should be minimal.
- Active range of motion is continued at all the joint of the affected extremity.
- Continue strengthening exercises to the wrist musculature.
- Resisted exercises for the forearm muscles are initiated.
- Gentle isometrics to biceps and triceps are instituted at the end of six weeks.
- No heavy lifting is allowed on the affected extremity.

Eight to Twelve Weeks:

- Full weight bearing is allowed on the affected extremity.

- Passive range of motion exercises are initiated at shoulder and elbow if the range is still limited.
- Progressive resistive exercise with gradual increase in resistance should be instituted at shoulder and elbow.
- Light lifting is allowed with affected extremity.
- No heavy contact sports are allowed.

Complications

- Nerve injury: Radial nerve is commonly injured in fracture shaft humerus (Fig. 2.17).
- Delayed union (Fig. 2.18).
- Malunion (Fig. 2.18).

SUPRACONDYLAR FRACTURE OF HUMERUS

The supracondylar fracture of humerus is an extra articular fracture with fracture line extending transversely through the distal metaphysis of humerus just above the condyles (Fig. 2.19). The fracture is most common among the children. The fracture is potentially dangerous with greater risks due to serious complications like injury to nerve and artery.

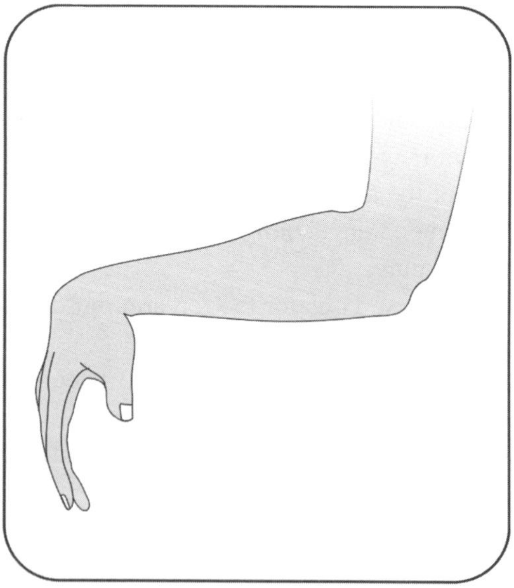

Fig. 2.17: Radial nerve palsy

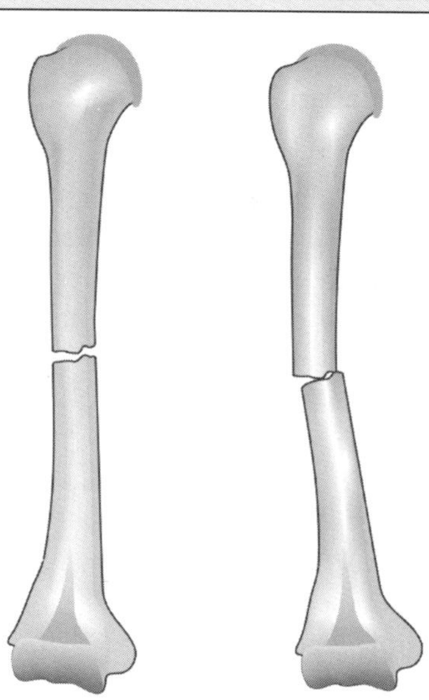

Fig. 2.18: Delayed union and malunion

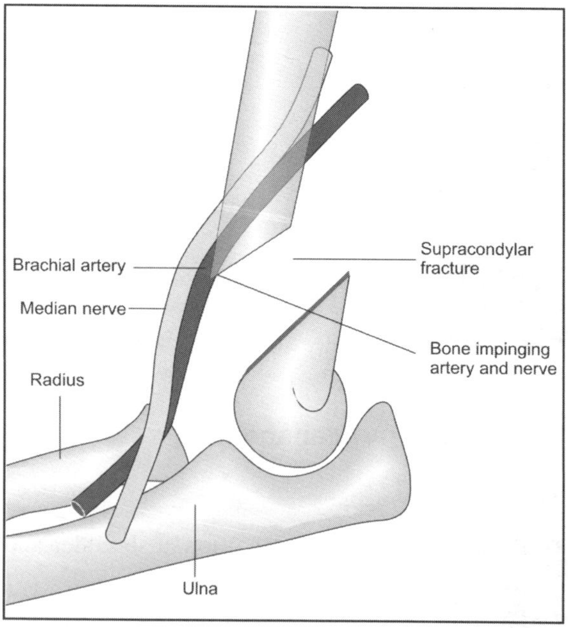

Fig. 2.19: Supracondylar fracture of humerus

Mechanism of Injury

The supracondylar fracture of humerus can occur due to any of the following mechanism:

- Fall on the elbow.
- Direct blow over the posterior aspect of elbow.

- Fall on outstretched hand, forcing the elbow into hyperextension resulting in fracture above the condyles.

Types of Fracture

The supracondylar fracture of humerus is basically divided into two categories depending upon the positioning of distal fractured segment. The two types of supracondylar fracture of humerus are as follows:

Flexion type supracondylar fracture (Fig. 2.20): The distal fractured segment is forward tilted, i.e., appears to be flexed in respect to the proximal fractured segment.

Extension type supracondylar fracture (Fig. 2.21): The distal fractured segment is tilted backward, i.e., extended in relation to proximal segment.

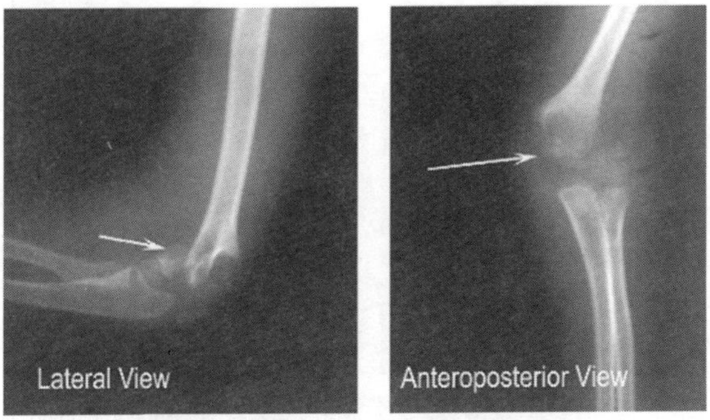

Fig. 2.20: Flexion type supracondylar fracture

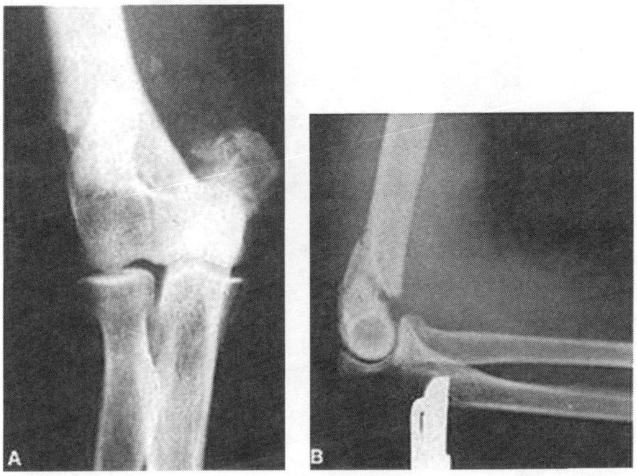

Fig. 2.21: Extension type supracondylar fracture

The extension type supracondylar fracture of humerus is most common of the two types, so while dealing with the supracondylar fractures, extension type of the fracture is commonly dealt with.

Displacement

In supracondylar fracture (Extension type) the distal fragment is displaced from its original position in any of the following ways:

- Posterior or backward shift.
- Posterior or backward tilt.
- Posterior shift.
- Medial or lateral shift.
- Medial tilt.
- Internal rotation.

Clinical Features

The clinical features presented by patient with supracondylar fracture humerus depend upon the severity of swelling around the elbow. The patients present with history of injury or fall after while he/she was unable to use the affected extremity elbow joint. Pain and deformity are usually present.

In cases where patient presents early, before significant swelling has occurred, there is an unusual prominence of elbow due to backward tilt of distal fragment.

Radiological Diagnosis

The supracondylar fracture of humerus is easily diagnosed on a radiograph due to marked displacement. In cases of undisplaced fracture comparative radiograph of opposite elbow is also taken in order to differentiate. Usually an antero-posterior and a lateral view of the elbow are obtained.

- *Antero-posterior view:* AP view on radiograph demonstrates proximal shift, medial or lateral shift, medial tilt and rotation of distal fragment.
- *Lateral view:* The lateral view demonstrates proximal shift, posterior shift, posterior tilt and rotation of distal fragment.

Treatment

Objectives of orthopedic treatment:
- Accurate alignment of distal humerus.
- Stability of fractured segment.

The treatment of the supracondylar fracture of humerus depends upon the nature of the fractured segment, i.e., either undisplaced or displaced.

Undisplaced fracture: In case of supracondylar fracture of humerus where the fractured segments are in their position, i.e., they are undisplaced, the only treatment required is immobilization in an above elbow plaster slab with elbow in 90° flexion. The immobilization period is of 3 weeks.

Displaced fracture: The displaced supra-condylar fracture of humerus can be treated either conservatively or surgically depending upon the extent of the fracture:

- Closed reduction *(manipulation and immobilization)* (Fig. 2.22):

  The displaced fractured segments are reduced by traction and manipulation in order to reduce the displacement and bring about the correct alignment of the segments. Traction is applied with elbow in 30°-40° of flexion, applying countertraction at the arm. While in traction the elbow is gradually extended and forearm is fully supinated. While maintaining the traction, the elbow is now flexed slowly. While the above maneuver is continued, the thumb above the olecranon process presses it forward into flexion. Traction is maintained as the elbow is flexed beyond 90°. The elbow is immobilized in plaster with the elbow flexed a little more acutely than the right angle for 3 weeks.

- *Open reduction and internal fixation (Fig. 2.23):*

  In cases of unstable fracture when it is impossible to reduce the fracture by closed manipulation, open reduction and internal fixation by k-wire is necessary.

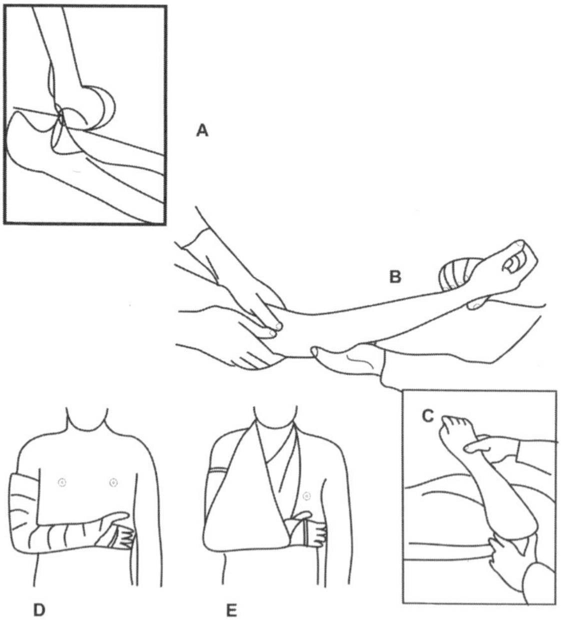

Fig. 2.22: Technique of closed reduction following displaced supracondylar fracture of humerus

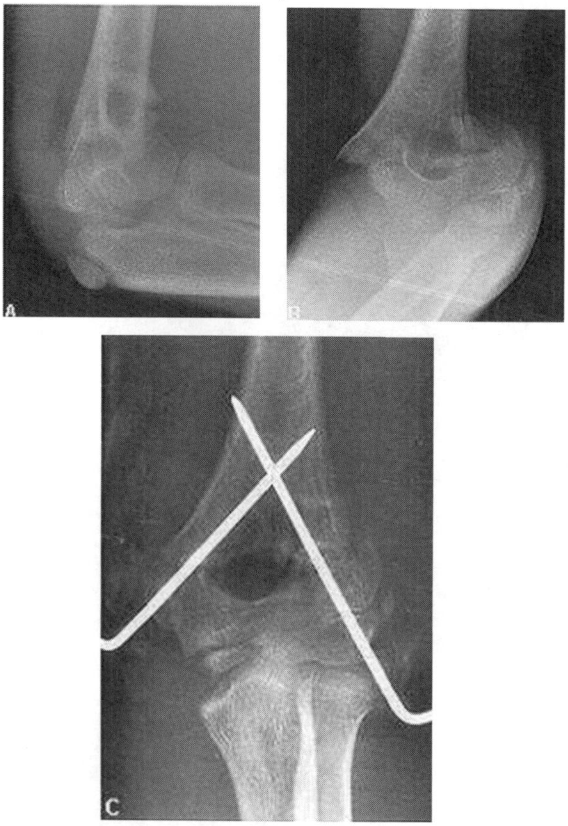

Fig. 2.23: Open reduction and internal fixation

- *Continuous traction:*
  Continuous traction is a mode of treatment in cases marked with intense swelling or open wounds. The methods used are as follows:
  - Traction given with k-wire passed through olecranon process, i.e., Smith's traction.
  - Below elbow skin traction, i.e., Dunlop's traction.

Complications

As already discussed the fracture is potentially dangerous due to large number of post-fracture complications which would arrive at any point of time during the course of the treatment. Therefore the complications are divided into following categories:

Immediate complications:
- Injury to the brachial artery.
- Injury to nerves.

Early complications:
- Volkmann's ischaemia.

Late complications:
- Malunion.
- Myositis ossificans.
- Volkmann's ischaemic contracture.

Physiotherapy Management

The physiotherapy management follows the same guidelines in both the cases whether the fracture is treated either conservatively or surgically. The only difference being the therapist has to be more careful with the incision site and internal fixator device while dealing with the patient treated surgically.

Goals of Physiotherapy Treatment

- To reduce pain and inflammation.
- To increase range of motion at elbow and forearm.

Physiotherapeutic Intervention during Immobilization

- Free range of motion exercise to all the free joints of the affected limb must be instituted so that the future complication can be reduced.

Physiotherapeutic Intervention during mobilization

- *To reduce pain and inflammation.* Various physiotherapeutic adjuncts like hot packs, paraffin wax bath are used to reduce pain before and after the exercise regime. These adjuncts not only reduce pain but also provides comfort to the patient along with the increase in local circulation. This aids in proper relaxation of the involved area.
- *To increase range of motion at elbow joint.* The main movements at the elbow joint are flexion and extension. Both the movements must be concentrated during the exercise regime. The regime should begin with active-assisted exercises, followed by active exercises and manual mobilization.

Active-assisted exercises for elbow

- Both flexion and extension at the elbow joint can be practised by holding a wand in both the hands. The shoulder joint and arm must be positioned carefully so as to have isolated flexion-extension at elbow joint.
- Use of roller skate could also be practised in gaining flexion-extension at the elbow. The patient is made to sit on a chair while the affected forearm is positioned on the table with roller skate in the hand. The roller skate is moved by the patient as performing flexion-extension at the elbow while the therapist stabilizes the arm.

The active-assisted movements performed either using a wand or a roller skate must be in gravity-eliminated position.

Active exercises for the elbow

- The active exercises for gaining flexion-extension at elbow must be initiated as free swinging of the forearm producing flexion and extension at the elbow.

Manual mobilization for the elbow

Once the patient is able to perform active elbow flexion and extension, manual mobilization is initiated in the form of stretching to gain further range of motion. It should always be kept in mind that the passive stretching should be gentle and pain-free. Even if the range of motion is not progressive vigorous passive mobilization must not be practised as it could lead to development of myositis ossificans.

- *To increase range of motion of supination-pronation:* The supination-pronation exercise goes hand in hand with elbow flexion-extension. Supination should be practised with elbow flexion and pronation with elbow extension.

INTERCONDYLAR FRACTURE OF HUMERUS

Intercondylar fracture of humerus is more common amongst adults, sustaining the injury after having fall on point of elbow.

Mechanism of Injury

After falling on the elbow, the olecranon process pushes itself into the condyles of the humerus separating them from each other.

Types of Fracture

The intercondylar fracture of humerus can be divided into various types depending upon the location of fracture line:

- T- type intercondylar fracture of humerus (Fig. 2.24).
- Y- type intercondylar fracture of humerus (Fig. 2.24).
- Comminuted fracture.

Clinical Features

The patient presents with a definite history of fall or hitting the elbow severely, along with following signs and symptoms:

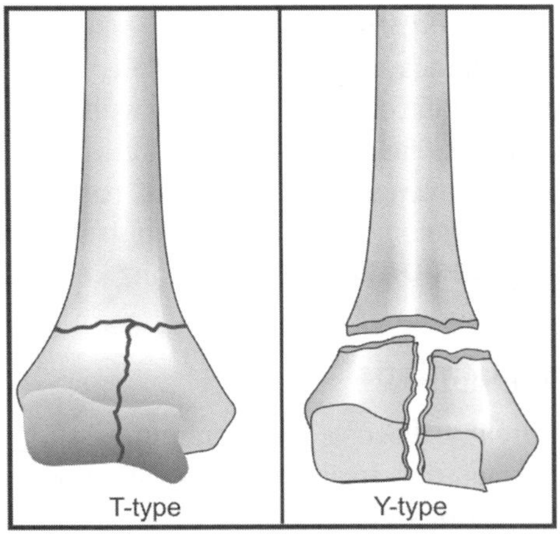

Fig. 2.24: Intercondylar fracture of humerus

- Severe pain.
- Swelling.
- Ecchymosis.
- Crepitus.

Radiographic Examination

The diagnosis is confirmed by the radiographic examination of the area further detailing the extent of damage along with type of fracture.

Treatment

The management of the intercondylar fracture of humerus depends upon the nature of the fracture, i.e., whether displaced, undisplaced or comminuted.

Undisplaced Fracture

In cases of undisplaced intercondylar fracture of humerus, the only treatment required is immobilization of the affected extremity in an above elbow plaster cast for 3-4 weeks.

Displaced Fracture

Displaced intercondylar fracture of humerus are difficult to treat conservatively. They are best managed by open reduction and internal fixation of fractured segments.

Comminuted Fracture

These cases are treated by traction. Early in the treatment course traction through olecranon is used to reduce the fracture and after reduction it is used for its maintenance.

Complications

- Stiffness around the elbow joint.
- Osteoarthritis.
- Malunion.

Physiotherapy Management

The intercondylar fracture of humerus is treated on the same lines as described for the supra condylar fracture of humerus. The prognosis and outcome is poor in this fracture as the whole joint is disturbed due to fracture along with massive soft tissue injury. The patient with intercondylar fracture of humerus do not gain full range of motion at elbow, therefore it is advisable to stuck to functional use of hand beyond a certain range.

In these cases more emphasis must be laid on supination-pronation exercises at elbow as flexion-extension are more difficult to gain.

The functional outcome is better in surgically treated cases.

FRACTURE OF OLECRANON PROCESS

Olecranon process forms the proximal part of ulna, which articulates with trochlea of the distal humerus. Its fracture could either be extra-articular or intra-articular (Fig. 2.25). It usually occurs in adults.

Mechanism of Injury

The fracture of olecranon process may result from any of the following reasons:

- Direct injury as in fall on point of elbow.
- Fall on outstretched hand with elbow in flexion.
- Road traffic accidents.

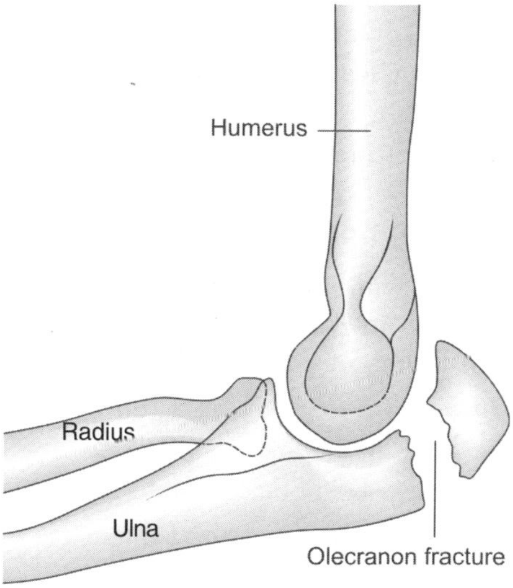

Fig. 2.25: Olecranon fracture

Pathoanatomy

The proximal fractured fragment is pulled by the triceps muscle thus creating a gap at the fractured site.

Classification

The fracture of the olecranon process is classified into three types depending on the extent of the injury (Fig. 2.26):

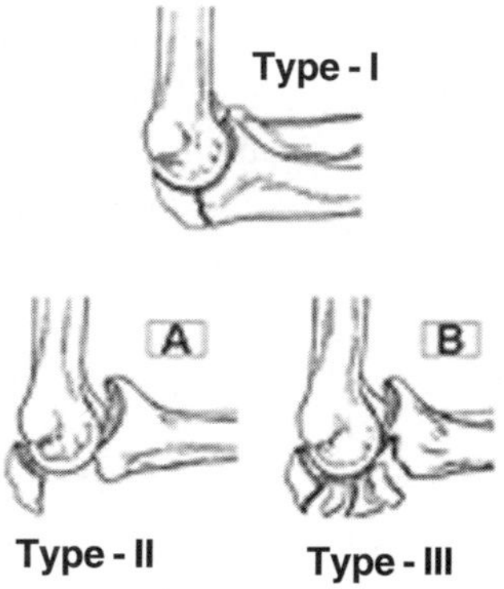

Fig. 2.26: Classification of olecranon fracture

- Type-I: Crack without displacement of fractured fragment.
- Type-II: Clean break with separation of the fragment.
- Type-III: Comminuted fracture.

Clinical Features

The patient with fractured olecranon process may present with following signs and symptoms with obvious history of injury:

- Pain.
- Swelling.
- Tenderness being maximum at point of elbow.
- Crepitus between fractured fragments.
- Active extension of elbow on clinical feature.

Radiograph

The radiographic evaluation is necessary in order to confirm the diagnosis based on clinical features.

Management

Objectives of orthopaedic treatment:

- Restoration of articular alignment.
- To maintain stability of the elbow joint.

The orthopaedic management of fractured olecranon process depends upon the type of the fracture depending upon the above-mentioned classification:

- *Type-I–Crack without displacement:* If the olecranon is fractured without displacement, i.e., if fractured fragments are still in contact with each other, the only treatment required is immobilization of the affected limb. The affected limb is immobilized in an above elbow plaster cast with elbow in flexion varying from 30°-90°.
- *Type II–Clean break with separation:* This type of fracture is treated by open reduction and internal fixation. The internal fixation can be done with help of cancellous screws or tension band wiring. It is better to go for surgical intervention because conservative management in plaster cast can further distract the fractured segment due to action of triceps muscle.
- *Type III–Comminuted fracture:* This type of fracture is best treated by excision of the fractured fragments. With availability of best facilities, this type of fracture can be treated by internal fixation of fractured fragments. The surgical intervention is always followed by repair of triceps mechanism.

Complications

- Non union.
- Malunion.
- Osteoarthritis.
- Elbow stiffness.

Physiotherapy Management

Objectives:

- To maintain the range of motion at shoulder and wrist.
- To restore and improve range of motion at the affected elbow.
- To improve the strength of all muscles around the elbow like biceps, triceps, supinators, pronators, wrist extensors and wrist flexors.
- To restore and normalize the activities of daily living.

Intervention:

Day of Injury to One Week:

- The affected limb should be kept in elevation in order to reduce the oedema, retrograde massage will also help.
- Active range of motion exercises should be started at the shoulder joint.
- If the patient is treated conservatively no exercises are allowed at elbow and wrist.
- No weight bearing is allowed at the affected extremity.

- Active flexion and extension of the digits along with the gripping exercises are encouraged to maintain the strength.
- After 3-4 days of the injury, gentle isometrics to the wrist can be started.
- No strengthening exercises are initiated for the elbow.

Second to Fourth Week:

- Patient has to continue with active range of motion exercises to the shoulder and wrist.
- Weight bearing is still not allowed on the affected extremity.
- Gentle isometrics exercises to the biceps are initiated.
- Isotonic exercises to the digits along with the gripping exercise are continued.
- Elbow extension should not be attempted even in cases treated by surgical intervention and no strengthening exercises for the extensor mechanism of the elbow are initiated.

Four to Six Weeks:

- Active assistive exercise should be initiated at shoulder, elbow and wrist.
- No passive exercises are permitted at any of the upper limb joint, especially at elbow.
- Isometric exercise to the biceps must be enhanced at this stage.
- Isometeric exercise to the triceps has to be initiated at this stage.
- Isotonic exercise to the long flexors and extensors of the wrist has to be continued.
- Weight bearing is still not allowed on the affected extremity.
- Patient can start using the affected extremity for basic activities of daily living like grooming.

Six to Eight Weeks:

- Full range of motion exercises, both active and active-assisted should be performed at the elbow joint till satisfactory results are not obtained.
- Patient may progressively bear weight on the affected extremity.
- Resistive exercises are initiated for biceps and triceps in to order to strengthen the elbow muscul-ature.
- The patient must be advised to do self-resistive exercise for biceps and triceps. In this case the uninvolved extremity could be used as the resistive device.

Eight to Twelve Weeks:

- Full weight bearing is allowed on the affected extremity.
- The patient might experience some limitation in the extension at the elbow joint, in order to overcome it passive stretching may be necessary.
- A dynamic splint may also be used for passive elbow stretch.
- Progressive resistive exercise to wrist and elbow, gradually increasing the resistance.
- Graded weights are used for strengthening exercises.

FRACTURE OF HEAD OF RADIUS

Fracture of head of radius is a common fracture of upper extremity occurring in adults (Fig. 2.27).

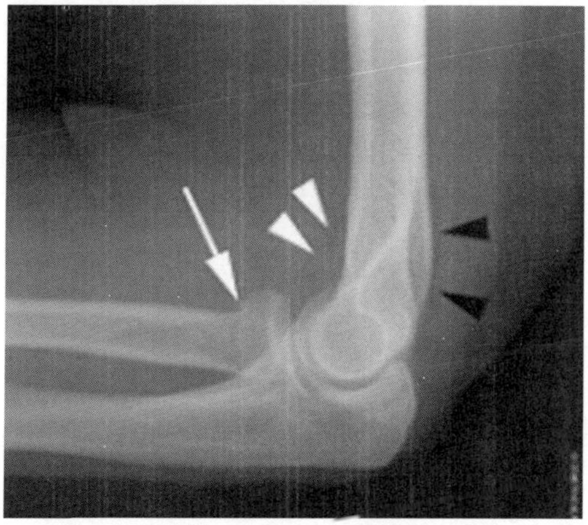

Fig. 2.27: Fracture of head of radius

Mechanism of Injury

- Valgus injury to the elbow causing the impaction of capitulum into radial head.
- Fall on the outstretched hand, transmitting the force axially along the radius shaft causing impaction of radial head into capitulum.

Pathoanatomy

The fracture of radius varies from the simple crack to a badly comminuted fracture. This fracture also cause the bruising of cartilage covering of the articular surface.

Types of Fracture

The fracture of head of radius is divided into the following categories (Fig. 2.28):

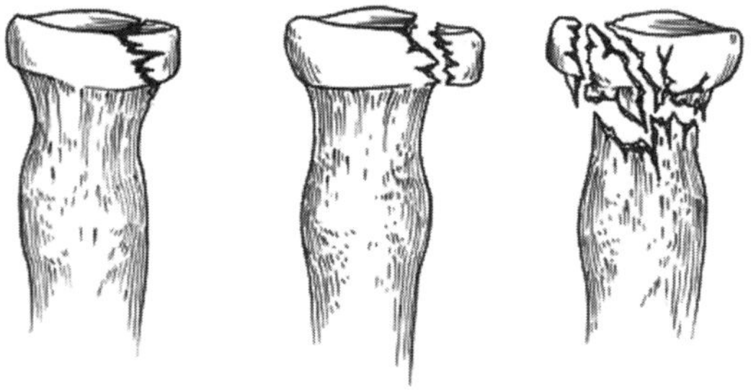

A Undisplaced crack fracture B Displaced fracture C Comminuted fracture

Fig. 2.28

- Undisplaced crack fracture.
- Displaced fracture: A segment of disc shaped radius head is broken and depressed below the plane of articular surface. The broken fragment may be:
  - Fragment < 1/3.
  - Fragment > 1/3.
- Comminuted fracture.

Clinical Features

The patient presents with the history of injury with minimal symptoms:

- Mild pain.
- Minimal swelling at lateral aspect of the elbow.
- Marked local tenderness over the head of the radius.
- Restriction of elbow movement especially of forearm rotations.
- Severe pain at the end range of forearm rotation.

Radiological Examination

The fracture could be easily diagnosed on the radiograph.

Management

The treatment of fracture head of radius depends upon the extent of damage and its severity.

Conservative Treatment

The conservative treatment in case of fracture head of radius is indicated in cases of undisplaced fracture. The elbow is immobilized in an above elbow plaster cast with elbow at 90° of flexion and forearm midway between pronation and supination. The immobilization period is of 2-3 weeks. A plaster cast is always preferred over the cuff and collar sling as the plaster providing rigid immobilization and eliminates pain allowing free movement at shoulder and wrist.

Surgical Treatment

- *Excision of fractured segment:* If the fractured segment is lying loose in the joint cavity causing difficulty in movement, its excision is indicated.
- *Open reduction and internal fixation:* It is indicated in slightly displaced fracture with gross comminution. It prevents proximal migration of radius. The internal fixation can be achieved by either of the following:
  - Miniature plate.
  - Herbert dual pitch headless screw.
- *Excision of radial head:* The head of the radius has to be excised in case of severely comminuted fractures.

Complications

- Joint stiffness.
- Osteoarthritis.

Physiotherapy Treatment

Once the immobilization period is completed, the affected elbow must be rehabilitated with the help of proper physiotherapy protocol so as to gain range of motion, strength and better functional outcome. The movement of supination and pronation must be emphasized.

Day 1 to Week 2:

Aims:

- To decrease pain and inflammation.
- To regain range of motion at wrist and elbow.
- To retard muscle atrophy.

Physiotherapeutic Intervention:

- Range of motion exercises must begin as active-assisted and active exercise for the elbow joint along with pronation-supination.
- Gripping exercise must be initiated.
- Isometric exercise for the elbow joint muscles must be started.
- The muscles at the wrist joint are strengthened using isotonic exercise regime.

Week 3 to Week 6:

Aims:

- To maintain full range of motion at the elbow.
- Elbow strengthening exercises.
- Functional exercises.

Physiotherapeutic Intervention:

- Strengthening of shoulder musculature is done with special emphasis over rotator cuff muscles.
- Range of motion exercise at the elbow must be continued.
- Strengthening exercise at the elbow should be done with light weight cuffs.
- Passive range of motion exercise for gaining supination-pronation must be initiated around week 6 beginning.

Week 7 to Week 12:

This is the period of gaining more strength and practising sports activities.

Aims:

- To enhance strength, power and endurance.
- To practice sports activities.

Physiotherapeutic Intervention:

- Eccentric exercises for the elbow joint.
- Continue isotonic exercise regime for shoulder, forearm and wrist.
- Plyometric exercises.

COLLE'S FRACTURE

Colle's fracture is the fracture of distal end of radius, with fracture line running transversely at cortico-cancellous junction (Fig. 2.29). The fracture is common in all age groups but mostly affects women above 40 years of age due to post-menopausal osteoporosis.

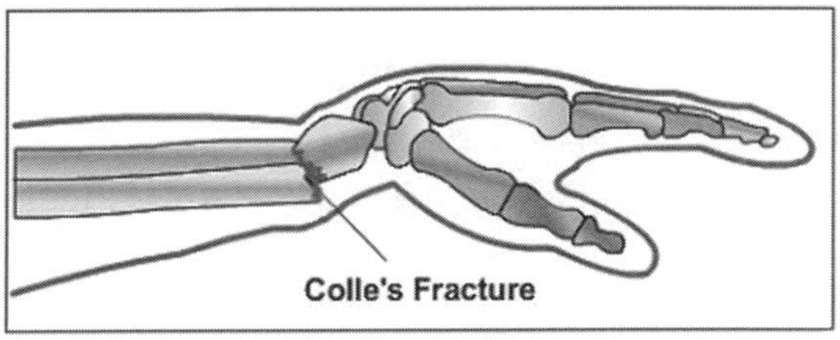

Fig. 2.29: Colle's fracture

Mode of Injury

The fracture results after fall on outstretched hand (Fig. 2.30).

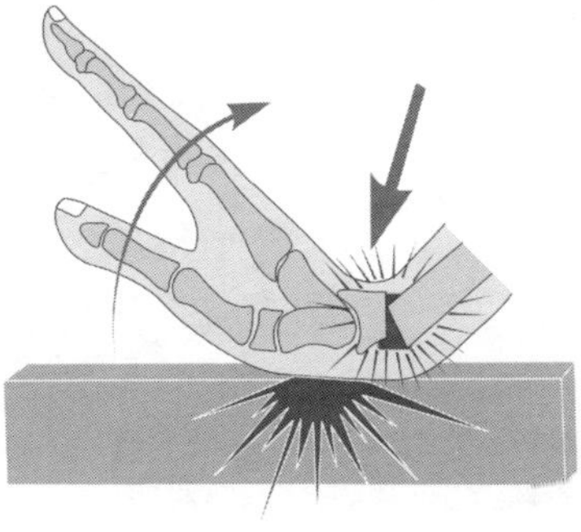

Fig. 2.30: Fall on outstretched hand causing Colle's fracture

Clinical Features

- Pain.
- Swelling.
- Deformity.

On Examination

- There is marked tenderness over the distal end of radius.
- There is abnormal irregularity of lower end of radius.
- The ulnar and radial styloid process comes to lie at the same level or radial styloid process attains a slightly higher position than ulnar styloid.
- On the dorsal aspect of lower third forearm there is hollow or depression proximal to fracture site.
- The lower fracture fragment is displaced backwards producing a marked prominence immediately below the hollow.

Types of Colle's Fracture

There are two classical types of fracture observed:

- Crack fracture without displacement (Fig. 2.31).

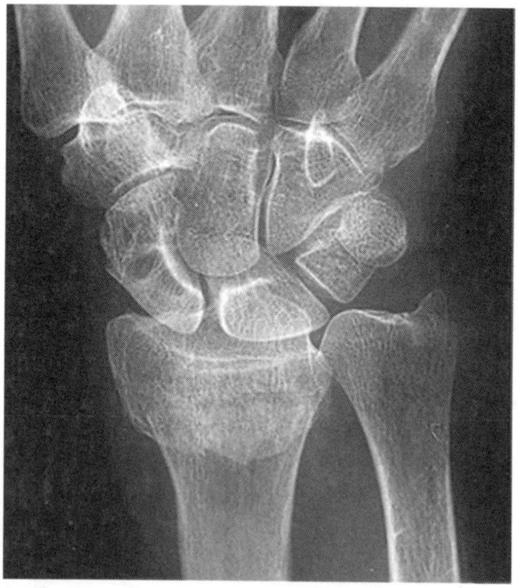

Fig. 2.31: Crack fracture witout displacement

- Displaced C olle's fracture: This is the most common type (Fig. 2.32).

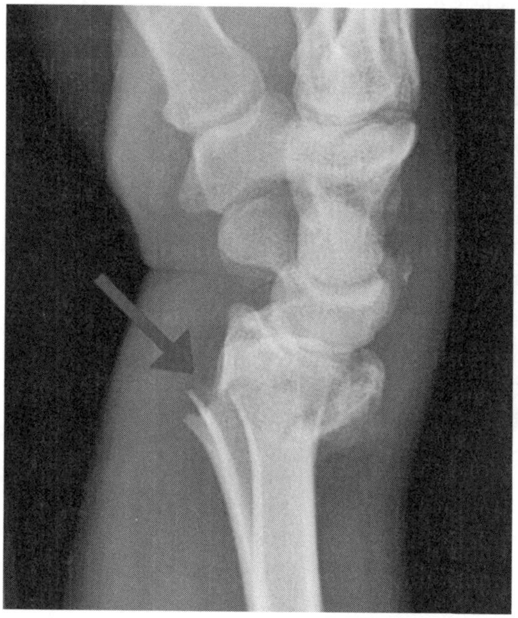

Fig. 2.32: Displaced Colle's fracture

The following displacements are observed:

- Impaction of fragments.
- Dorsal displacements.
- Dorsal tilt.
- Supination.
- Lateral tilt.
- Lateral displacement.

Associated Injury

The following injuries are associated with colle's fracture:

- Fracture styloid process of ulna.
- Rupture of ulnar collateral ligament.
- Rupture of triangular cartilage of ulna.
- Rupture of interosseous radioulnar ligament.

Management

The selected methods of treatment depend upon the type of the fracture and age of the patient.

Undisplaced Fracture: The undisplaced Colle's fracture is immobilized in below elbow plaster cast (Colle's cast) for a period of six weeks (Fig 2.33).

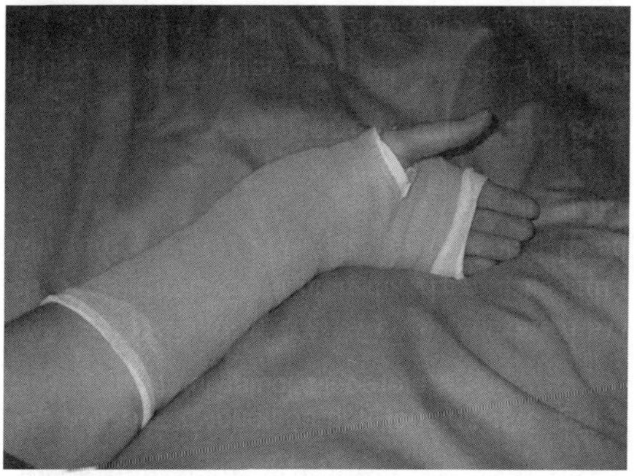

Fig. 2.33: Colle's cast

Displaced Fracture: The displaced colle's fracture is reduced by closed reduction followed by immobilization in Colle's cast.

Young Patients: In case of young patient having displaced colle's fracture or severely comminuted fracture external fixation of the fractured fragment is required.

Complications

- Joint stiffness.
- Malunion.
- Subluxation of inferior radioulnar joint.
- Carpal tunnel syndrome.
- Sudeck's osteodystrophy.
- Rupture of extensor pollicis longus tendon.

Physiotherapy Management of Colle's Fracture

During Immobilization: When the forearm is immobilized in a plaster cast, the therapist must check that it allows full range of movement at the metacarpophalangeal joint of thumb and fingers.

Aims of Physiotherapy during Immobilization:

- To increase circulation.
- To reduce pain and swelling.

To increase circulation: Elbow and the shoulder joint of the ipsilateral hand must be moved through full range of motion. The fingers must be strongly exercised for the active movement.

To reduce pain and swelling:

- The affected hand must be elevated above the level of the heart, this elevation will reduce swelling.
- Wrapping the digits and the hand with self-adhesive elastic tapes provides a compression effect and thus reduces oedema.
- Various physiotherapy adjuncts like cryotherapy, moist hot packs, infra-red and TENS can be used to combat pain and swelling.
- Full range active movements at all the free joints of the affected extremity must be encouraged.

During Mobilization: The main goal of physiotherapy treatment during mobilization is to achieve full range of movement at wrist and forearm along with the strengthening of forearm muscles. Prior to the range of motion exercise, the affected area must be prepared for the exercise by inducing relaxation using paraffin wax bath or the hydrocollatoral packs.

The range of motion exercises at wrist and forearm must be initiated as active-assisted exercises:

- The patient must be instructed to perform free movements at the wrist in the available range to gain flexion and extension.
- Gravity assisted flexion and extension can be initiated by placing the patient's forearm on the table and the hand hanging freely. Flexion at wrist is achieved by placing the forearm in pronation and extension by placing the forearm in supination.
- Wand exercises provide good means of assistance in increasing flexion and extension at wrist and forearm supination and pronation.

The patient must be encouraged to do the exercises to gain grip strengthening either by using springs, therabands or clay.

Passive mobilization of the wrist and forearm are initiated, once the healing is well established. The technique of passive mobilization is as mentioned below:

The patient is in sitting position with forearm supported on the treatment table and wrist over edge of the table. The therapist grasps the patient's forearm around the styloid process to fix radius and ulna, and uses the other hand to grasp the distal row of carpals. The therapist applies a pull in the distal direction with respect to arm to provide joint distraction and performs the various glides to improve the restricted range of motion:

- Dorsal glide to increase flexion.
- Volar glide to increase extension.
- Radial glide to increase ulnar deviation.
- Ulnar glide to increase radial deviation.

Along with these basic glides to improve the range of motion the movement must be attempted simultaneously.

In the early stage of the treatment, if swelling and pain persist even after an exercise session, the use of intermittent sling must be encouraged.

Day 0 - Week 1:

- Full active range of motion of digits at metacarpophalangeal joint.
- Full opposition of the thumb.
- Attempt isometric exercises to the intrinsic muscles of the hand.
- No supination and pronation of the involved extremity.
- No weight bearing on the involved extremity.

Week 2 - Week 4:

- Full range of motion of metacarpophalangeal and interphalangeal joints.
- Attempt gentle active range of motion of wrist if treated by open reduction and internal fixation.
- Isometric exercises to intrinsic muscles of the hand and wrist flexors and extensors.
- No weight bearing on affected extremity.

Week 4 - Week 6:

- Full active range of motion of wrist, metacarpophalangeal and interphalangeal joints.
- Encourage supination and pronation, along with active ulnar and radial deviation.
- Gentle resisted exercise to the digits.
- Isometric exercises to the wrist flexors, extensors, radial and ulnar deviators.
- Use of involved extremity as stabilizer in two-handed activities. Attempt self-care with involved extremity.
- Avoid weight bearing until the end of week 6.

Week 6 - Week 8:

- Full range of motion at all joints of upper extremity.
- Emphasis on supination and ulnar deviation.
- Initiate active assistive to passive range of motion.
- Gentle resistive exercises to digits and wrist.
- Improve power grip.
- Weight bearing on involved extremity as tolerated.

Week 8 - Week 12:

- Full active and passive range of motion in all planes to wrist and digits.
- Stress on supination and ulnar deviation.
- Progressive resistive exercises to all muscle groups of wrist and digits.
- Full weight bearing as tolerated on involved extremity.

SCAPHOID FRACTURE

The fracture of scaphoid bone is common in young adults. The fracture line runs through the waist of scaphoid, therefore the proximal and distal fractures fragment are of equal sizes.

Mode of Injury

Fall on outstretched hand (Fig. 2.34).

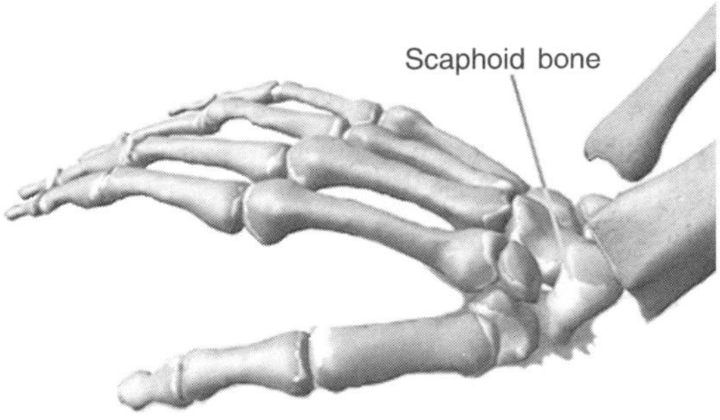

Fig. 2.34: Scaphoid fracture

Types of Scaphoid Fracture

- *Crack Fracture:* There occurs no displacement and the fractured fragments lie in close opposition (Fig. 2.35).
- *Displaced Fracture:* There occurs development of step between fractures fragment (Fig. 2.36).

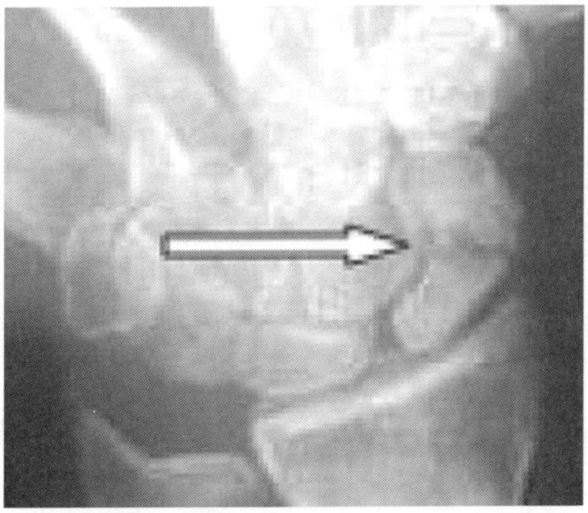

Fig. 2.35: Crack fracture

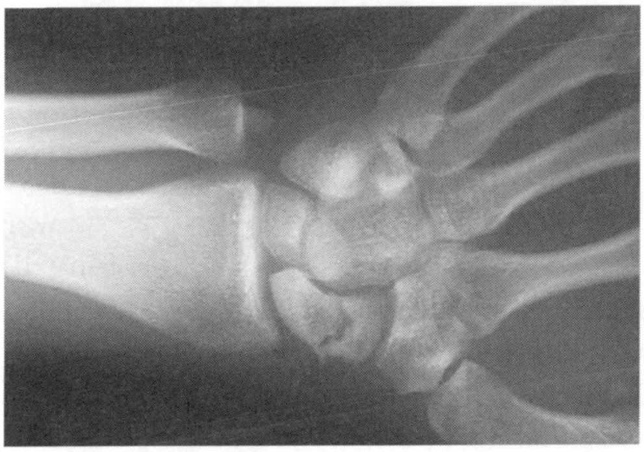

Fig. 2.36: Displaced scaphoid fracture

Clinical Features

- The patient complains of pain and swelling on the radial aspect of wrist.
- On examination, tenderness is elicited in the anatomical snuff box (Scaphoid fossa).
- The wrist movements are impaired.

Radiological Examination

The fracture of scaphoid can be missed if only AP and lateral views of the wrist are taken. Oblique view of the wrist joint is required.

Management

Conservative Treatment (Fig. 2.37)

It is used in patient with crack fracture. The fractured extremity is immobilized in scaphoid cast for 3-4 weeks.

Surgical Treatment (Fig. 2.38)

The treatment is recommended in cases of displaced scaphoid fracture. Open reduction and internal fixation is required.

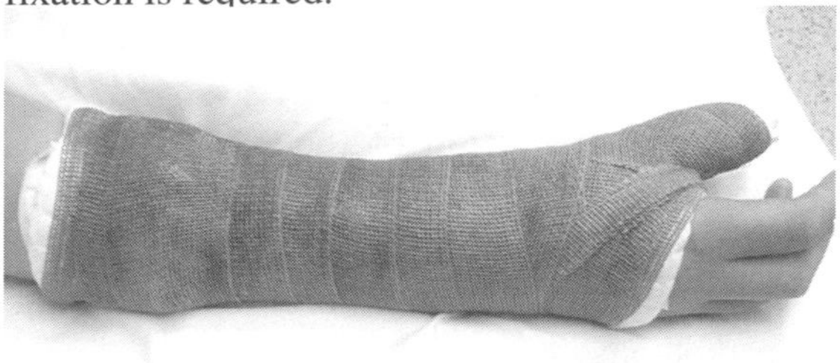

Fig. 2.37: Scaphoid cast

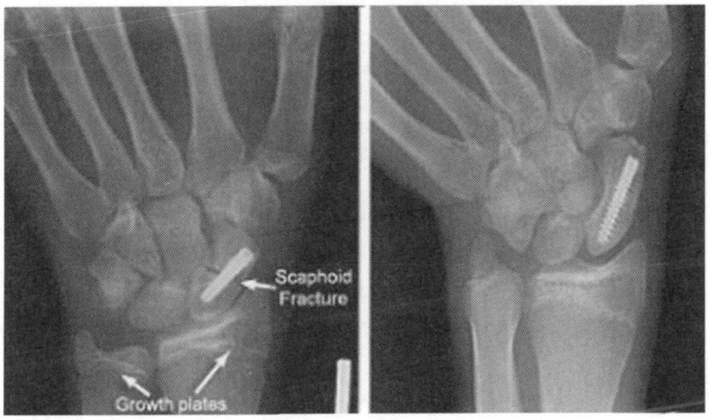

Fig. 2.38: Open reduction and internal fixation of displaced scaphoid fracture

Complications

- Avascular necrosis.
- Delayed and non union.
- Wrist osteoarthritis.

Physiotherapy Management

During Immobilization:

- Active movements at the shoulder joint are encouraged.
- All the metacarpophalangeal and interphalangeal joints from second to fifth digit are checked and encouraged for the full range of movements.
- Active flexion-extension and supination-pronation at the elbow and forearm are initiated.

During Mobilization:

- Immediately after the removal of the plaster cast the primary aim is to reduce pain. To reduce pain various physiotherapeutic adjuncts like ultrasound, TENS, hot packs may be employed.
- Removable thumb spica splint is used for two weeks after the removal of plaster cast.
- Gentle mobilization of the wrist (flexion-extension, ulnar-radial deviation) and the thumb (at MCP and IP) must be initiated.
- Grip strengthening exercises must be incorporated.
- The patient is allowed to use wrist for all the movements.

Day 0 - Week 1:
- No range of motion exercise to thumb and wrist.
- Gentle active range of motion exercise to all the digits, elbow and shoulder.
- Avoid supination and pronation.
- No strengthening exercises to the thumb, wrist and elbow.
- Initiate isometric exercises to the deltoid, biceps and triceps.
- No weight bearing is allowed on the affected extremity.

Week 2 - Week 4:
- No range of motion exercise to thumb and wrist.
- Active and passive range of motion to the digits.
- Gentle active elbow flexion and extension.
- Active and active assisted range of motion at shoulder.
- No strengthening exercise to thumb, wrist and elbow.
- Isometric exercise to deltoid, biceps and triceps.

Week 4 - Week 6:
- Gentle active range of motion exercise to wrist and thumb. Hydrotherapy can be utilized to improve range of motion.
- Gentle active range of motion to elbow in flexion and extension. No supination-pronation is allowed.
- Active and passive range of motion to all digits and shoulder.
- Isotonic exercise to the elbow flexors is initiated.

Week 8 - Week 12:
- In cases treated conservatively, gentle active range of motion to all joints of thumb and wrist.
- In cases treated surgically, regain full range of motion at all joints of thumb and wrist using active, active assisted and passive range of motion exercises.
- At the end of 12 weeks, initiate resisted exercises to the long flexors end extensors of thumb and wrist.
- Resisted exercises to the elbow flexors, extensors, supinators and pronators.
- Encourage patients to use affected extremity for stabilization purposes and certain self-care activities.
- Weight bearing on the affected extremity is allowed after 12 weeks.

Week 12 - Week 16:
- Active-assisted and passive range of motion of wrist and thumb.
- Initiate progressive resistive exercises to the musculature of wrist and thumb.
- Full weight bearing on the affected extremity is allowed.

BARTON'S FRACTURE

The Barton's fracture extends from distal articular surface of radius to anterior or posterior cortices.

Mode of Injury

Fall on back of hand, i.e., with wrist flexed.

Types of Fracture

Barton's fracture exhibits two types:

- Anterior marginal type: Volar Barton's fracture (Fig. 2.39).
- Posterior marginal type: Dorsal Barton's fracture (Fig. 2.40).

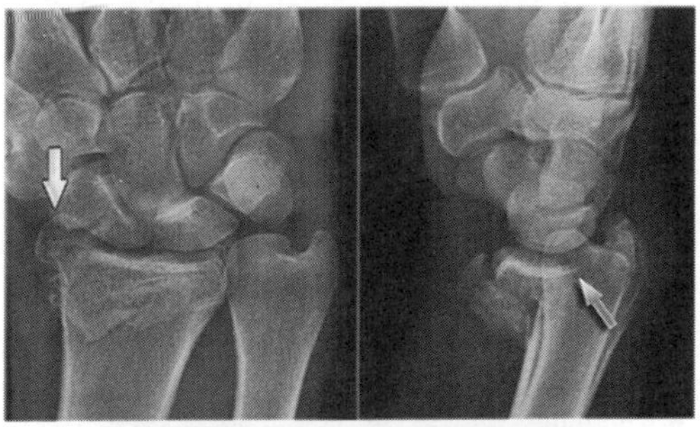

Fig. 2.39: Volar Barton's fracture

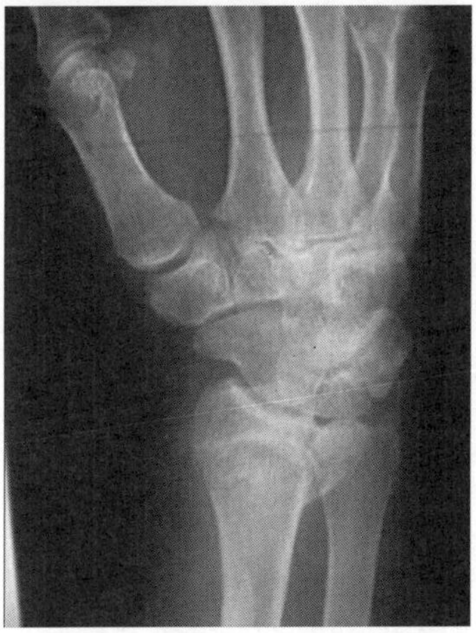

Fig. 2.40: Dorsal Barton's fracture

Treatment

Closed reduction and immobilization in a plaster cast is required. If it fails, open reduction and internal fixation of fractured fragments is required.

FRACTURE OF METACARPAL BONE

This is a common fracture usually encountered in all age groups.

Mode of Injury

- Fall on hand.
- Blow on knuckles.
- Crushing of hand under heavy object.

Position of Fracture (Fig. 2.41)

Fracture of base of metacarpal: The fracture can be transverse or undisplaced.

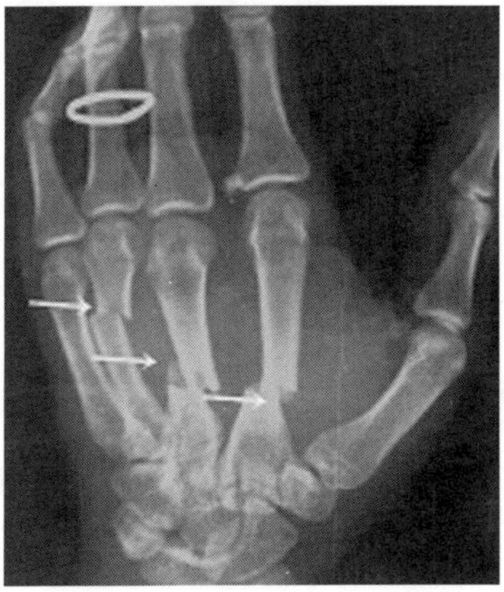

Fig. 2.41: Fracture of metacarpal bone

Fracture through shaft of metacarpal: The fracture can be transverse or oblique. The fracture through shaft of metacarpal is usually undisplaced due to splinting effect of interossei and adjacent metacarpals. When more than one metacarpal shaft is fractured, auto-immobilization or splinting advantage is lost thus making the fracture unstable.

Fracture through neck of metacarpal: This fracture is common in fifth metacarpal known as Boxer's fracture. In this the distal fractures fragment is tilted forwards.

Management

Conservative Treatment:

It is used for stable fractures in which the hand is immobilized in dorsal slab for three weeks. Closed reduction is recommended if the fractured fragments are displaced or angulated.

Surgical Treatment:
It is only recommended in the unstable fracture through shaft of metacarpal in which the fractured fragments are internally fixed using k-wires.

Physiotherapy Management

Day 0 - Week 1:
- No passive range of motion is allowed.
- Active range of motion to non-splinted digits.
- Prescribe isometric exercises within the cast of non-splinted fingers.

Week 2 - Week 4:
- No passive range of motion to the affected digit.
- In cases treated with rigid fixation, active range of motion exercise to the affected digits can be initiated.
- Active, active assisted and passive range of motion to the non-splinted digits.

Week 4 - Week 6:
- Full active range of motion exercises to all digits and wrist.
- Gentle ball squeezing and silly putty exercises.
- Gentle adduction and abduction resistive exercises to the digits.
- Bimanual activities are encouraged at week 6.

Week 6 - Week 8:
- Active, active assistive and passive range of motion to all digits.
- Resistive exercise to all digits and wrist.
- Full weight bearing on affected extremity.

Week 8 - Week 12:
- Full active and passive range of motion to all digits and wrist.
- Progressive resistive exercises to the digits and wrist.

FRACTURE OF BASE OF FIRST METACARPAL

The fracture of base of first metacarpal is common in boxers.

Cause: Longitudinal violence applied to thumb.

Types of Fracture

- Extra-articular fracture of base of first metacarpal.
- Intra-articular fracture of base of first metacarpal.

Bennett's Fracture-Dislocation (Fig. 2.42)

It is the intra-articular fracture-dislocation at base of first metacarpal. The fracture line is oblique with subluxation or dislocation of metacarpal. The fracture-dislocation is quite serious because of more chance of displacement of large distal fragment backwards and upwards upon the smaller proximal fragment.

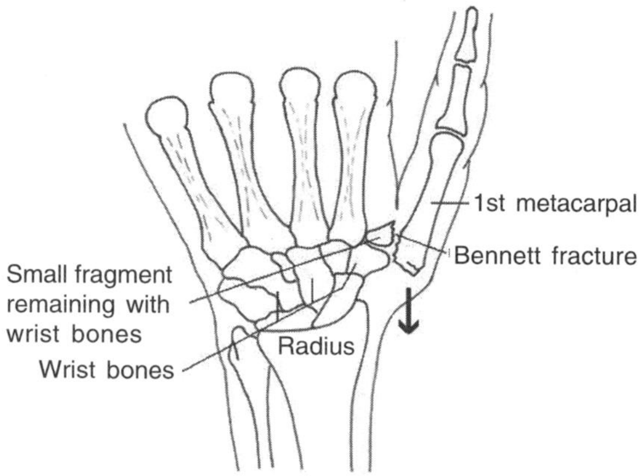

Fig. 2.42: Bennett's fracture-dislocation

Treatment

- In case of mild displacement, closed manipulation and immobilization in a plaster cast is recommended.
- Closed reduction and internal fixation is also practised.
- Open reduction and internal fixation with k-wire or screw is recommended in severely displaced fracture.

Complications

- Redisplacement is common.
- Osteoarthritis.

Rolando's Fracture (Fig 2.43)

It is the extra-articular fracture of the base of first metacarpal. The fracture is not serious in nature.

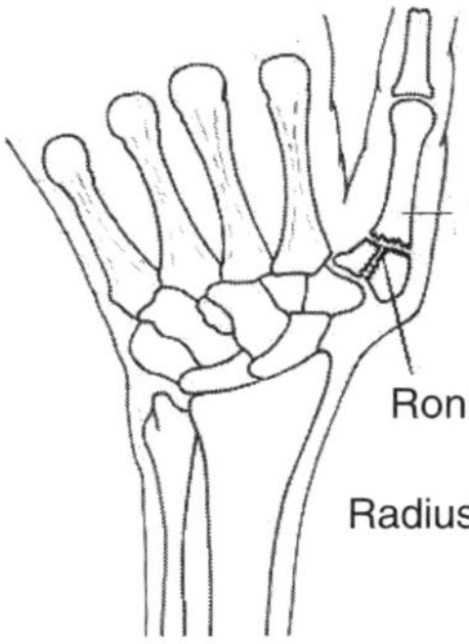

Fig. 2.43: Rolando's fracture

Treatment

The affected extremity is immobilized in thumb spica for a period of three weeks after reduction of the fracture.

FRACTURE OF PHALANGES

Mode of Injury

- Fall of a heavy object on finger.
- Crush injury

Patterns of Fracture of Phalanges

- Long spiral fracture of shaft.
- Oblique fracture of base.
- Transverse fracture of shaft.
- Comminuted fracture.

Management

Fracture of phalanges readily unites irrespective of splintage or immobilization.

Undisplaced Fracture: Splintage using adhesive strapping to the corresponding segment of adjacent finger is done. The splintage is needed to prevent redisplacement and to control pain. The period of immobilization is of two weeks.

Displaced Fracture: In cases where the fractures fragments are displaced closed reduction and immobilization in malleable aluminum splint for three weeks is required. If closed reduction fails, open reduction and internal fixation using k-wires or percutaneous fixation is required.

Comminuted Fracture: In case of comminuted fracture no special treatment is required and special attention is needed for accompanying soft tissue injury.

Physiotherapy Management

Day 0 - Week 1:

- No range of motion to the affected digit in case of unstable fracture.
- Active range of motion exercise to the unaffected digits and to the affected digit in case of stable fracture.
- Initiate isometric exercise to the intrinsic muscles of the unaffected digits.

Week 2 - Week 4:

- No range of motion to the splinted joint.
- Active range of motion to all non-splinted joint and digits.
- Isometric strengthening to the intrinsic muscles.

Week 4 - Week 6:

- No passive range of motion to the affected joint.
- Full active and active assistive range of motion to all the digits.
- Isometric and isotonic exercises for all the muscles of the digits.
- Bimanual activities using involved extremity are encouraged for self-care.
- Weight bearing on involved extremity as tolerated by patient.

Week 6 - Week 8:

- Use night splint if required.
- Active, active assisted and passive range of motion to all digits.
- Gentle resistive exercise to all digits.
- Use involved extremity for self-care.
- Full weight bearing initiated on involved extremity.

Week 8 - Week 12:

- Full active and passive range of motion exercises to all digits.
- Progressive resistive exercises to all digits.

CHAPTER 3

DISLOCATIONS OF UPPER EXTREMITY

DISLOCATION OF STERNOCLAVICULAR JOINT

Dislocation of sternoclavicular joint (Fig. 3.1) is a rare injury. In this type of injury the medial end of clavicle is usually displaced forwards. Backward dislocation is rarely seen. The backward dislocation of medial end of clavicle is known as reterosternal dislocation.

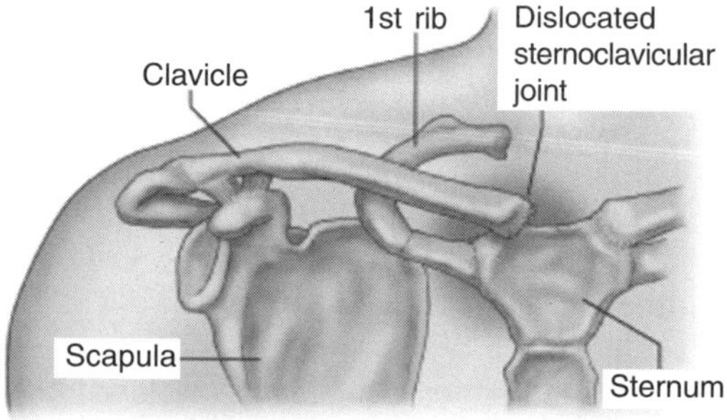

Fig. 3.1: Dislocation of sternoclavicular joint

Diagnosis

The diagnosis of sternoclavicular dislocation is more often made clinically rather than radiographic visualization.

Treatment

In anterior displacement (Fig. 3.2(a)): The anterior displacement of sternoclavicular joint is reduced by direct pressure over the medial end of clavicle while shoulders are arched forwards. Reduction is maintained in figure of eight bandage after applying a pad over the front of joint. The sling has to be worn atleast for two weeks.

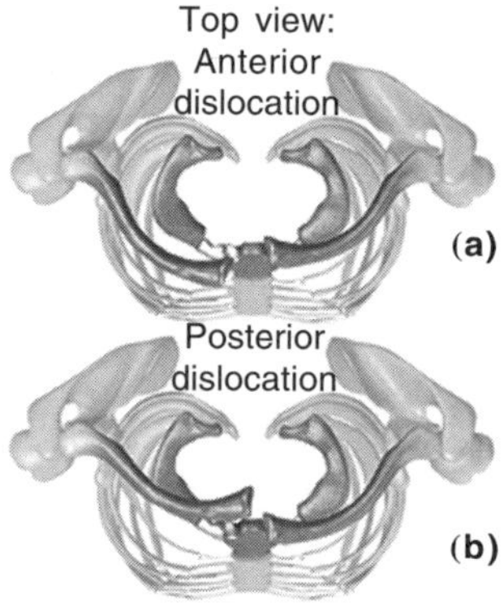

Fig. 3.2: Anterior and posterior dislocation of sternoclavicular joint

In retrosternal/posterior displacement (Fig. 3.2(b)): In this case, early surgical intervention is needed. The displaced bone is pulled forward into place with hook.

Physiotherapy Management

In both types of displacement, active shoulder exercises are encouraged after two weeks.

Complications

In case of retrosternal dislocation, the medial end of clavicle may press dangerously upon the trachea or great vessels.

RECURRENT DISLOCATION OF STERNOCLAVICULAR JOINT

Recurrent dislocation of sternoclavicular joint is evident when the medial end of clavicle projects out each time the shoulders are braced. There occurs self reduction with the medial end clicking back into position when the shoulders are arched forwards.

Treatment

The treatment is needed only if repeated dislocations are causing any sort of problem.
Surgical stabilization of joint is necessary and is done by constructing a new retaining ligament from tendon of subclavius muscle or from a strip of fascia lata.

DISLOCATION OF ACROMIOCLAVICULAR JOINT

Mode of Injury

Fall on the outer prominence of shoulder.

Pathology

The integrity of acromioclavicular joint depends upon acromioclavicular and coracoclavicular ligaments. Injury to the joint may cause either subluxation or dislocation depending upon the severity of injury. The acromion is displaced slightly downwards from the lateral end of clavicle (Fig. 3.3).

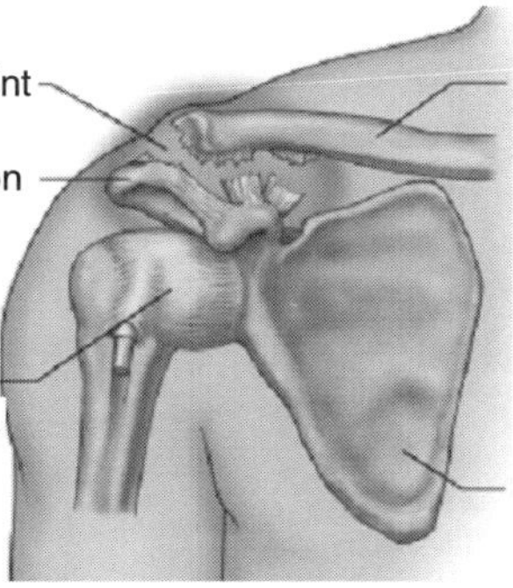

Fig. 3.3: Dislocation of acromioclavicular joint

Thus the severity of injury classifies the acromioclavicular joint injury into 3 grades (Fig. 3.4):

Grade	*Severity of injury*	*Pathoanatomy*
Grade 1	Minimal strain	Rupture of joint capsule
Grade 2	Moderate strain	Rupture of acromioclavicular ligament with joint capsule
Grade 3	Maximum strain	Rupture of joint capsule, acromioclavicular and coracoclavicular ligament

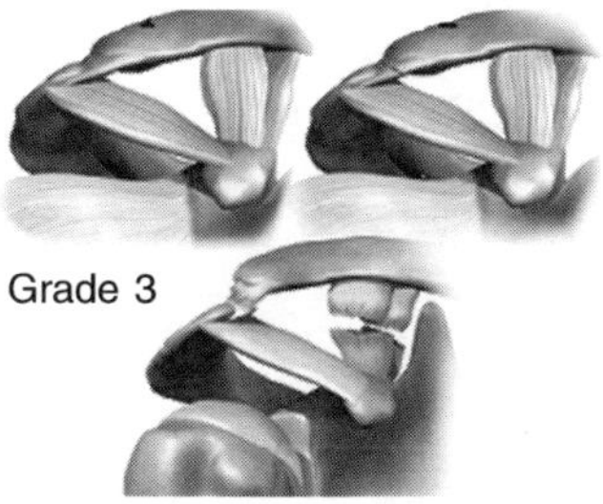

Fig. 3.4: Classification of acromioclavicular joint injury

Clinical Features

All the signs and symptoms pertaining to injury is localised to the acromioclavicular joint:
- Pain.
- Swelling.
- Tenderness.
- Difference in level of outer end of clavicle and acromion.

Treatment

In case of subluxation: Subluxation of acromioclavicular joint is treated by conservative management. Either of the following methods could be employed:
- Strapping of joint for three weeks.
- Support to the limb for two weeks.

In case of dislocation: Dislocation of acromioclavicular joint is managed by open reduction and internal fixation, i.e., surgical intervention is necessary. Internal fixation of joint is done either with the help of screw or wire. The screw or wire should be removed after 10 or 12 weeks.

In some severe cases, reconstruction of the coracoalvicular ligaments is necessary.

Physiotherapy Management

In case of conservative treatment:

Immobilization period: It is of three weeks. Following is to be done during immobilization:
- Careful checking of immobilization.
- Full range of movements to elbow, forearm, wrist and fingers.
- Isometrics to the shoulder.

Mobilization Period

- Pendular swinging movements at the shoulder are initiated, while the limb is still supported in the sling.
- Passive mobilization of the joint is initiated with the patient in supine lying. The emphasis is given on abduction–elevation, horizontal abduction and horizontal adduction. These movements put stretch on AC joint.
- Acromioclavicular joint plays an important role in abduction-elevation beyond 135°. Thus active assisted movement of abduction beyond 90 is emphasized.
- In order to relieve pain and induce relaxation, thermotherapy adjuncts can be used.
- Self resistive regime of movements is initiated with graduated dumbbell exercises.

Regainment of strong active function within full range takes 6-8 weeks.

In case of surgical treatment:

Immobilization period: 4 weeks:
- Careful checking of immobilization is necessary.
- Full range of active movements to be initiated at the joints free from immobilization.

During mobilization period:

- To relieve pain and reduce the patient's reluctance, thermotherapy adjuncts are used before and after exercise regime.
- Strengthening of coracoclavicular ligament is initiated by self resisted isometric exercises of shoulder horizontal abduction and horizontal adduction.
- Rest of treatment is same as for conservative management.

Active range of shoulder is regained within 8–10 weeks.

SHOULDER DISLOCATION

The glenohumeral joint is the most common joint to be dislocated either anteriorly, posteriorly or inferiorly. The dislocation is more common in adults as compared to children.

Mechanism of Injury

For anterior disolcation:
- Fall on outstretched hand with shoulder in abduction and external rotation.
- Direct force pushing the humerus out of glenoid cavity.

For posterior dislocation:
- Direct blow on front of shoulder.
- As a consequence of electric shock or an epileptiform convulsions.

Classification

The glenohumeral dislocation is classified into three types depending upon the position of dislocated humeral head:
- Anterior dislocation.
- Posterior dislocation.
- Inferior dislocation.

Anterior dislocation (Fig. 3.5): It is the most common of all glenohumeral dislocation. In this type of dislocation, the humeral head comes out

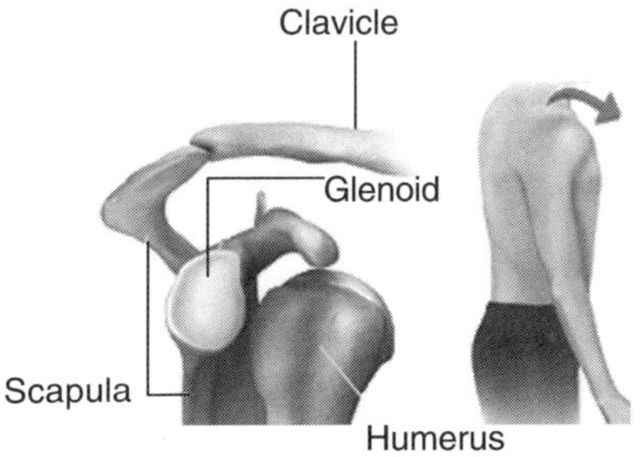

Fig. 3.5: Anterior dislocation

of glenoid cavity to lie in anterior position. The anterior dislocation is further categorised into following categories:

- Preglenoid anterior dislocation–The humeral head lies in front of glenoid cavity.
- Subcoracoid anterior dislocation–The humeral head lies below the coracoids process.
- Subclavicular anterior dislocation–The humeral head lies below the clavicle.

Posterior dislocation (Fig. 3.6): In this type of dislocation the humeral head lies posteriorly behind the glenoid cavity.

Inferior dislocation (Fig. 3.7): It is also known as Luxatio erecta and the position of the humeral head is subglenoid, i.e., the head lies beneath the glenoid cavity. This is a rare type of dislocation.

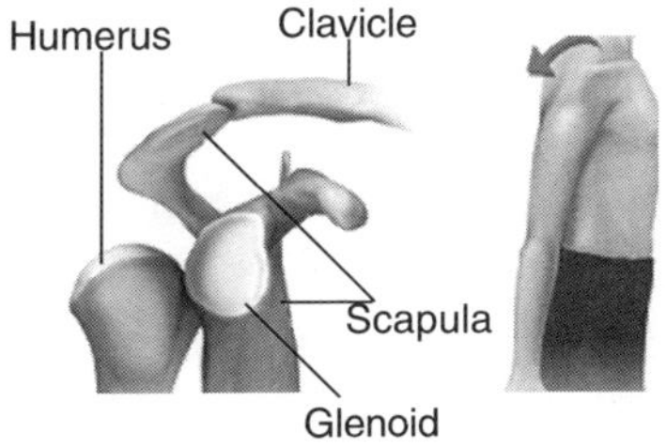

Fig. 3.6: Posterior dislocation

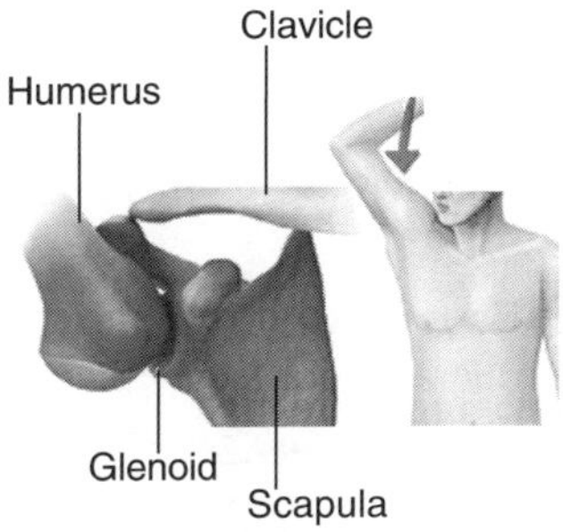

Fig. 3.7: Inferior dislocation

Clinical Features

Anterior Dislocation:

- The affected arm is in abduction.
- Severe pain.
- Restricted movements of the shoulder joint.
- Flattened contour of the shoulder.
- Fullness is experienced below the clavicle due to position of dislocated glenohumeral joint.

Posterior Dislocation:

- The affected arm is fixed in medial rotation.
- Anterior flattening of the shoulder below the front of acromion.

Diagnosis

Special tests for anterior dislocation:

- *Dugas test:* Patient is not able to touch his/her opposite shoulder.
- *Hamilton ruler test:*If we place a ruler on lateral side of arm, acromion and lateral humeral condyle can be touched simultaneously due to flattening of shoulder.
- *Callaway's test:* In case of dislocated shoulder, ventral circumference of the axilla is increased compared to normal extremity.

Radiographic examination: The characterstic feature of dislocation may be masked by the soft tissues in case of obese patients hence the radiographic evaluation is always necessary. The following radiographic views are to be taken:

- Anteriorposterior view.
- Axillary view.
- Oblique Wallace-Hellier view.

Treatment

The basic aim of treatment is to reduce the dislocated humeral head back to its position and thus maintaining it.

Reduction of Dislocation in case of Anterior Dislocation:

- *Kocher's manoeuvre*–In this method traction is applied to the long head of humerus with the elbow flexed to 90^0. The arm is rotated externally and is then adducted by carrying the elbow across the body towards the midline. Then the arm is rotated medially so that the hand of the affected extremity falls across the opposite shoulder.
- *Hippocrate's manoeuvre*–In this method the patient lies supine on the floor with the affected arm semi-abducted. On this semi-abducted arm the surgeon applies a firm and steady traction. He keep his foot in the axilla against the chest wall. The head of the humerus is levered back into position using the foot as fulcrum.

Reduction of Posterior Dislocation:

Longitudinal traction is applied on the affected arm while rotating it laterally. Direct forward pressure may also be applied over the displaced humeral head.

In both types of dislocation, reduction is carried out under sedation or general anaesthesia.

Maintenance of Reduction:

- *In anterior dislocation*–The reduced glenohumeral joint immobilized for a period of three weeks by strapping the arm to the trunk.
- *In posterior dislocation*–Immobilization period in case of posterior glenohumeral dislocation is of 2-3 weeks in a sling.

Physiotherapy Management

During Immobilization

- Checking of immobilization as to ensure proper circulation to the limb.
- Full range strong resistive movements to all the free joints of the immobilized extremity.
- Isometric contractions, i.e., self resistive exercises to the deltoid, biceps and triceps.

During Mobilization

Aims of physiotherapy treatment:

- Reduction of pain.
- Regaining range of motion at shoulder joint.
- Strengthening of the shoulder muscles.

Reduction of pain:

Pain during mobilization period can occur either due to the muscular spasm developed during the period of immobilization or due to the incorporated shoulder exercises. In order to relieve pain and muscle spasm following measures could be taken:

- Thermotherapy adjuncts: Hot packs, short wave diathermy.
- Ultrasound therapy.
- Interferential therapy.

Range of motion exercises:

- Full range active movements to the elbow.
- Pendular movements to the shoulder joint: The patient stands in forward stoop position with the arm hanging loosely by the side. The movement of flexion-extension is initiated with the arm hanging to the side.
- In order to achieve the movements of abduction, adduction and shoulder rotations, different regime has to be undertaken for anterior and posterior dislocations.

In case of anterior dislocation:

- Adduction and internal rotation of the arm can be initiated freely.
- Abduction and external rotation may cause the redislocation of the joint and thus needs to be taken care of.
- Abduction is initiated as relaxed passive movement upto 45° with the patient lying supine. The movement is done with the arm in internal rotation.
- External rotation is initiated as a relaxed passive movement in supine lying with arm adducted to the side of the body.

In case of posterior dislocation:
- Abduction and external rotation of the arm can be initiated freely.
- The redislocation of the joint may be caused by the movement of adduction and internal rotation.
- The movement of adduction should be done with shoulder in external rotation.
- The movement of internal rotation should be done with shoulder in abduction.

In both anterior and posterior dislocation, self assisted relaxed movements with wand in supine lying are also helpful at this stage.

Strengthening exercises:
- Self resisted isometric exercises.
- Isotonic movements.
- Dumbbells as resistive devices could be used.

Complications of Glenohumeral Dislocation

- Fracture of greater tuberosity or surgical neck of humerus.
- Supraspinatus tendinitis.
- Rotator cuff injury.
- Recurrent anterior dislocation of shoulder.
- Injury to axillary nerve.

RECURRENT ANTERIOR DISLOCATION OF SHOULDER

The shoulder is the most common joint in the body to undergo recurrent dislocation. The injury tends to occur with increasing frequency and decreasing violence.

Causes

- Marfan's syndrome: Anatomically unstable joint.
- Inadequate treatment of preceding episode of anterior dislocation.
- Improper healing of soft tissues.
- Epileptic patients.

Mode of Injury

Recurrent anterior dislocation of shoulder occurs as a result of abduction, extension and lateral rotation.

Pathology

The pathological changes occurring in case of recurrent anterior dislocation of shoulder can be described as:
- *Bankart's lesion:* The joint capsule is stripped from anterior margin of glenoid rim (Fig. 3.8).
- *Hill Sach's lesion:* The articular surface of humeral head is dented in its postero-lateral quadrant (Fig. 3.9).

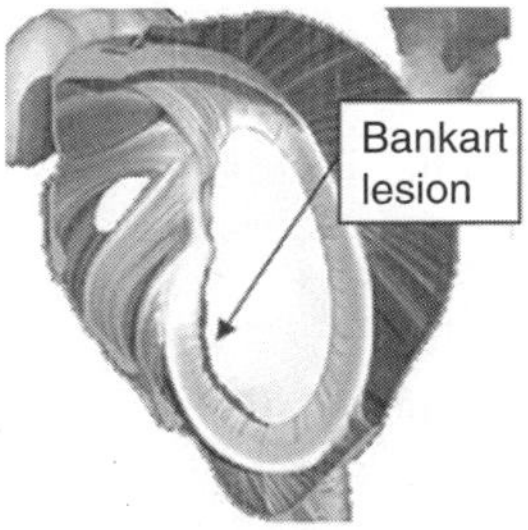

Fig. 3.8: Bankart's lesion

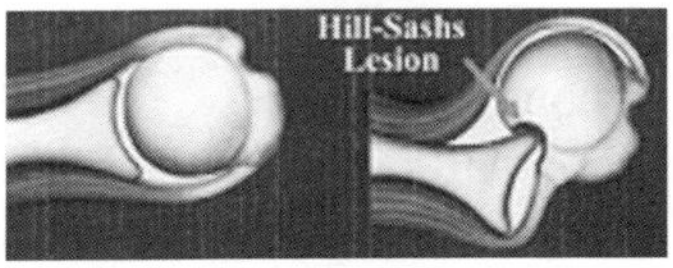

Fig. 3.9: Hill Sach's lesion

- Roundening of anterior glenoid rim occurs due to recurrent dislocation of humeral head over it.

Management

In cases where disability is troublesome, surgical intervention is required. Following surgical techniques are usually undertaken:
- *Putti-Platt surgery:* In order to prevent external rotation and abduction, the subscapularis tendon is double breasted.
- *Bankart's surgery:* The glenoid labrum and capsule are reattached to the front of glenoid rim.
- *Bristow's surgery:* Osteotomization of the coracoid process along with its attatched

muscles at its base and fixation to lower half of anterior margin of glenoid.
- Arthroscopic bankart repair.

Physiotherapy Management

The physiotherapy plays an important role in dealing with the cases of recurrent anterior dislocation of shoulder. The main aspects of physiotherapy regime are:
- Preventive physiotherapy regime.
- Post-surgical physiotherapy regime.

Preventive Physiotherapy Regime:

Objectives:
- Strengthening of ligament and muscles crossing the shoulder joint.
- Regaining full range of motion.

Strengthening Regime

Strengthening regime of ligament and muscles crossing the shoulder joint incorporates several repetitions of one movement.
Position of patient: Standing or sitting.
- Self resisted eccentric exercises.
- Isometric contractions.
- Self resisted small range reversal technique for various agonists and respective antagonist groups.
- Progression is done by using weighted dumbbells or weight cuffs.

Range of Motion Regime

- Passive range of motion exercises with the patient in supine lying.
- Adequate stabilization of shoulder girdle.
- Active-assisted movements.
- Active range of motion to all the shoulder movements with more emphasis on terminal ranges.

Post-Surgical Physiotherapy Regime

The post-surgical physiotherapy regime proceeds on the same line as for anterior dislocation. Post-surgically a functional shoulder can be achieved within 10-12 weeks; however the extreme range of external rotation may remain deficient in some cases.

DISLOCATION OF ELBOW

The dislocation of elbow is fairly common injury both in children and in adults (Fig. 3.10).

Mode of Injury

The elbow dislocation is caused by falling on the outstretched hand with the elbow slightly flexed.

Classification of Elbow Dislocation

- Posterior dislocation–The ulna and radius are displaced backwardly in comparison to humerus (Fig. 3.11).

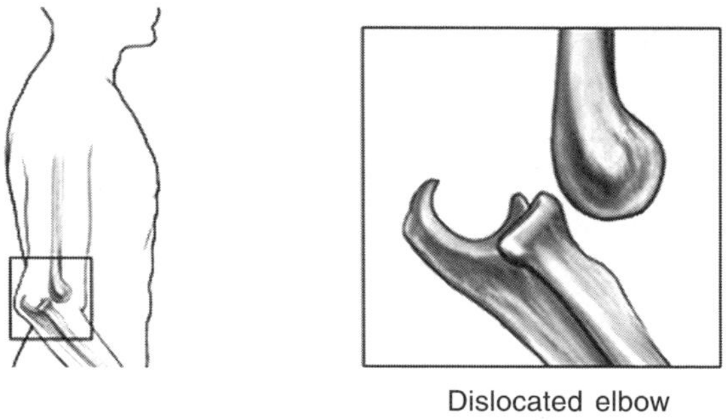

Fig. 3.10: Dislocation of elbow

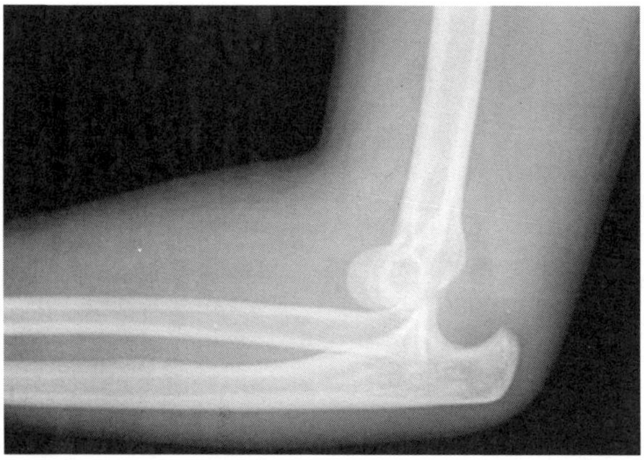

Fig. 3.11: Posterior elbow dislocation

- Posteromedial dislocation (Fig. 3.12).
- Posterolateral dislocation (Fig. 3.13).
- Divergent dislocation–The radius and ulna are diverged in lateral and medial directions respectively (Fig. 3.14).

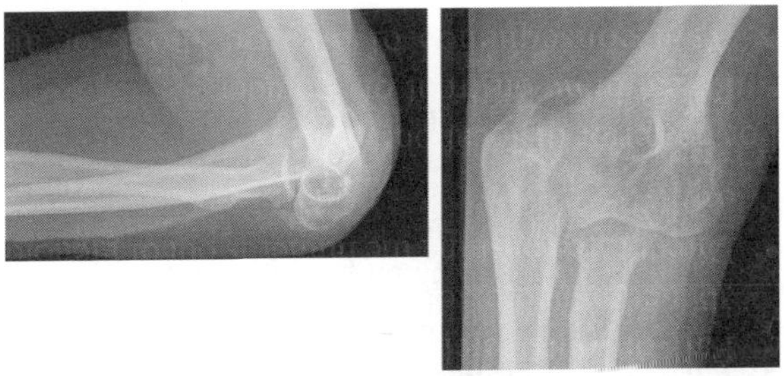

Fig. 3.12: Posteromedial elbow dislocation

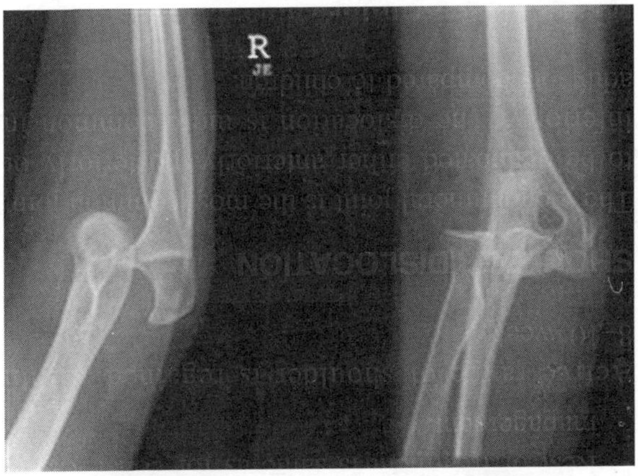

Fig. 3.13: Posterolateral elbow dislocation

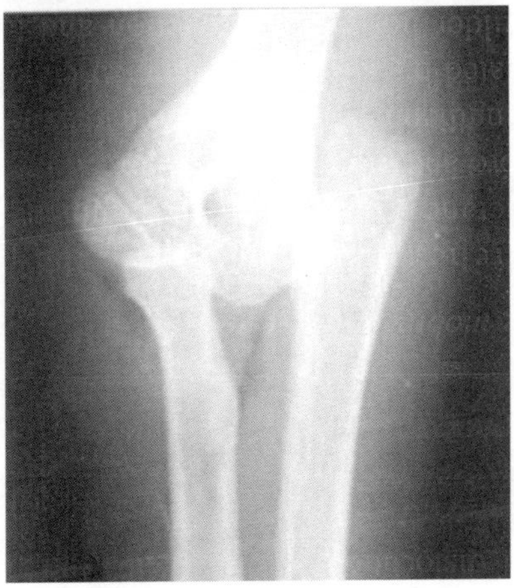

Fig. 3.14: Divergent elbow dislocation

Amongst all types of elbow dislocation, posterior dislocation is the one which is encountered most often in clinical practice.

Posterior Dislocation

The pushing back of radius and ulna results in rupture of periosteum from the lower end of humerus along with the injury to brachialis muscle from coronoid process.

Clinical Features

- Severe pain at the elbow.
- Bowstringing of triceps tendon, i.e., triceps tendon stands out prominently.
- Reversal of three point bony relationship of the elbow.
- Associated median nerve palsy.

Diagnosis

Radiographic examination confirms the clinical diagnosis.

Treatment

The dislocation is reduced under anaesthesia.

Procedure of reduction: The forearm is pulled steadily with the elbow semi-flexed and direct pressure is applied behind the olecranon.

Immobilization: The elbow is immobilized in 90° of flexion in an above elbow plaster slab for 3 weeks. The forearm is held in supination.

Surgical Management

- Open reduction may be necessary in cases where closed manipulation fails and in late cases.
- In neglected cases of elbow dislocation, excisional arthroplasty of the elbow may be done.

Physiotherapy Management

The physiotherapy management in cases of dislocated elbow is needed both during the period of immobilization and mobilization.

Immobilization period: 3 weeks.

Physiotherapy during immobilization period:

Aims:

- To reduce swelling.
- To maintain range of motion.
- Guiding the exercise regime during the period of mobilization.

Intervention:

- Careful checking of plaster cast to ensure proper circulation and freedom of movement to all the free joints.
- To reduce swelling
  - Elevation of the limb.
  - Strong and vigorous movements of all the free joints.
- To maintain range of motion
  - Free active movements to all the free joints, i.e., shoulder, wrist and hand.
- Guiding the exercise regime for the period of mobilization.
  - The complete exercise regime is guided to the patient on the normal extremity to facilitate the exercises on the affected extremity in a proper scheduled manner during mobilization.

Physiotherapy during the period of mobilization:

Aims:

- Evaluation of the post-injury and post-immobilization status of the patient.
- To decrease pain and swelling.
- To increase range of motion at elbow and forearm.

Intervention:

- Evaluation of patient
  - Evaluation of degree of pain and swelling has to be done.
  - Careful examination of range of motion at elbow and forearm, i.e., flexion-extension and pronation-supination.
- To reduce pain and swelling: In order to reduce pain and swelling, suitable thermotherapy adjuncts and other electrotherapy equipments may be used.
  - Paraffin wax bath.
  - Hot saline water.
  - Ultrasound therapy.
- To increase range of motion at elbow and forearm
  - Relaxed and rhythmical active assisted mobilization of elbow and forearm are initiated. Following assistive devices can be used:
    - o Roller skates.
    - o Wand.
    - o Whirlpool bath.
  - Pronation and supination to be initiated in forearm lap position.

Contraindication during mobilization:

- Vigorous passive movements.
- Passive stretching.
- Massage.

Functionally acceptable results can be achieved by 6-8 weeks.

Complications

- Elbow stiffness.
- Myositis ossificans.
- Vascular or nerve injury.

PULLED ELBOW

It is the name given to the subluxation of the head of the radius in young children.

Mode of Injury

Sudden lifting of the child by pulling the wrist (Fig. 3.15).

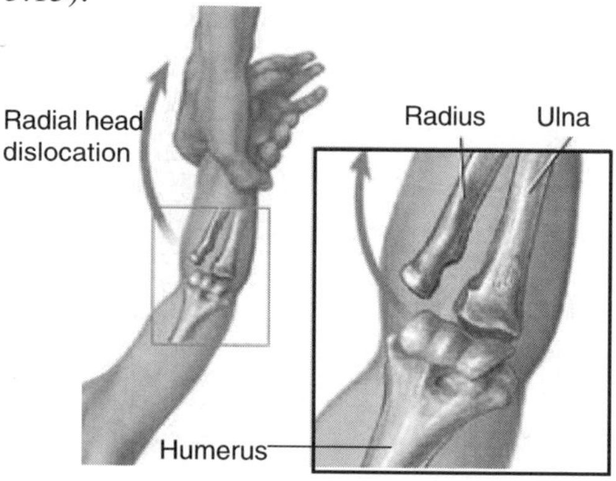

Fig. 3.15: Pulled elbow

Pathology

The head of the radius is pulled partly out of the annular ligament. The radial head is subluxated in an anterior direction (Fig. 3.16).

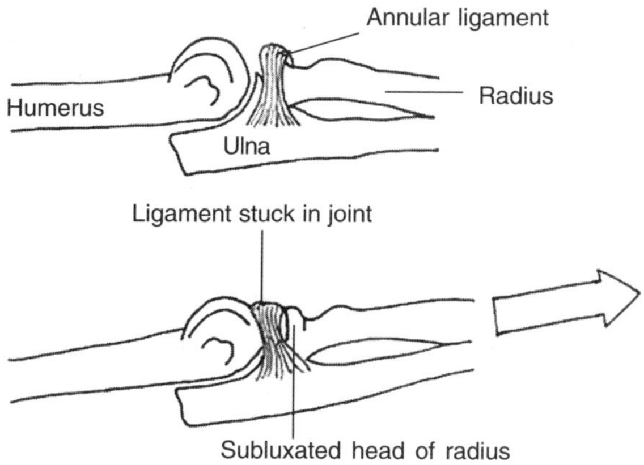

Fig. 3.16: Subluxated radial head

Clinical Features

- Continuously crying child.
- The forearm lies in an attitude of pronation.
- There is mild swelling.
- Localised pain.
- Restricted movements of the elbow.

Radiographic Examination

The subluated radial head being cartilaginous is not visible on a radiograph. Radiograph is taken to rule out any bony injury.

Treatment

The head is reduced by fully supinating the forearm and applying direct pressure over the head of radius.

MONTEGGIA FRACTURE DISLOCATION

This is characterized by the fracture of upper third of the ulna with dislocation of head of radius (Fig. 3.17). It is also referred to as hyperpronation injury.

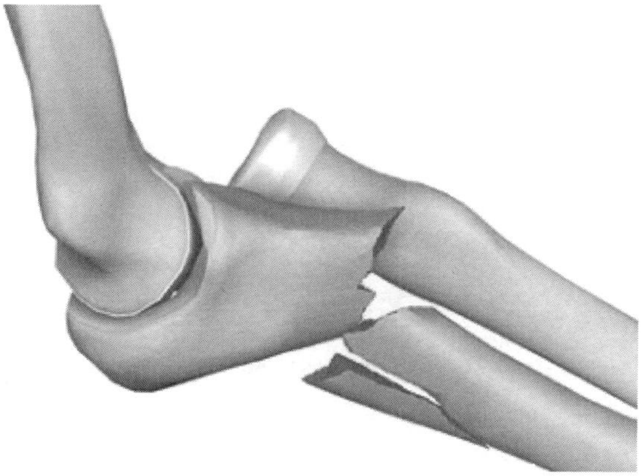

Fig. 3.17: Monteggia fracture dislocation

Mode of Injury

- Fall on outstretched hand with forearm forced into excessive pronation.
- Direct blow on back of upper forearm.

Classification

- *Extension type*: Fractured ulna angulates anteriorly with anterior dislocation of radial head. It is more common type (Fig. 3.18).

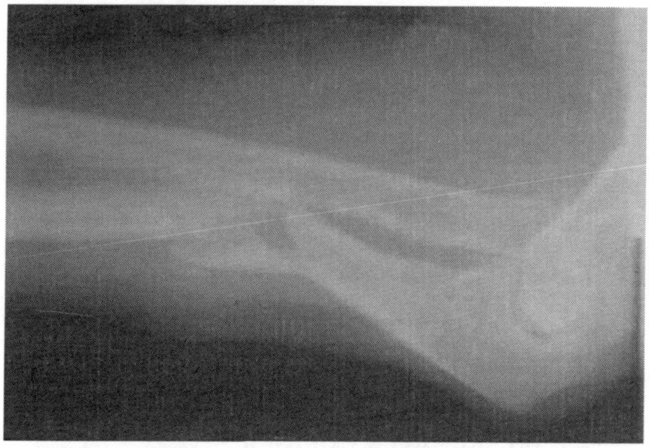

Fig. 3.18: Extension type Monteggia fracture dislocation

- *Flexion type:* Fractured ulna angulates posteriorly with posterior dislocation of radial head (Fig. 3.19).

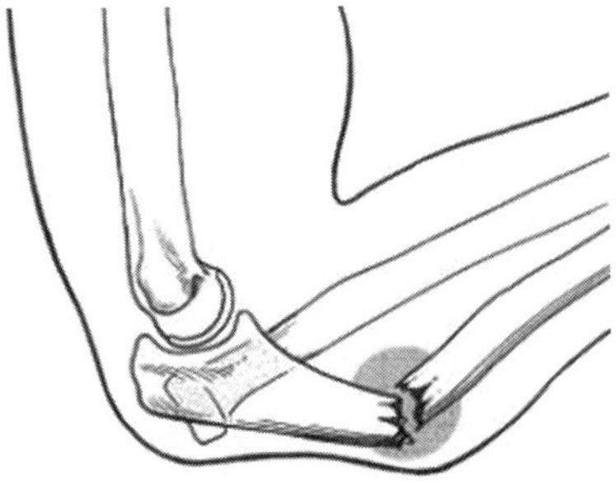

Fig. 3.19: Flexion type Monteggia fracture dislocation

Treatment

- *Closed manipulation*: It is usually done in children. Reduction is done by bringing the forearm into full supination. Then the reduced extremity is immobilized in a plaster cast with elbow flexed to 90° and forearm supinated for about 12 weeks.
- *Open reduction and internal fixation:* It is practised in following cases:
  - Where closed manipulation fails.
  - Redisplacement in plaster cast.
  - Late neglected cases.

Physiotherapy Management

In cases treated conservatively:

During Immobilization:

- Checking of plaster cast.
- Strong and full range movement of all the free joints.

During Mobilization:

- Measures to relief pain, swelling and inflammation are undertaken.
- Range of motion exercises to facilitate.
  - Elbow flexion – extension.
  - Forearm pronation – supination.

In cases treated surgically:

The physiotherapy follows the same guidelines as for conservatively treated cases but the exercise progression should be slow and rhythmic.

GALEAZZI FRACTURE DISLOCATION

In this injury there occurs fracture of lower one-third of the radius along with dislocation or subluxation of distal radio-ulnar joint (Fig. 3.20).

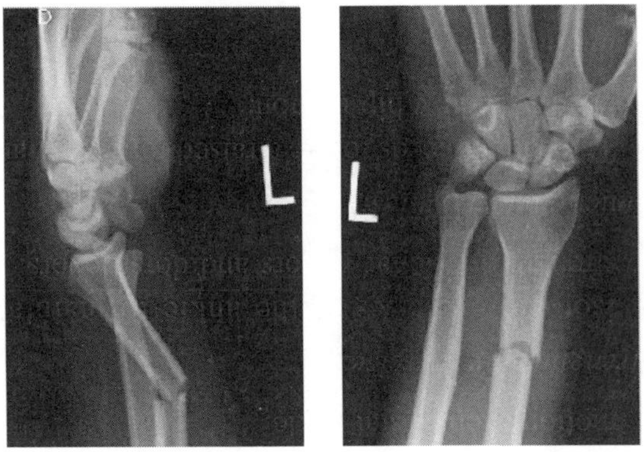

Fig. 3.20: Galeazzi fracture dislocation

Mode of Injury

Fall on outstretched hand.

Pathology

The ligaments surrounding the inferior radio-ulnar joint are ruptured resulting in the subluxation or dislocation of the inferior radio-ulnar joint.

Displacement

The fractured radius angulates anteromedially and distal end of ulna is dislocated dorsally.

Treatment

The treatment of Galeazzi fracture dislocation is done by both conservative and surgical methods.

Physiotherapy Management

The physiotherapy regime runs on the same lines as for Monteggia fracture dislocation. Special concentration is provided on range of motion exercises for:

- Elbow flexion–extension.
- Forearm pronation–supination.
- Wrist flexion–extension.

BENNETT'S FRACTURE DISLOCATION

It is an unstable fracture dislocation which is intra-articular at the base of first metacarpal with subluxation or dislocation of the metacarpal.

Mode of Injury

Longitudinal force applied to the thumb as in boxing.

Displacement

The distal fragment is displaced backwards and upwards upon the proximal fragment.

Treatment

The treatment in this type of fracture dislocation has to be done very accurately either by conservative or surgical means.

Conservative Treatment

The closed manipulation is practised in the mild cases. It is always done under anaesthesia and a well-moulded plaster cast is employed for immobilization. The cast extends from forearm, wrist and should hold the metacarpal well extended at carpo-metacarpal joint. Check radiographs are always taken to ensure the correct position and healing.

Surgical Treatment

- Closed reduction and percutaneous fixation by kuschner wire.
- Open reduction and internal fixation by k-wire or screw.

Physiotherapy Management

During Immobilization:

- Immobilization period is of usually 4-6 weeks.
- Careful range of motion exercises to all the free joints.

During Mobilization:

- Reducing pain and swelling:
  - Diapulse.
  - Ultrasound.
  - Paraffin wax bath.
- Increasing range of motion for all the movements of thumb.
- Improving the strength and endurance of all the muscles crossing the first metacarpal and carpo-metacarpal joint.
- Scar remodelling after surgical intervention is necessary.
- *Use of splints:* Dynamic flexion splint is used.

The involved thumb should regain function by 10-12 weeks.

Complications

- Malunion.
- Stiffness of hand.
- Osteoarthritis of carpo-metacarpal joint.

DISLOCATION OF METACARPOPHALANGEAL JOINT

The disolocation of metacarpophalangeal joint is an uncommon injury.

Mode of Injury

Hyperextension of metacarpophalangeal joint.

Commonly Affected Joint

Metacarpophalangeal joint of index finger is most commonly affected.

Button-hole Injury

The distal segment is displaced backwards from the proximal. The head of metacarpal bone is driven forwards through rent in volar capsule and phalan is dislocated backwads.

Treatment

Open reduction and internal fixation is usually required.

CHAPTER 4
FRACTURES OF LOWER EXTREMITY

FRACTURE OF NECK OF FEMUR

A femoral neck fracture is a fracture occurring proximal to the intertrochanteric line in the intra-capsular region of the hip (Fig. 4.1).

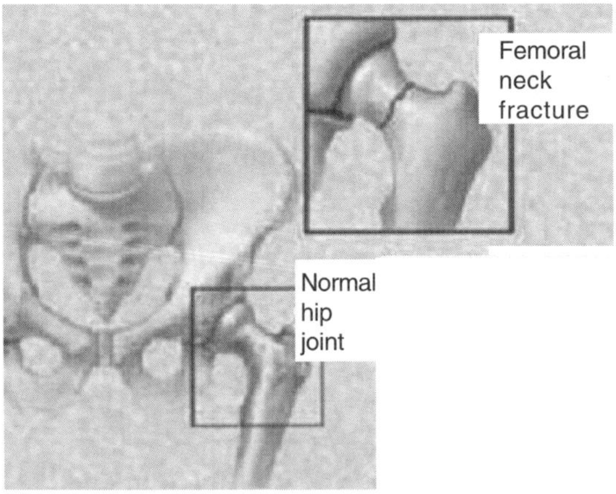

Fig. 4.1: Fracture of neck of femur

Mechanism of Injury

The fractures of femoral neck are common in elderly population especially in women above 60 years of age suffering from osteoporosis. This fracture can occur in elderly even with low-energy trauma. The causative injury is often stumble or a fall.

In younger population high-energy trauma is required for the occurrence of femoral neck fracture.

Classification

Garden's classification (Fig. 4.2) of femoral neck fracture:

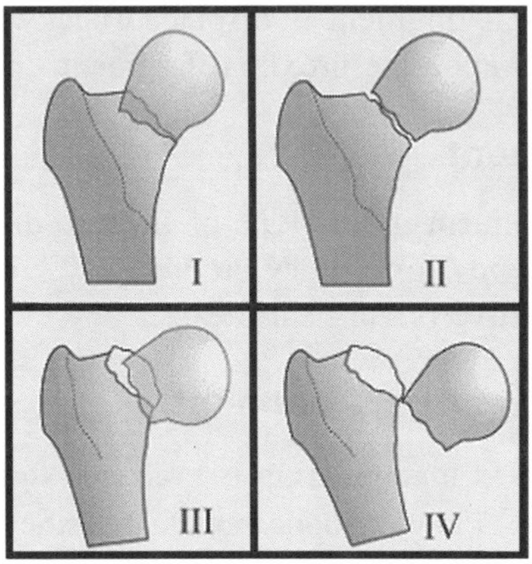

Fig. 4.2: Garden's classification

- *Type 1*– An incomplete impacted femoral neck fracture in valgus position. The femoral head is tilted in postero-lateral direction so that there is an obtuse angle laterally at trabecular stream.
- *Type 2*– A non-displaced complete femoral neck fracture with break in trabecular stream with little angulation.
- *Type 3*– A complete and displaced femoral neck fracture. The distal fragment is externally rotated causing internal rotation of femoral head. The trabecular stream at the fracture site in broken and displaced. There is often disruption of joint capsule.
- *Type 4*– A completely displaced femoral neck fracture with significant external rotation of distal fragment. The head loses contact with distal segment and springs back to its original position.

There is normal alignment of trabecular stream of head and acetabulum while there is no contact between head and neck.

Types

There are two types of femoral neck fractures seen clinically:
- Displaced fracture.
- Impacted abduction fracture.

Displaced Fracture:

In majority of the cases (approx. 95%) there is marked displacement with the distal fragment being rotated laterally and displaced upwards (Fig. 4.3).

Impacted Abduction Fracture:

The two fragments are firmly impacted together with slight abduction of distal fragment upon the proximal (Fig. 4.4).

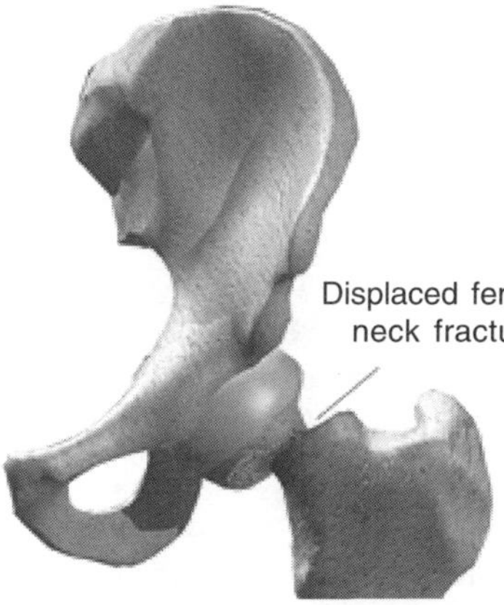

Fig. 4.3: Displaced femoral neck fracture

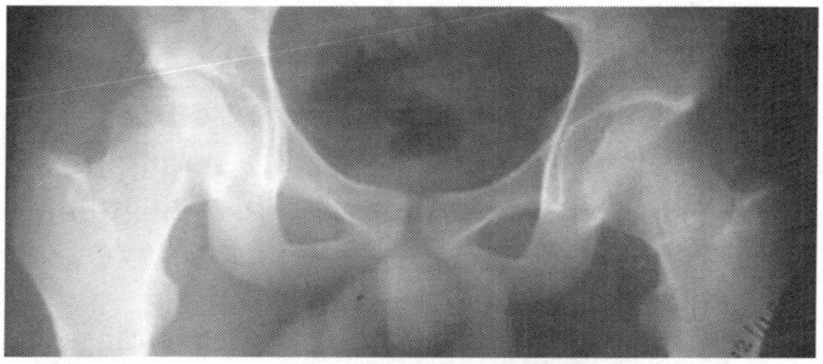

Fig. 4.4: Impacted abduction fracture of femoral neck

Clinical Presentation

Displaced Fracture:

The patient is usually of an elderly age group giving history of fall after which he/she was unable to get up again unaided. The patient is not able to bear weight on the affected extremity.

On Examination:

- There is marked lateral rotation of the extremity with patella and foot facing laterally.
- The affected limb is shortened by 2-3 cms.
- There is marked tenderness in the groin.
- Any movement attempted at hip is extremely painful and is associated with severe spasm.

Impacted Abduction Fracture:

The patient with impacted abduction fracture may have been able to pick herself after falling and may even have walked a few steps afterwards with assistance or the patient could even come walking with only complain of little bit pain in the groin.

On Examination:

- No rotational deformity is noted.
- There may be mild or no shortening of the affected limb.
- Patient is able to move the hip through moderate range without severe pain.

Radiological Features

X-ray of pelvis with both hips is usually taken so that comparison could be made between the affected and non-affected side. Both antero-posterior and lateral views are taken. Following features should be noted:
- Break in medial cortex of neck.
- External rotation of femur is evident.
- Lesser trochanter appears to be more prominent.
- Overriding of greater trochanter, so that it lies at level of femoral head.
- Break in the trabecular stream.
- Break in shenton's line.

Treatment

Conservative Treatment:

The conservative treatment in fracture femoral neck is indicated in children and impacted abduction fracture. The various methods of conservative treatment that can be utilized are as follows:

- Skin traction for a period of 4-6 weeks.
- Hip spica is used in children for a period of 6 weeks.
- Derotation bar, i.e., plaster of paris boot and bar is given for 4-6 weeks.
- In elderly patients with impacted fracture, below knee plaster boot with horizontal bar to prevent rotation of limb is used.

All the cases treated by the conservative treatment is immobilized for a period of six weeks but the weight bearing on the affected extremity is allowed only after complete healing of the fracture i.e. after 10-12 weeks.

Surgical Treatment:

Surgical treatment usually aims towards early union and proper fixation especially in case of elderly. Following methods are usually implied:

- Internal fixation.
- Joint replacement.

Internal fixation: Various surgical implants can be used as internal fixators, some of them are as following:

- Multiple cancellous screws.
- Dynamic hip screw.
- Multiple knowle's pins/Moore's pin.
- Smith Peterson nail.

Joint Replacement: Joint replacement is preferred over internal fixation in elderly population as the prosthesis could permit early weight bearing providing functional independence and also the failure of internal fixation is high in elderly. So in order to prevent complications and allow early weight bearing joint replacement is preferred. It could be either hemi-replacement arthroplasty or total hip replacement arthroplasty.

Rehabilitation Objectives

- To improve and restore range of motion of knee and hip.
- To improve the strength of the muscles affected by the fracture.
- To normalize the patient's gait.

Physiotherapy Following Conservative Treatment:

During Immobilization

- Emphasis should be laid on correct positioning of the limb especially avoidance of rotation.
- Adequate chest physiotherapy to avoid respiratory complications.
- Resistive movements to ankle and toe.
- Isometric exercises to quadriceps, hamstrings, abductors and hip extensors to maintain muscle physiology and avoid any muscular weakness or atrophy.
- Initiation of sitting in the bed should be made at the earliest with proper back support.

During Mobilization:

- Maximum concentration and emphasis should be laid on proper range of motion exercises for hip and knee joint. Efforts should be made to achieve maximum possible ROM at hip and knee as soon as possible.
- Progressive passive stretchings are done at hip and knee joint aiding in improving range of motion.
- Strengthening exercises especially for glutei and quadriceps are essential.
- Pre-weight bearing exercises:
  - Four-point kneeling.
  - Knee walking.
- Weight transfers and single limb standing to allow brief periods of full weight bearing on the affected leg.
- Guided and gradually progressed supported squatting and cross-leg sitting with back supported.

Physiotherapy Following Surgical Treatment

- To avoid respiratory complications deep breathing and coughing manoeuvres are to be started immediately.
- Vigorous frequent ankle toe movements.
- Isometric contractions of quadriceps, hamstrings and glutei.
- The limb should be kept in the elevated position to avoid oedema of the affected limb.
- Proper positioning of the limb avoiding any rotations.

Day of injury–Week 1:

Range of motion:

- Active range of motion exercise to the hip to be instituted.
- Gentle active flexion-extension of knee is performed.
- Patient is instructed to perform full range of motion exercises at ankle.

Strengthening exercises:

- Isotonic exercises to the ankle to maintain strength of plantar flexors and dorsiflexors.

Functional activities:

- The patient needs to use a raised toilet seat and chair to reduce hip flexion.

Ambulation:

- The gait and transfers by the patient is done with the help of assistive devices such as walker or crutches. Three-point gait is usually preferred.

Weight bearing:

- Stable fracture could be allowed to bear partial weight but unstable fractures remain non-weight bearing to toe touch weight bearing.
- In case of replacement surgery weight bearing is tolerated within first few days.

Week 1–Week 4:

Range of motion:

- Active or active assistive range of motion exercises to hip.
- Active range of motion exercises to knee and ankle.
- Avoid internal rotation and adduction past midline in cases treated with hemi-arthroplasty.

Strengthening exercises:

- Isometric exercise to quadriceps and glutei.

Gait:

- Three-point gait with the use of assistive devices like crutches.

Week 4 – Week 6:

Range of motion:

- The hip should have achieved 90° of flexion by now. Active exercises to the hip should be continued.

Strengthening exercises:

- Isotonic strengthening of hip abductors, flexors and extensors should be practised.
- Quadriceps strengthening is continued.

Functional activities:

- Patient should be independent and functional in his/her activities of daily living (ADLs).

Week 6–Week 12:

Range of motion:

- Passive range of motion exercises are instituted at hip as the fracture site is stable by this time.
- Stretching of hip flexors and extensors are initiated to improve range of motion.

Strengthening Exercises:

- Isometric exercises to the glutei.
- Resistive exercises to be initiated.
- Isokinetic exercises to strengthen quadriceps and hip musculature.

Functional activities:

- Use of affected extremity during transfers and ambulation.
- Use of raised toilet seat and chair is minimized.

Gait:

- Four point gait with crutches bearing more weight on the affected limb.

Weight bearing:

- The patient is allowed to bear full weight in the affected extremity.

Week 12–Week 16:

By this time the patient is allowed to bear full weight and range of motion is within the normal limits. The emphasis is laid towards muscle strengthening by isotonics, isokinetics and progressive resistive exercises along with normalization of gait.

Complications

- *Avascular Necrosis:* The blood supply to the head of femur is precarious. When the neck of femur is fractured the nutrient vessels within the bone are necessarily severed. Thus the viability of femoral head may depend entirely upon blood supplied through ligamentum teres, which is insufficient to keep the head alive. Fracture may fail to unite. Depending upon the degree of ischaemia, avascular changes may be total or partial.
- *Non-Union:* Various causes of non-union like avascular necrosis, incomplete immobilization or flow of synovial fluid between the fracture surfaces may prevent the formation of haematoma and of bone forming tissue. When the fracture fails to unite, the neck of the femur undergoes progressive absorption.
- *Ostearthritis:* Arthritis may arise from:
  - Mechanical damage to the articular cartilage at time of injury.
  - Impaired blood supply.
  - Faulty alignment.

FRACTURES OF TROCHANTERIC REGION

Fracture of trochanteric region refers to any fracture in the region that lies approximately between greater and lesser trochanter. These fractures are always extra-capsular (Fig. 4.5). These fractures unite readily.

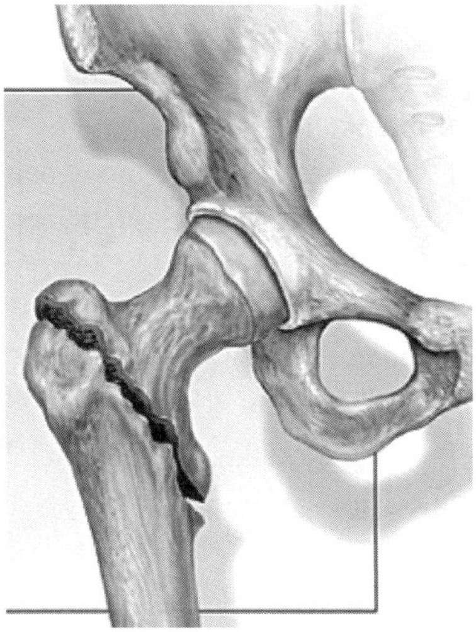

Fig. 4.5: Fracture of trochanteric region

Mechanism of Injury

The fracture is common amongst elderly population especially women suffering from post-menopausal osteoporosis. A stumble or fall can cause this injury. In younger population, high-energy trauma results in this type of injury.

Pathoanatomy

The distal fragment rides up reducing the femoral neck-shaft angle resulting in coxa-vara. The fracture is usually comminuted and displaced.

Clinical Features

The patient gives history of fall after which he/she was not able to get up without assistance and weight bearing on the affected limb is not possible. The patient shows following features:

- Marked pain over the trochanteric region.
- There is marked tenderness over the greater trochanter.
- Presence of swelling in region of hip.
- Limb length discrepancy is evident.
- The limb is in a position of external rotation.

- Visible ecchymosis often appears at back of thigh after a day or two of the injury.

Radiographic Examination

Antero-posterior and lateral radiographs are required so that fractures even without displacement may not be overlooked.

Treatment Objectives

When dealing with the fractures of trochanteric region, the main objectives of an orthopaedician are:

- Restoring, the normal neck shaft angle to 127°.
- Stability of the fracture site.

Treatment

The fractures of trochanteric region unite readily, so conservative means of treatment mainly in the form of traction is used. In case of elderly patients internal fixation is the preferred treatment because conservative treatment by traction needs a prolonged period of recumbancy, which could be deteriorating for the elderly patients bringing about respiratory complications.

Conservative Treatment:

The following methods of treatment can be used:

- Russell's traction is used for 10-12 weeks until the fracture is united soundly.
- Skeletal traction in Thomas splint.
- Plaster spica or plaster splint is used in case of children.
- Plaster of paris derotation bar is used in elderly in whom surgery is contraindicated due to medical problems.

Surgical Treatment:

The fracture treated by surgery is internally fixed under X-ray control. The various internal fixators that can be used are:

- Smith Peterson nail.
- Ender's nail.
- Dynamic hip screw.

Rehabilitation Objectives

- To improve and restore the range of motion at hip joint.
- Improve the strength of the muscles around the hip.
- To restore normal gait pattern and independent ambulation.

Physiotherapy Management

Day 1 - Week 1:

Weight Bearing:

- Protected toe touch to partial weight bearing should be initiated.

Range of motion:

- Active range of motion exercises should be practised at hip within the available range.
- Full range active exercises are allowed at hip joint.

Muscle strength:

- No strengthening exercises to quadriceps or hamstrings.
- Isometric exercises to glutei are initiated.
- Isotonic ankle exercises.

Ambulation and transfers:

- Two or three point gait with crutches or walker is taught to the patient.
- Walker or crutches should be used for support and stability during transfers.

Week 2 – Week 4:

Weight Bearing:

- Weight bearing as tolerated by the patient

Range of Motion:

- Active, active assistive to gentle passive range of motion to hip in flexion and extension.
- Range of motion exercise to the knee should be continued.

Muscle strength:

- Isometric glutei strengthening exercises.
- By the end of two weeks isometrics to quadriceps and hamstrings are initiated.

Ambulation and transfers:

- Patient has to still use the assistive devices like crutches or walker for ambulation and transfers.

Week 4 – Week 8:

Weight bearing:

- Weight bearing as tolerated by the patient

Range of motion:

- Continue active range of motion exercise at hip and knee.
- Active range of motion of hip abduction and adduction is to be initiated.

Muscle strength:

- Isometric exercises to quadriceps and glutei are continued.
- Isometric exercises to hamstrings are initiated in sitting position.

Ambulation:

- For ambulation and transfers patients can start using cane at the end of six weeks.

Week 8 – Week 12:

Weight bearing:

- By this time fracture have sufficient bone healing and callus to allow full weight bearing.

Range of motion:

- By this time the patient should have achieved full range of motion at the hip joint; else passive exercises must be practised.

Muscle strength:

- Isometric exercises to glutei hamstrings and quadriceps.
- Resistive exercises to quadriceps and hamstrings can be initiated by 10 weeks.
- Isometric strengthening to hip abductors and adductors.

Ambulation and transfers:

- Standing should be improved to allow dynamic unilateral balance and single limb weight shifting.
- Proper gait pattern should be emphasized.

Week 12 – Week 16:

By now the patient is almost bearing equal weight on both the limbs having a proper gait pattern. Stretching can be used to treat the residual tightness of muscle groups in order to enhance range of motion. Isotonic and isokinetic strengthening for all muscle groups of lower limb are advocated.

Complications

- Failure of fixation devices.
- Malunion.
- Osteoarthritis.

FRACTURE OF SHAFT OF FEMUR

The fracture of shaft of femur is a diaphyseal fracture, which never extends upto metaphyseal or articular region. It is equally common in upper, middle and lower thirds of femoral shaft. It can occur in any age group.

Mechanism of Injury

The fracture of femoral shaft can be caused either by high-energy trauma such as a direct forceful blow to the thigh or an accident or low energy trauma, as in case of elderly population whose bones are usually osteopenic.

Fractures caused by high-energy trauma are often associated with significant soft tissue trauma and at times open wounds.

Types of Fracture

The fracture of femoral shaft could either be transverse, oblique, spiral or comminuted depending upon the fracturing forcec (Fig. 4.6).

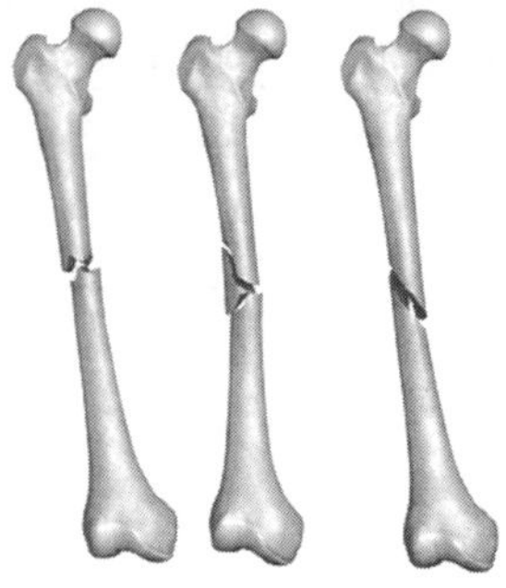

Fig. 4.6: Fracture of shaft of femur

Displacement

- The fractured segments do not show a great amount of displacement in case of children.
- In adults the fracture could either be displaced or undisplaced. In displaced fractures, the proximal fragment is flexed, abducted and externally rotated while the distal fragment is adducted. The displacements are due to the pull of the attached muscles.

Clinical Features

The patient presents with the history of severe trauma along with classic signs and symptoms of fracture like:

- Pain.
- Swelling.
- Abnormal mobility.
- Inability to bear weight.
- Deformity.

Radiological Examination

The radiographs are obtained for the whole length of femur along with the pelvis (Fig. 4.7).

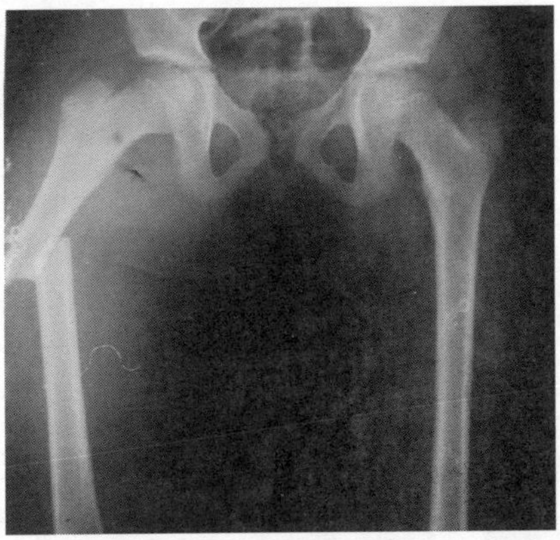

Fig. 4.7 Radiograph showing fracture of shaft of femur

Treatment

The fracture of shaft of femur can be managed both by conservative and surgical means depending upon the age of the patient and the extent of fracture.

Conservative Treatment:

The principles of this method are to reduce the fracture by traction and manipulation and to support the limb in Thomas or Povey's splint.

- *From birth to two years:* Children under the age of 2 years having fracture of shaft of femur are treated by Gallow's traction.
- *Older children (From two years to sixteen years):* Different methods of skin traction are used to maintain the fragments into proper alignment. Once the callus formation starts, immobilization can be provided in Thomas splint or POP hip spica.
- *In adults:* In adults the fracture is reduced by skeletal traction.

Surgical Treatment:

Surgical intervention is the treatment of choice whenever the facilities are available as it reduces the period of recumbancy and provides early mobilization. Closed or open reduction and internal fixation is the treatment of choice. Various methods of internal fixation used are:

- Closed intra-medullary nailing.
- Interlocking nailing.
- Kuntscher's cloverleaf intra-medullary nail.
- Plating.

Complications

Early complications:

- Shock
- Fat embolism
- Injury to femoral nerve
- Injury to femoral artery
- Injury to sciatic nerve
- Infection
- Simultaneous dislocation of hip

Late Complications:

- Delayed union.
- Non-union.
- Malunion.
- Knee stiffness.

Physiotherapy Management

Objectives:

- To restore and maintain full range of motion of knee and hip.
- To improve the strength of the muscles those are affected by the fracture like quadriceps and hamstrings.
- To restore normal gait pattern.

Intervention:

Day of injury to Week 1:

- In case of internal fixation by nail toe touch to partial weight bearing is allowed during ambulation and transfers but if internal fixation is done with help of plate non-weight bearing to toe-touch weight bearing with crutches or walker is preferred. If external fixator has been applied no weight bearing is allowed.
- The limb should be kept in elevated position in order to reduce oedema.
- Active range of motion exercises are initiated at all joints of lower limb–hip, knee and ankle.
- Active ankle foot exercises (dorsi flexion-plantar flexion) should be started in order to increase venous return and prevent venous stasis.
- In order to prevent plantar flexion contracture, stretching to the gastrocsoleus muscle.
- Isometric exercises to quadriceps and glutei are instituted.
- The patient uses the walking aids like crutch or walker for ambulation. In case of non-weight bearing two-point gait and in case of partial weight bearing three-point gait is taught to the patients.
- No stair climbing is allowed.

Week 2 – Week 4:

- Weight bearing status of the patient is same as in the initial stages depending upon the type of treatment.
- Active-assisted range of motion exercise should be done at hip and knee.
- In order to prevent adhesion of quadriceps muscle at the fracture site it is important to achieve full knee flexion and extension as soon as possible.
- Special emphasis should be made on quadriceps-hamstrings mechanism in order to prevent the extension lag.
- Straight leg raising exercises should be initiated depending on the patient's tolerance.
- Repetitive knee movements, i.e., flexion-extension to strengthen the quadriceps and hamstrings.
- Isometrics to the glutei and hamstrings should be continued.
- Isotonic exercises to the ankle musculature.
- The patient should use assistive devices for transfers and ambulation which depends upon the weight bearing status of the patient.
- Patient could ascend or descend the stairs using assistive devices.

Week 4 – Week 6:

- By this time full weight bearing is allowed for stable fractures and partial weight bearing for unstable fractures.
- Passive range of motion exercises are initiated at hip and knee joint.
- Strengthening exercises to the quadriceps and hamstrings are initiated using weight cuffs tied at the ankle, which could be increased progressively.
- Patient has to continue with two-point or three-point gait depending upon the weight bearing status of the patient.

Week 8 – Week 12:

- In case of intramedullary nail fixation, weight bearing is as per tolerated by the patient but if plate is used as an internal fixator patient can bear full weight of the affected limb. In case of external fixator partial or non-weight bearing is allowed to the patient.
- Passive exercises are continued at hip and knee to avoid any restriction in the motion.
- Progressive resistive exercises for quadriceps and hamstrings are done in order to strengthen them with increasing repetitions.

- Once the full weight bearing is permitted to the patient, the patient could be weaned from the assistive devices during transfers and ambulation.
- Gait pattern of the patient has to be normalized following the proper movement pattern.
- Weight shifting and balance exercises are initiated once the patient is allowed full weight bearing.

Week 12 – Week 16:
- Patient is allowed to bear full weight on the affected extremity.
- Passive exercises are continued in order to prevent any tightness in the knee musculature.
- Patient has to concentrate on weight shifting exercises and normalizing the gait pattern.

FRACTURES OF PATELLA

Patella is the largest sesamoid bone in the human body, present in the tendon of quadriceps muscles. It is also regarded as the knee cap. Fracture of patella is the common fracture to occur.

Mechanism of Injury

- Direct blow to anterior aspect of knee.
- Fall on knee cap.
- Sudden violent contraction of quadriceps muscle.

Types of Patellar Fracture (Fig. 4.8):

There are two types of patellar fractures that are diagnosed clinically:
- Two-part fracture.
- Comminuted fracture.

Two-Part Fracture:

It is a type of transverse fracture caused due to sudden violent contraction of quadriceps muscle as if in case of passive flexion of knee, sudden extension of knee is attempted. The transverse line runs across the patella.

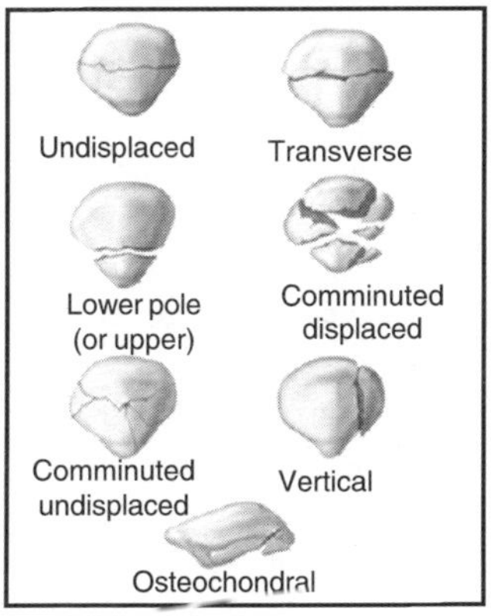

Fig. 4.8: Types of patellar fracture

Comminuted Fracture:

This type of fracture is always traumatic in nature. The patella fractures into many pieces. It is also known as stellate fracture.

Pathoanatomy

The fracture of the patella may be displaced or undisplaced depending on the force of contraction of quadriceps muscle. The fractured fragments may remain undisplaced due to intact prepatellar expansion of quadriceps tendon in front and by patellar retinaculae on both the sides. The displacement occurs due to tearing of patellar retinaculum.

Clinical Features

- Pain.
- Swelling.
- Tenderness.
- Crepitus is felt in case of displaced fracture.
- Gap is felt between the fractured fragments in case of displaced fracture.
- Extension lag is present, i.e., patient is not able to lift his leg with knee in full extension.
- Haemarthrosis may be seen.

Radiological Diagnosis

Various radiographic views are necessary to diagnose the fracture of the patella:

- Anteroposterior (AP) view.
- Lateral view.
- Skyline view.

Treatment

The treatment of fracture patella depends upon many factors such as:

- Type of the fracture.
- Age of the patient.

Undisplaced Fracture

Aims of Treatment:

- To relieve pain.
- To preserve and restore function.

Treatment Plan:

Cylindrical plaster cast extending from groin to just above the malleoli with knee in extension. The period of immobilization is of three weeks.

Aspiration of blood is necessary in case of painful tense haemarthrosis.

Two-Part Fracture (Clean Break with Fragment Separation)

The proximal fragment of fractured patella is pulled away by the pull of quadriceps muscle. Thus approximation is not possible conservatively and surgical intervention is always required.

- *If age of patient is under 45 years:* Internal fixation of the fractured fragment is done either by tension band wiring or by using bolt and screw. Extensor retinaculum is to be repaired simultaneously. The period of immobilization is 4-6 weeks.
- *If age of patient is more than 45 years:* With increasing age there is difficulty in regaining full range of motion at knee joint after internal fixation therefore it is wiser to excise the patella which could either be partial or complete. The period of immobilization is 5-6 weeks.

Comminuted Fracture

In case of comminuted fracture the fractured fragments are always excised irrespective of age of patient, i.e., patellectomy is the treatment of the choice. The period of immobilization is 5-6 weeks.

Physiotherapy Management

The best of the physiotherapy management is required both during the period of immobilization and mobilization.

Aims of physiotherapy treatment

- To relieve pain.
- To increase the strength of quadriceps muscle.
- To regain range of motion of knee joint.

Physiotherapy following conservative treatment

Following the conservative treatment of the fractured patella, the period of immobilization is 3-4 weeks.

During immobilization:

- Vigorous ankle toe movements are ensured so as to maintain perfect circulation and reduce any type of swelling.
- The limb is to be kept in an elevated position.
- Static quadriceps exercise is to be initiated.
- Assisted SLR with hold of 10 seconds at terminal range. POP slab provides assistance as well as the resistance.
- Crutch walking is initiated on the second day of the immobilization.

During mobilization:

- To relieve pain
  Proper thermotherapy adjunct should be used to relieve the pain in the period of immobilization. These thermotherapy adjuncts not only relieve the pain but also make the mobilization easier. Some of the thermotherapy adjuncts used are:
  - Short wave diathermy.
  - Paraffin wax bath.
  - Hot packs.
- To increase muscular strength:
  - Static quadriceps exercises.
  - Straight leg raises (SLR) with knee in full extension till 30° of hip flexion is to be progressed from assisted to active to resisted.

  - Once the range of knee flexion reaches 90°, quadriceps strengthening is to be initiated in high sitting.
- To increase range of motion:
  The range of knee flexion has to be increased with re-establishment of proper extensor mechanism. The patellar mobility has to be regained.
- To improve ambulation:
  Correct weight bearing and gait pattern has to be re-educated and re-established to avoid limp. Full function is regained by 8-12 weeks.

Physiotherapy following Tension Band Wiring (TBW)

Pre-operative Regime

The pre-operative regime of the patient with fractured patella includes the evaluation and education of the patient.

Pre-operative Evaluation:
- Pain assessment.
- Extent of swelling.
- Any external trauma marks: Haemarthrosis, bruises.
- Range of motion.

Sometimes the accurate evaluation is not possible in the presence of extensive haemarthrosis and pain.

Pre-operative Education:
The patient has to be educated about the following before surgery:
- The surgical procedure.
- Post-operative physiotherapy management.

Post-operative Regime

Immobilization Techniques:
- Posterior plaster cast.
- Pressure bandage.

First 10 days:
- Elevation of the limb is necessary. The elevated limb should be fully supported from ankle to thigh using pillows.
- For pain relief, diapulse can be used even on the posterior cast or the bandage.
- Vigorous ankle toe movements to be initiated immediately.
- Passive movements of the hip should be given.
- Indirect isometerics can be initiated by pushing down the whole leg against the mattress.

Glide	*Indication*	*Position of patient*	*Mobilising force*
Joint traction (TF joint)	Pain control Geneal mobility	Sitting, supine or prone beginning with knee in resting position	Pull on long axis of tibia to separate joint surfaces
Posterior glide (TF joint)	To increase flexion	Supine with foot resting on table	Extend your elbows and lean your body weight forward, push tibia posteriorly with thumbs
Posterior glide progression (TF joint)	To increase flexion	Sitting with knee flexed over edge of treatment table, beginning in resting position and progressing to near 90°	Extend your elbow and lean your body weight onto tibia, gliding it posteriorly
Distal glide (PF joint)	To increase patellar mobility for knee flexion	Supine with knee extended	Glide the patella in a caudal direction parallel to femur.
Medial-lateral glide (PF joint)	To increase patellar mobility	Supine with knee extended	Glide the patella in medial or lateral direction against restriction

- After 3-4 days assisted SLR to be initiated if it is not painful.
- Non weight bearing crutch walking to be initiated as soon as possible.

After 10 days:

- To increase range of motion:
  Knee flexion range has to be increased. In order to initiate continuous passive motion (CPM) machine is to be used. It could be used till the knee flexion reaches 90° along with passive knee mobilization as discussed earlier.
- To increase patellar mobility:
  The patellar mobility has to be regained for proper functional knee joint. So passive patellar mobilization has to be emphasized.
- To improve quadriceps muscle strength:
  - Strong isometerics to the quadriceps to be initiated.
  - Assisted SLR progressing to active and then to resisted.
- Ambulation:
  Gradual weight bearing is to be initiated after 6 weeks in parallel bars. Correct weight bearing, weight transfers and proper gait pattern to be taught. The progression to the cane is made.
  Adequate knee range of motion is acquired within 6-8 weeks and full ROM is gained by 8-12 weeks. Mild extensor lag way continue for about six months.

Physiotherapy following Patellectomy

First Week:

- The limb is to be kept in elevation.
- Strong ankle and toe movements to be initiated.
- Mild indirect contractions to the quadriceps.
- Re-education of quadriceps contraction by electrical stimulation.
- Assisted SLR to be initiated if it is pain-free.

Second Week:

- Controlled CPM is used to initiate knee flexion.
- Effective passive knee movements to be started.
- Deep friction massage around the stitches is done to break adhesions.
- Pulsed ultrasound is used to relieve pain.
- Gradual knee mobilization in small range has to be begun.
- Partial weight bearing is started.

Third Week Onwards:

- Active assisted movements to be initiated.
- Hydrotherapy is an effective measure to achieve mobility and strength.
- Various structures around the knee like quadriceps, hamstrings and ligaments have to be strengthened using progressive resistive exercises.
- Proper gait training and functional positions are guided. Graduated weight bearing is to be progressed.

The patient usually gains adequate range of motion and strength by 8-12 weeks post-surgically.

Complications

- Knee stiffness.
- Extensor mechanism weakness.
- Osteoarthritis.
- Infection to the knee joint.

FRACTURE OF SHAFT OF TIBIA AND FIBULA

Both the bones of the leg, i.e., tibia and fibula are usually fractured together either by direct or indirect violence. The fracture usually occurs in the diaphysis of the bones neither affecting the metaphysis nor the articular surfaces. The fracture could occur at any level on the shaft, i.e., upper, middle or lower (Fig. 4.9).

Mechanism of Injury

- *Direct Injury:* The direct injury to both bones of the leg occurs usually in a road traffic accident or by direct blow to the leg. In case of direct injury both the bones are fractured at the same level.

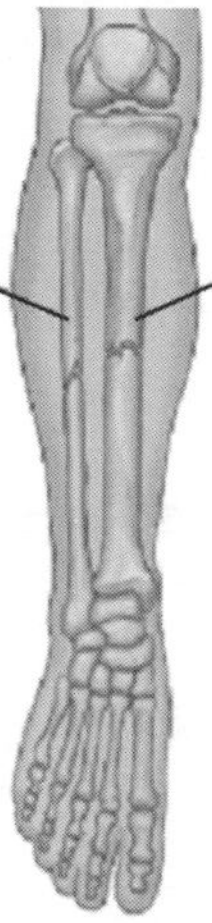

Fig. 4.9: Fracture of shaft of tibia and fibula

- *Indirect Injury:* It may be either by an angulatory or rotational force. Fractures resulting from angulatory force occur at the same level on both the bones which is usually transverse or of short oblique type. Fractures from rotational force are spiral in nature and occurs at two different levels on both the bones.

Pathoanatomy

The tibia being a subcutaneous bone throughout its length is poorly protected by the muscles. The fracture is usually of open type.

Displacement

The fracture of tibia and fibula are occasionally undisplaced. In younger children, displacement is rare. If displacement occurs it could be sideways, rotational or angulatory.

Clinical Features

The patient presents with history of injury to the leg followed by classical signs and symptoms of the fracture like pain, marked swelling, deformity, inability to use the limb in functional position.

Radiological Features (Fig. 4.10)

The fracture can be evaluated on a radiograph describing the extent of fractures bones,

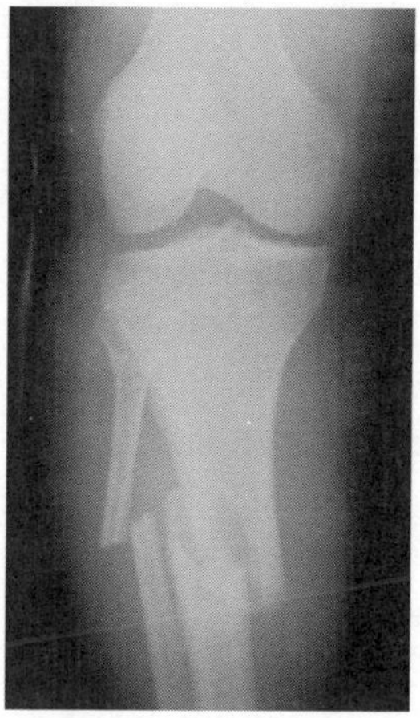

Fig. 4.10: Radiograph showing fracture of tibia and fibula

Management

The fractures of shaft of tibia and fibula are treated either by conservative or surgical means. The choice of treatment depends upon the type of fracture, which could be either open or closed.

Closed Fracture: Treatment of closed fracture is by:

- Closed reduction under anesthesia followed by above knee plaster cast.
- Open reduction and internal fixation is used in case of displaced and unstable fractures.

Open Fracture: In case of open fracture, the main aim of treatment is to convert it into a closed fracture by taking good care of the wound.

Methods of treatment:

Conservative Treatment-The conservative treatment of fracture shaft of tibia and fibula is always initiated by closed reduction of the fracture by an orthopaedician followed by the maintenance of reduction by immobilization techniques.

Closed Reduction: The patient lies supine over the couch with knees flexed to 90° over the end of the couch. The orthopaedician seated on stool faces the injured leg. The leg is kept in traction around the ankle. The fracture ends are manipulated and good alignment is achieved.

Immobilization Techniques:

- *Plaster of paris cast:* The limb is immobilized in full length plaster cast with knee slightly flexed and the ankle at right angle. The plaster may need to change after 1 or 2 weeks as the initial soft tissue swelling subsides.
- *Functional cast:* The plaster of paris cast can be replaced by functional patellar tendon bearing cast after 4-6 weeks. This allows early weight bearing and renders the knee free for mobilization.
- *Skeletal Traction:* It is often employed in cases where patient is confined to bed due to various multiple injuries. Sustained skeletal traction through lower tibia or calcaneum is applied with the limb resting upon Braun's frame.

Surgical Treatment – Surgical treatment is indicated in cases where conservative treatment fails to achieve satisfactory results or the fracture site is severely infected. The various methods of surgical treatment that can be employed are open reduction and internal fixation (ORIF) and external fixation.

- *Open reduction and Internal Fixation (ORIF):* Open reduction and internal fixation is used in cases where closed reduction of the fracture fails or it is impossible to maintain the reduction by plaster cast. Various internal fixators that can be used are as follows:
  - Plate and screws
  - Intermedullary nailing
  - Oblique transfixation screws
- *External Fixation:* It is usually indicated in cases of severely comminuted fractures with extensive soft tissue damage. It is often prescribed for open fractures having high risk of infection or already infected fracture, which makes the internal fixation delayed or impossible. The method facilitates the wound care.

Complications

- Infection.
- Injury to major vessels and nerves.
- Malunion.
- Non union.
- Delayed union.
- Compartment syndrome.
- Knee stiffness.

Physiotherapy Management

Objectives:

- To restore and maintain the range of motion at knee and ankle joints of the affected extremity at least to functional limits.
- To improve the strength of the muscles affected by the injury: plantar flexors, dorsiflexors, invertors and evertors.
- To normalize the gait pattern of the patient.

Intervention:

Day of Injury to Week 1:

- The patient's limb should be kept in an elevated position in order to prevent or subside the oedema (if already exists).
- The patient is instructed to do active ankle-foot exercises in an elevated position (if ankle joint is free from immobilization) in order to maintain circulation and subside the existing swelling.
- In cases where the affected limb is immobilized in a plaster cast along with knee and ankle immobilization, the patient must be instructed to do isometric exercise for quadriceps, tibialis anterior and gastro-soleus.
- In cases where knee and ankle are free from immobilization as in surgically treated patient, the patient can begun with active knee and ankle exercise in the available range.
- Isotonic exercises to the ankle should always be in accordance with the patient's tolerance to pain.
- By the end of first week, as the soft tissue swelling subsides patient treated with cast immobilization is allowed to bear partial weight on the affected extremity; toe touch to partial

weight bearing in case of internal fixation; non weight bearing in case of external fixation.

- Ambulatory aids like crutches or walker are used for transfers and ambulation.
- The patient must be taught either a two-point or three-point gait pattern according to the weight bearing status of the patient.

Week 2 – Week 4:

- Patient should perform active range of motion exercises at the hip joint of the affected extremity.
- The knee and ankle should be actively exercised depending upon the type of fixation and extremity.
- Isometric exercises to the quadriceps muscle.
- Ankle should be strengthened by both isometric and isotonic exercises.
- Ambulation and transfers depends upon the weight bearing status of the patient along with the walking aid used.
- It has been studied that cyclical loading secondary to weight bearing has been shown to produce osteogenesis. Therefore it is advised to bear weight on the affected extremity in accordance with the stability of the fracture site.
- No rotatory movements with the foot on the ground are allowed at the affected extremity.

Week 4 – Week 6:

- Active range of motion to knee and ankle if not immobilized.
- Isometric and isotonic exercise to the knee and ankle.
- For unstable fractures: Stand/pivot transfers and non-weight bearing ambulation with assistive devices.
- Weight bearing as tolerated along with partial to full weight bearing transfers and ambulation with assistive devices.

Week 8 – Week 12:

- Active, active-assisted and passive range of motion exercises to ankle and knee.
- Gentle progressive resistive exercise to quadriceps, dorsiflexors and plantar flexors.
- Patient may still need assistive devices for transfers and ambulation.
- Encourage weight bearing as tolerated.

ANKLE FRACTURES

It includes fracture of medial and lateral malleoli as well as distal articular surface of tibia and fibula.

Classification of Ankle Fractures

- Isolated lateral malleolar fracture which is extra articular in nature (Fig. 4.11).
- Bimalleolar fracture which is intra articular in nature (Fig. 4.12).

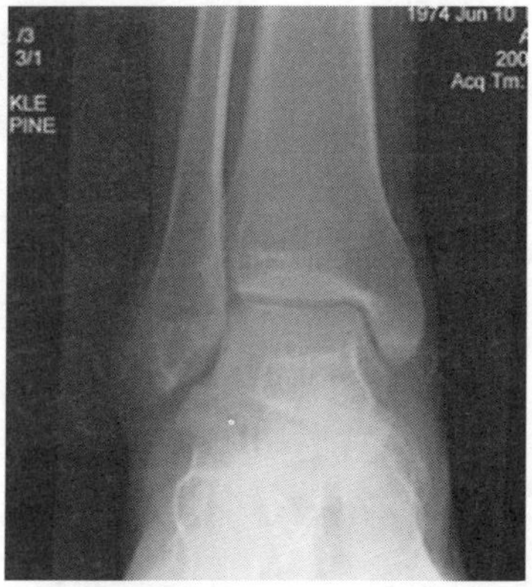

Fig. 4.11: Isolated lateral malleolar fracture

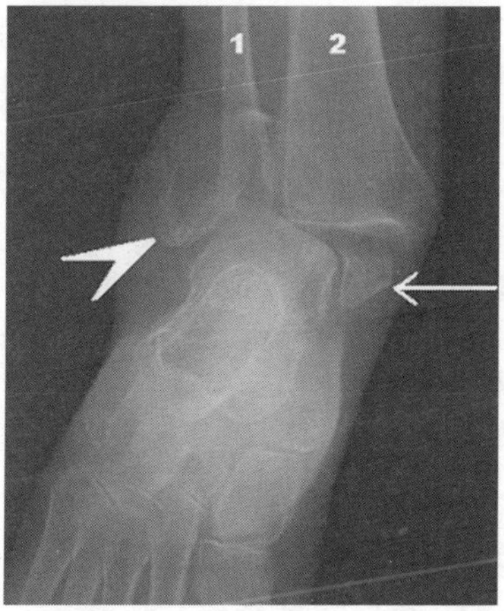

Fig. 4.12: Bimalleolar fracture

- Medial malleolar fracture which is intra articular in nature.
- Bimalleolar equivalent fracture which is intra articular in nature. In this lateral malleolus is fractured and medial side of ankle mortise is widened.
- Trimalleolar fracture with fracture of posterior aspect of tibial plafond (Fig. 4.13).

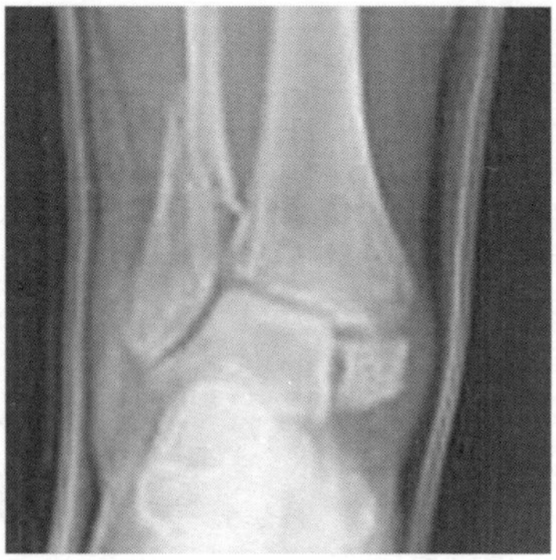

Fig. 4.13: Trimalleolar fracture

Mechanism of Injury

- Ankle fracture can occur due to low energy forces as in tripping or twisting.
- Motor vehicle accident.

Pattern of Injury

The pattern of ankle injury depends on position of foot at time of injury, which can either be supination or pronation. Combination of foot position and deforming forces provide characteristic pattern of ankle fracture.

Deforming Forces

- Supination/external rotation.
- Pronation/external rotation.
- Supination/Adduction.
- Pronation/Abduction.

Treatment

Conservative Treatment:

Cast is the treatment of choice and is indicated in the following conditions:

- Non-displaced or minimally displaced malleolar fracture.
- Isolated fracture of distal fibula.
- Minimal to moderately displaced fracture in patients who are amenable to surgical intervention.

Surgical Treatment

Open reduction and internal fixation using K-wires, screws, and plates is done and is indicated in following conditions:

- Displaced malleolar fracture.
- Syndesmotic disruption involving significant subluxation or dislocation of tibiotalar joint.
- Anatomically unstable fracture.
- Failure of conservative treatment.

Physiotherapeutic Intervention

Day 0 – Week 1:

Range of motion:

- For rigidly fixed fractures, active range of motion at metatarsophalangeal and knee joint to be initiated but ankle movements are not permitted.
- For non-rigidly fixed fractures, initiate range of motion exercises at metatarsophalangeal joints. No range of motion exercises at ankle or knee.

Muscle strength:

- Initiate quadriceps isometric exercises as tolerated.
- No strengthening exercises to ankle or foot.

Functional activities:

- Non-weight bearing stand/pivot transfers and ambulation with assistive devices.

Weight bearing:

- No weight bearing is allowed.

Week 2 – Week 4

Range of motion:

- For rigidly fixed fractures, active range of motion at metatarsophalangeal and knee joint to

be initiated but ankle movements are not permitted.
- For non-rigidly fixed fractures, initiate range of motion exercises at metatarsophalangeal joints. No range of motion exercises at ankle or knee.

Muscle strength:
- For rigidly fixed fractures, isometric exercises of dorsiflexors and plantar flexors of the toes and ankle.
- For non-rigidly fixed fractures, no strengthening exercises.
- Continue quadriceps strengthening exercises in both cases.

Functional activities:
- Non-weight bearing stand/pivot transfers and ambulation with assistive devices.

Weight bearing:
- Toe-touch weight bearing for rigidly fixed fractures.

Week 4 – Week 6:
Range of motion:
- For rigidly fixed fractures, active range of motion at metatarsophalangeal, ankle and knee joints.
- For non-rigidly fixed fractures, active range of motion exercises at metatarsophalangeal joints. Range of motion exercises at ankle and knee as immobilization device allows.

Muscle strength:
- For rigidly fixed fractures, isometric and isotonic exercises to dorsiflexors, plantar flexors, invertors and evertors of ankle and foot.
- For non-rigidly fixed fractures gentle isometric exercises to dorsiflexors and plantar flexors within the cast.
- Continue with quadriceps strengthening in both the cases.

Functional activities:
- Non-weight bearing stand/pivot transfers and ambulation with assistive devices for fractures with little evidence of healing.
- Toe-touch to partial weight bearing with assistive devices for fractures showing evidence of healing.

Weight bearing:
- Partial weight bearing for fractures that are non-tender to palpation and appear stable on a radiograph.

Week 6 – Week 8:
Range of motion:
- For rigidly fixed fractures, active, active assistive and passive range of motion in all planes to the ankle and sub-talar joints.
- For non-rigidly fixed fractures, initiate active and active assisted range of motion to the ankle and subtalar joints.

Muscle strength:
- Initiate resistive exercise to the dorsiflexors, plantar flexors, invertors and evertors of the ankle in both the cases.

Functional activities:
- For rigidly fixed fractures, partial to full weight bearing with assistive devices for fractures showing evidence of healing. Use assistive devices as necessary.
- For non-rigidly fixed fractures, toe-touch to partial weight bearing using assistive devices for transfers and ambulation.

Weight bearing:
- Partial to full weight bearing.

Week 8 – Week 12:
Range of motion:
- For rigidly fixed fractures, active, active assistive and passive range of motion in all planes to the ankle and sub-talar joints.
- For non-rigidly fixed fractures, initiate active and active assisted range of motion to the ankle and subtalar joints.

Muscle strength:
- For rigidly fixed fractures, initiate progressive resistive exercises to plantar flexors, dorsiflexors, invertors and evertors.

- For non-rigidly fixed fractures continue gentle resistive exercises.

Functional activities:
- For rigidly fixed fractures, progress from partial to full weight bearing as tolerated for transfers and ambulation, using assistive devices if necessary.
- For non-rigidly fixed fractures, initiate partial weight bearing. Assistive devices are required for transfers and ambulation.

Weight bearing:
- Partial to full weight bearing.

TALAR FRACTURES

Talus can fracture at any of the following positions:
- Fracture of talar neck (Fig. 4.14).
- Fracture of talar body (Fig. 4.15).
- Fracture of talar head (Fig. 4.16).
- Osteochondral fracture (Fig. 4.17).
- Fracture of lateral process (Fig. 4.18).

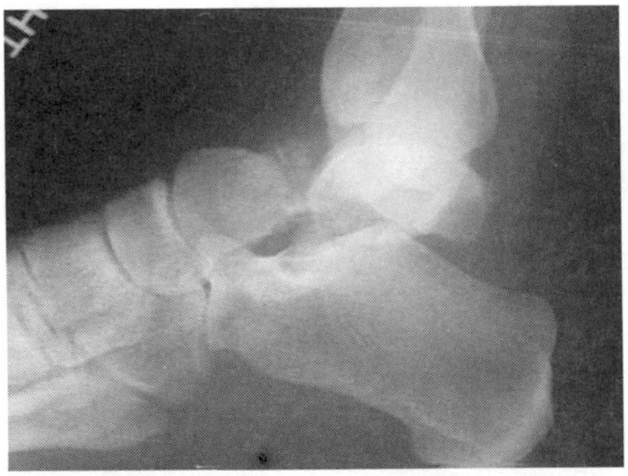

Fig. 4.14: Fracture of talar neck

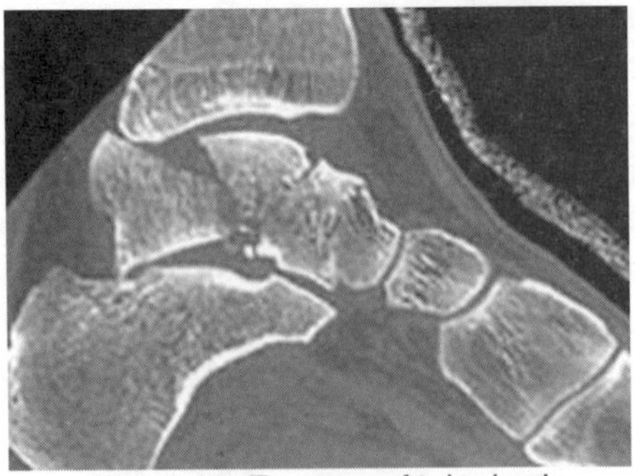

Fig. 4.15: Fracture of talar body

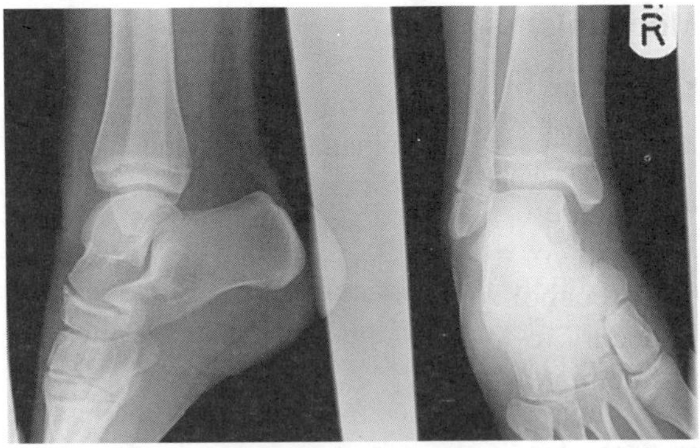

Fig. 4.16: Fracture of talar head

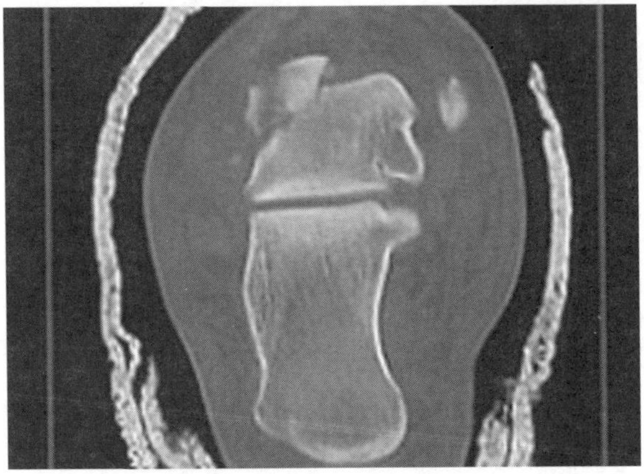

Fig. 4.17: Osteochondral fracture

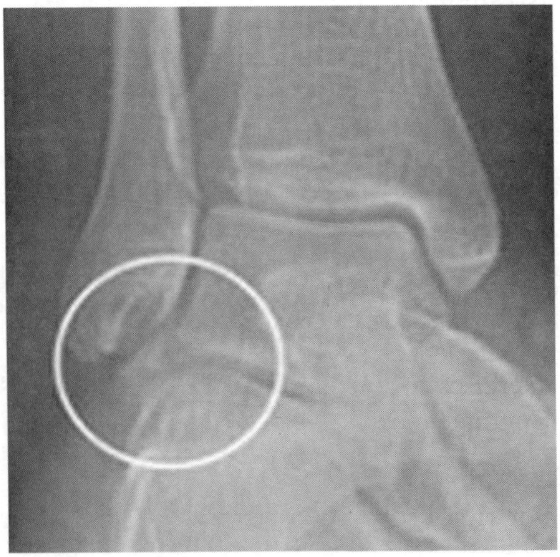

Fig. 4.18: Fracture of lateral process

Mechanism of Injury

- Fracture of body or neck of talus occurs as a result of high energy injuries such as in motor vehicle accidents.
- Fracture of posterior aspect of talus occurs as a result of axial load.
- Osteochondral and lateral process fracture occurs following ankle or subtalar sprain or fracture/dislocation of subtalar joints.

Treatment

Conservative Treatment

Cast is applied in non-displaced or minimally displaced fracture of talar neck.

Surgical Treatment

Open reduction and internal fixation using multiple screws is optioned in displaced talar fracture.

Physiotherapeutic Intervention

Day 0 – Week 1:

Range of motion:

- Active range of motion of the toes, metatarsophalangeal and knee joints.

Muscle strength:

- No strengthening exercises to ankle and foot.

Functional activities:

- Non-weight bearing stand/pivot transfers and ambulation with assistive devices.

Weight bearing:

- No weight bearing is allowed.

Week 2 – Week 4:

Range of motion:

- Initiate active ankle and sub-talar range of motion exercises for rigidly fixed talar fractures.
- Continue metatarsophalangeal joint exercises.

Muscle strength:

- For rigidly fixed fractures, initiate isometric exercises to dorsiflexors, plantar flexors, invertors and evertors.

Functional activities:

- Toe-touch weight bearing transfers with assistive devices for rigidly fixed fractures.

Weight bearing:

- Initiate toe touch weight bearing for rigidly fixed fractures.

Week 4 – Week 6:

Range of motion:

- Continue active range of motion at the metatarsophalangeal, tibiotalar and sub-talar joints for rigidly fixed fractures.
- Continue active range of motion at only metatarsophalangeal joint for non-rigidly fixed fractures.

Muscle strength:

- For rigidly fixed fractures, initiate isometric exercises to dorsiflexors, plantar flexors, invertors and evertors.
- No strengthening exercises for non-rigidly fixed fractures.

Functional activities:

- For rigidly fixed fractures, continue partial weight bearing stand/pivot transfers and three point gait.

Weight bearing:

- Continue toe-touch to partial weight bearing for rigidly fixed fractures.
- No weight bearing is allowed for non-rigidly fixed fractures.

Week 6 – Week 8:

Range of motion:

- Initiate active assistive range of motion for dorsiflexors, plantar flexors, invertors and evertors at ankle and sub-talar joints for rigidly fixed fractures.
- For non-rigidly fixed fractures active range of motion exercises at metatarsophalangeal, ankle and sub-talar joints.

Muscle strength:

- For rigidly fixed fractures, continue isometric

exercises to dorsiflexors, plantar flexors, invertors and evertors.
- For non-rigidly fixed fractures, initiate isometric exercises to dorsiflexors, plantar flexors, invertors and evertors.

Functional activities:
- Rigidly fixed fractures continue partial weight bearing for transfers and ambulation with assistive devices.
- Non-rigidly fixed fractures continue non-weight bearing for transfers and ambulation.

Weight bearing:
- Rigidly fixed fractures initiate partial weight bearing as tolerated.
- Non-rigidly fixed fractures must remain non-weight bearing.

Week 8 – Week 12:

Range of motion:
- For rigidly fixed fractures active, active assistive and passive range of motion at ankle and sub-talar joints.
- For non-rigidly fixed fractures active range of motion exercises at metatarsophalangeal, ankle and sub-talar joints.

Muscle strength:
- Initiate gentle resistive exercises to the dorsiflexors, plantar flexors, invertors and evertors along with flexors and extensors of toes for rigidly fixed fractures.
- Isometric exercises of the ankle and sub-talar joints for non-rigidly fixed fractures. No resistive exercises are allowed.

Functional activities:
- Rigidly fixed fractures may progress to full weight bearing as tolerated for transfers and ambulation using assistive devices if necessary.
- Non-rigidly fixed fractures are either non-weight bearing or partial weight bearing. Assistive devices are required for transfers and ambulation.

Weight bearing:
- Rigidly fixed fractures are partial to full weight bearing.
- Non-rigidly fixed fractures are non-weight bearing to partial weight bearing.

CALCANEAL FRACTURES

Calcaneal fractures (Fig. 4.19) are often intra-articular (Fig. 4.20) involving sub-talar and sometimes the calcaneocuboid joints. Non-articular (Fig. 4.21) fracture of calcaneum usually involve the posterior beak (posterior aspect of calcaneum including bony insertion of Achilles tendon) and may or may not involve injury to Achilles tendon.

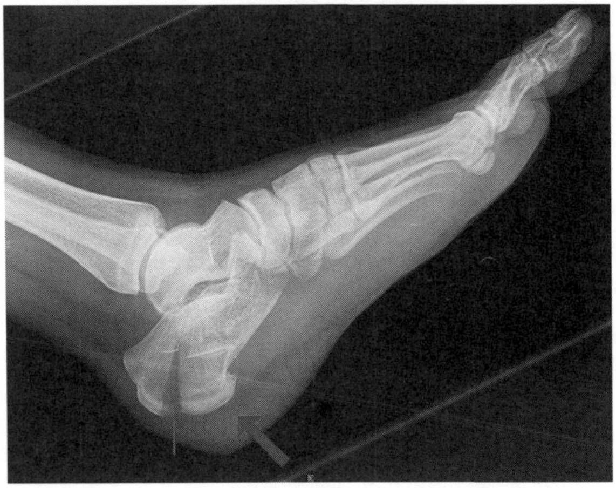

Fig. 4.19: Calcaneal fracture

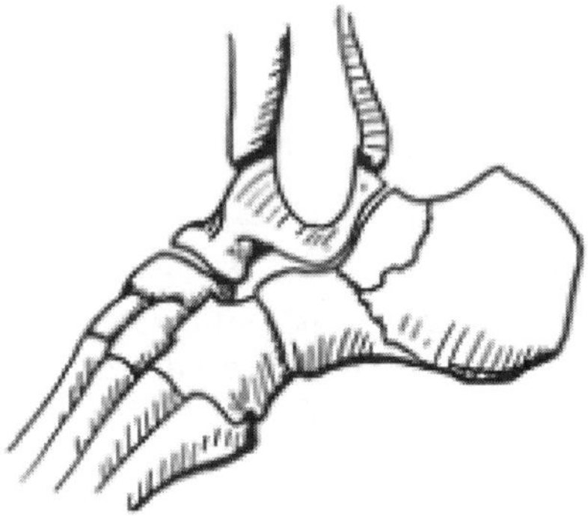

Fig. 4.20: Intra-articular calcaneal fractures

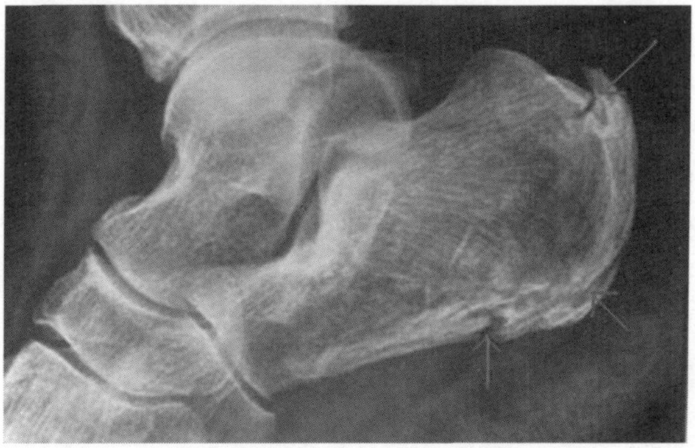

Fig. 4.21: Non-articular calcaneal fractures

Mechanism of Injury

Calcaneal fractures occur as a result of sudden high velocity impact on heel such as in motor vehicle accident or landing from a fall of 3 feet or more directly on to the heel.

Treatment

Conservative Treatment

Cast is the treatment of choice in following conditions:

- Minimally displaced non-articular fracture.
- Posterior beak fracture without the involvement of Achilles tendon.

Surgical Treatment

Open reduction and internal fixation using screw and plate fixation is opted in following conditions:

- Intra-articular calcaneal fracture involving facets of sub-talar jont.
- Large non-articular calcaneal fracture involving Achilles tendon.

Physiotherapeutic Intervention

Day 0 – Week 1:

Range of motion:

- Active range of motion of the toes, metatarsophalangeal and knee joints.

Muscle strength:

- No strengthening exercises to ankle and foot.

Functional activities:

- Non-weight bearing stand/pivot transfers and ambulation with assistive devices.

Weight bearing:

- No weight bearing is allowed.

Week 2 – Week 4:

Range of motion:

- Active range of motion of the toes, metatarsophalangeal and knee joints.

Muscle strength:

- Initiate isometric exercises for plantar flexors, dorsiflexors, invertors and evertors for rigidly fixed calcaneal fractures.

Functional activities:

- Non-weight bearing stand/pivot transfers.

Weight bearing:

- No weight bearing is allowed.

Week 4 – Week 6:

Range of motion:

- Active range of motion of the toes, metatarsophalangeal and knee joints for rigidly fixed fractures.
- Active range of motion only at metatarsophalangeal joint for non-rigidly fixed fractures.

Muscle strength:

- Continue isometric exercises for plantar flexors, dorsiflexors, invertors and evertors for rigidly fixed calcaneal fractures.
- No strengthening exercises for non-rigidly fixed fractures.

Functional activities:

- Initiate partial weight bearing stand/pivot transfers and three point gait for rigidly fixed fractures.

Weight bearing:

- Toe-touch to partial weight bearing for rigidly fixed fractures.
- No weight bearing is allowed for non-rigidly fixed fractures.

Week 6 – Week 8:

Range of motion:
- Continue active range of motion of the toes, metatarsophalangeal and knee joints for rigidly fixed fractures.
- Active range of motion only at metatar-sophalangeal joint for non-rigidly fixed fractures.

Muscle strength:
- Continue isometric exercises for plantar flexors, dorsiflexors, invertors and evertors for rigidly fixed calcaneal fractures.
- Initiate cfor non-rigidly fixed fractures.

Functional activities:
- Continue partial weight bearing stand/pivot transfers and three point gait for rigidly fixed fractures.
- Non-weight bearing transfers for non-rigidly fixed fractures.

Weight bearing:
- Partial weight bearing for rigidly fixed fractures.
- No weight bearing is allowed for non-rigidly fixed fractures.

Week 8 – Week 12:

Range of motion:
- Active, active-assistive and passive range of motion exercises at ankle and sub-talar joints for rigidly fixed fractures.
- Active range of motion only at metatar-sophalangeal joint for non-rigidly fixed fractures.

Muscle strength:
- Initiate gentle resistive exercises to dorsiflexors, plantar flexors, invertors and evertors along with flexors and extensors of toes for rigidly fixed fractures.
- No resistive exercises for non-rigidly fixed fractures. Continue isometric exercises of ankle and sub-talar joints.

Functional activities:
- Rigidly fixed fractures may progress to full weight bearing as tolerated for transfers and ambulation, using assistive devices if necessary.
- Non-rigidly fixed fractures are either non-weight bearing or partial weight bearing using assistive devices for transfers and ambulation.

Weight bearing:
- Rigidly fixed fractures are partial to full weight bearing.
- Non-rigidly fixed fractures are non-weight bearing to partial weight bearing.

MIDFOOT FRACTURES

Midfoot fractures involve the tarsometatarsal joint, cuneiforms, navicular bone and cuboid bone. Injuries to tarsometatarsal joint may or may not include fracture of metatarsal bone. Fracture of navicular bone includes cortical avulsion, fracture of tuberosity involving posterior tibial tendon, body fracture and stress fracture. Fracture of cuboid is called as nut cracker fracture.

The cuboid is cracked like a nut between fifth metatarsal and calcaneum as forefoot is forced in abduction.

Mechanism of Injury

- *Twisting of forefoot:* It can occur during motor vehicle accident when foot is forcefully abducted, or when forefoot is fixed and mid foot and hind foot twist around it as when a foot is caught in rung of a ladder.
- *Axial loading of a fixed foot:* Extensive axial compression applied to the heel as in fall on an extremely dorsiflexed foot or an extreme ankle equinus with axial loading from body weight as when stepping of a curve.
- Direct crushing blows to dorsum of foot usually occurs in industrial accidents. The foot must be evaluated for the compartment syndrome and injury to the dorsalis pedis artery in this type of injury.

Treatment

Tarsometatarsal joint injury:

- Cast is applied in cases of fracture or dislocation

of tarsometatarsal joint with preserved anatomic reduction. Immobilization is done with a short leg cast for six weeks.
- Open reduction and internal fixation is the treatment of choice in displaced fracture or dislocation of tarsometatarsal joint. Post surgically a non-weight bearing cast is given to the patient for six weeks.
- Closed reduction and percutaneous pinning is done when the injuries are bony in nature.

Navicular bone fractures:

- Cast is the treatment of choice in cortical avulsion fracture, tuberosity and non-displaced stress fracture. A short leg walking cast is given in cortical avulsion and tuberosity fracture for four to six weeks while a non-weight bearing cast is given in cases of stress fracture.
- Open reduction in internal fixation is done in cases of fracture body of navicular bone involving both talonavicular and naviculo-cuneiform joints, displaced stress fracture and non-united tuberosity fracture.

Cuboid and cuneiform fracture/dislocation

- A weight bearing cast is applied in cases of non displaced or minimally displaced avulsion fractures.
- Open reduction and internal fixation is preferred in compression injury, nut cracker fracture and displaced fractures.
- External fixator is applied if there is significant comminution or bone loss.

Physiotherapeutic Intervention

Day 0 to week 1:

Range of motion:
- Active range of motion to the toes and metatarsophalangeal joints is permitted.

Muscle strength:
- No strengthening exercises to the ankle and the foot.

Functional activities:
- Non-weight bearing stand/pivot transfers and ambulation with assistive devices is permitted.
- For some fractures of the navicular and cuboid bones partial weight bearing transfers and ambulation with assistive devices is permitted.

Weight bearing:
- In the first week all the fractures are non-weight bearing, except for some.
- Partial weight bearing for cortial avulsion and tuberosity fractures of navicular as well as avulsion or non displaced fractures of cuboid is allowed.

Week 2 to week 4

Range of motion:
- Active range of motion to the toes and metatarsophalangeal joints is permitted.

Muscle strength:
- Isometric exercises for the plantar flexors, dorsiflexors, invertors and evertors of ankle are performed in the cast.
- No resistive exercises to the long flexors and extensors of the toes and metatarsophalangeal joints is permitted.

Functional activities:
- Non-weight bearing stand/pivot transfers and ambulation with assistive devices depending on the type of fracture.
- Partial weight bearing to full weight bearing as tolerated with assistive devices for stable fractures of navicular and cuboid.

Weight bearing:
- Weight bearing as tolerated for stable fractures of the tarsal navicular and cuboid.

Week 4 to week 6

Range of motion:
- Active range of motion to toes and metatarso-phalangeal is initiated.
- Gentle active range of motion to ankle and sub-talar joint is permitted if they are out of the cast.

Muscle strength:
- Isometric exercises for the plantar flexors, dorsiflexors, invertors and evertors of ankle are performed in the cast.
- No resistive exercises to the long flexors and extensors of the toes and metatarsophalangeal joints are permitted.

Functional activities:
- Partial or non-weight bearing stand/pivot transfers and ambulation with assistive devices depending on type of fracture.

Weight bearing:
- No weight bearing is allowed for the patients with multiple cuneiform fractures, displaced stress fracture of tarsal navicular or if treated with open reduction and internal fixation.
- Partial weight bearing as tolerated for all other fractures including percutaneous pinning after hardware removal.

Week 6 to week 8

Range of motion:
- If ankle and subtalar joint are out of cast then gentle active to active assistive to gentle passive range of motion exercises as tolerated by the patient is permitted.

Muscle strength:
- Isometric and isotonic exercises to the ankle and sub-talar joint if out of cast.

Functional activities:
- Partial weight bearing is permitted during transfers except in fractures treated with open reduction and internal fixation.

Weight bearing:
- Partial to full weight bearing is allowed depending on tenderness at fracture site with the exception of fractures treated with open reduction and internal fixation.

Week 8 to week 12

Range of motion:
- Active, active assistive and passive range of motion exercises to the ankle and sub-talar joints.

Muscle strength:
- Gentle resistive exercises to dorsiflexors, plantar flexors, invertors, evertors, long flexors and extensors of the toes.

Functional activities:
- Partial to full weight bearing transfers and ambulation with or without assistive devices as healing permits.

Weight bearing:
- Partial to full weight bearing is allowed.

FOREFOOT FRACTURES

Forefoot fracture involves fracture of phalanges, metatarsals or sesamoid bones. Phalangeal and metatarsal fractures can either be intra or extra-articular and can involve neck, shaft or base of the bone. Metatarsal fractures can be stable or unstable. Unstable metatarsal fractures contributes to fracture of multiple metatarsals which can either be comminuted or displaced. They can complicate as compartment syndrome. Fracture of metatatarsal is known as Jones fracture. Sesamoid fractures occur as a result of splitting or fragmentation of one or both of the two small bones contain within the tendon of flexor hallucis longus. They are important because of their role in forefoot weight distribution.

Mechanism of Injury

Phalangeal fracture

- Fracture of first proximal phalanx can occur due to direct trauma or avulsion mechanism as when great toe is caught on table or chair leg.
- Fracture of lesser phalanges occur as a result of direct trauma.

Metatarsal fracture

- Fracture of first through fourth metatarsal occur as a result of direct trauma.
- Fracture of second through fifth metatarsal may occur as a result of twisting injury.
- Diaphyseal stress fracture are common in second through fourth metatarsal, commonly resulting from repeated trauma.
- Avulsion fractures of proximal apophysis and proximal shaft of fifth metatarsal may follow an inversion injury on a plantar flexed ankle.

Sesamoid fracture

- These fractures often occur secondary to impact of foot on hard surface while toes are dorsiflexed. Stress fracture occurs as a result of repeated impact and tension as seen in dancers and runners.

Treatment

Lesser phalanx fracture

- Splint or buddy taping is used in cases of diaphyseal fracture of proximal and middle phalanges.
- Open reduction and percutaneous pinning is done for open fractures. Post operatively a short leg cast that extends to toes is applied for two to three weeks.

Second, third and fourth metatarsal fracture

- A short leg walking cast is applied in cases of undisplaced or minimally displaced fracture of metatarsal shaft and stress fracture.
- Closed reduction and percutaneous pinning is done for closed, displaced or angulated metatarsal shaft fracture. Post operatively the limb is immobilized in a non weight bearing short leg cast for two to three weeks until the pins are removed.
- Open reduction and internal fixation is done for open displaced fracture. Post operatively a non weight bearing short leg cast is given for two to three weeks.

Fifth metatarsal fracture

- Cast or splint is treatment of choice in acute avulsion injury of apophysis and Jones fracture.
- Open reduction and internal fixation is done for avulsion fractures with greater than 2 mm displacement using tension band wiring or lag screw. Bone graft and intra medullary screw fixation is done in cases of delayed union and non union. Post operatively, a non weight bearing short leg cast is applied for six weeks.

Great toe phalanx fracture

- Non displaced extra articular fracture can be buddy taped and placed in non weight bearing short leg cast.
- Closed reduction and percutaneous pinning is done for displaced or intra articular fractures using K-wires.
- Open reduction and internal fixation is needed if closed reduction fails.

First metatarsal fracture

- A non weight bearing short leg cast is applied in non displaced fractures.
- Open reduction and internal fixation is done for displaced, intra articular or open fractures.

Sesamoid fracture

- Acute fracture or suspected stress fracture can be treated by placing a soft padding under the arch and first metatarsal head and strapping the metatarsophalangeal joint into neutral or slightly plantar flexed position. A short leg cast or alternatively a post operative bunion shoe may be used.
- Sesamoidectomy is done in cases of persistent pain or failure of conservative treatment. Toe is then splinted in a protected position for four to six weeks.

Physiotherapeutic Intervention

Day 1 – Week 1

Range of motion:

- Active range of motion to metatarsophalangeal joints for stable phalangeal fractures.

- No range of motion exercises for fractures of sesamoids, first phalanx and first metatarsal.

Strength:
- No strengthening exercises are advised.

Functional activities:
- For the fractures of sesamoid first phalanx, first and fifth metatarsal non weight bearing stand/ pivot transfers and ambulation with assistive devices is advised.
- For the stable fractures of metatarsals, lesser phalanges and lesser metatarsals allow weight bearing, transfers and ambulation as tolerated.

Weight bearing:
- For stable fractures of phalanges and lesser metatarsals weight bearing as tolerated.
- No weight bearing is allowed in case of fractures of sesamoid first phalanax, first and fifth metatarsal.

Week 2 - Week 4

Range of motion:
- Active range of motion to metatarsophalangeal joints for stable phalangeal fractures.
- No range of motion exercises for fractures of first metatarsal, Jones fracture, first phalanx and sesamoid.
- Active range of motion to metatarsal and interphalangeal joints for the fractures of lesser metatarsals.

Strength:
- No strengthening exercises in case of stable phalangeal fractures.
- Isometric strengthening exercises to the ankle musculature for metatarsal fractures.

Functional activities:
- For the fractures of sesamoid first phalanx, first and fifth metatarsal non weight bearing stand/ pivot transfers and ambulation with assistive devices is advised.
- For the stable fractures of metatarsals, lesser phalanges and lesser metatarsals allow weight bearing, transfers and ambulation as tolerated.

Weight bearing:
- For stable fractures of phalanges and lesser metatarsals weight bearing as tolerated.
- No weight bearing is allowed in case of fractures of sesamoid first phalanax, first and fifth metatarsal.

Week 4 – Week 6:

Range of motion:
- Full active range of motion exercises to the metatarsal joints for stable phalangeal fracture.
- Active range of motion exercises to metatarsal joints, active to active assistive range of motion exercises to ankle for metatarsal fractures out of cast.
- No range of motion exercises in case of fracture of sesamoid, first phalanx, first and fifth metatarsal.

Strength:
- Isotonic exercises to long flexors and extensors of toes for stable phalangeal fractures.
- Isometric and isotonic strengthening exercises to ankle musculature for metatarsal fractures.

Functional activities:
- Weight bearing transfers and ambulation for the stable fractures.
- Partial to non weight bearing transfers and ambulation for fractures of first phalanx, sesamoids, first and fifth metatarsals.

Weight bearing:
- For stable fractures of phalanges and lesser metatarsals weight bearing as tolerated.
- Non weight bearing to partial weight bearing is allowed in case of fractures of sesamoid first phalanx, first and fifth metatarsal.

Week 6 – Week 8

Range of motion:
- Active and active assistive to gentle passive range of motion exercises to all phalangeal, metatarsals and ankle joint.

Strength:
- Resisted isometric and isotonic exercises to the ankle musculature.

- Isotonic and isometric strengthening exercises to the long flexors and extensors of toes.

Functional activities:

- Weight bearing transfers and ambulation for the stable fractures.
- Partial to non weight bearing transfers and ambulation for fractures of first phalanx, sesamoids, first and fifth metatarsals.

Weight bearing:

- For stable fractures of phalanges and lesser metatarsals weight bearing as tolerated.
- Non weight bearing to partial weight bearing is allowed in case of fractures of sesamoid first phalanx, first and fifth metatarsal.

Week 8 – Week 12

Range of motion:

- Active, active assistive and passive range of motion exercises to metatarsophalangeal, interphalangeal and ankle joints.

Strength:

- Progressive resistive exercises to the ankle musculature, long flexors and extensors of the toes.

Functional activities:

- Full weight bearing transfers and ambulation is allowed.

Weight bearing:

- Full weight bearing is allowed.

CHAPTER 5

DISLOCATIONS OF LOWER EXTREMITY

DISLOCATION OF HIP

The dislocation of hip is categorised into three categories:
- Posterior dislocation.
- Anterior dislocation.
- Central fracture dislocation.

Posterior Dislocation (Fig. 5.1)

It is most common amongst all types of dislocations of hip. The head of the femur is pushed out of the acetabulum in a posterior direction. It is also known as dashboard injury.

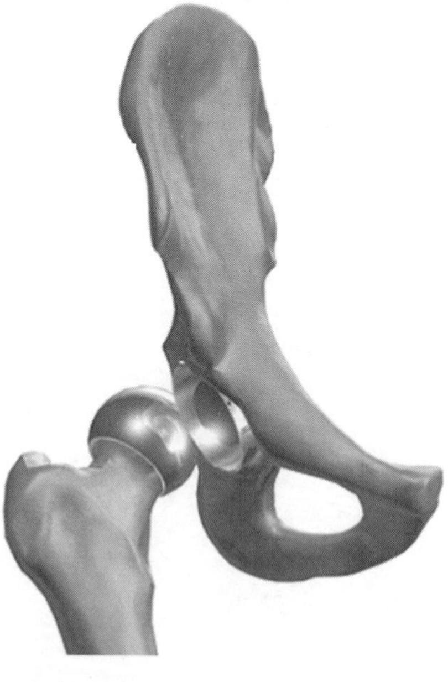

Fig. 5.1: Posteriorly dislocated hip

Mechanism of Injury

Moderately severe violent force directed along the femur when the hip is adducted and flexed as in case of car or motorbike accidents.

Associated Feature

Chip fracture of posterior lip of acetabulum.

Attitude of Dislocated Limb

Flexion, adduction and internal rotation (Fig. 5.2).

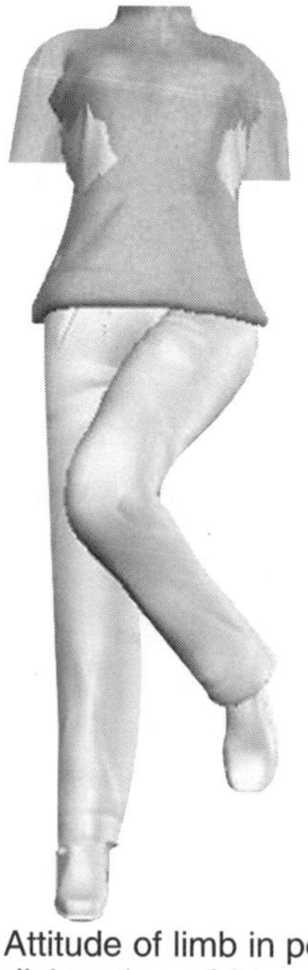

Fig. 5.2: Attitude of limb in posterior dislocation of hip

Clinical Features

- History of trauma reported by patient
- Pain.
- Swelling.
- Deformity.
- Shortening (apparent) of the leg by 2-3cms.
- *On palpation:* The head of the femur is felt in gluteal region.

Radiological Features (Fig. 5.3)

- Femoral head is out of acetabulum.
- Lesser trochanter becomes less prominent.
- Broken shenton's line.
- Bony chip from acetabulum lip must be looked upon carefully.

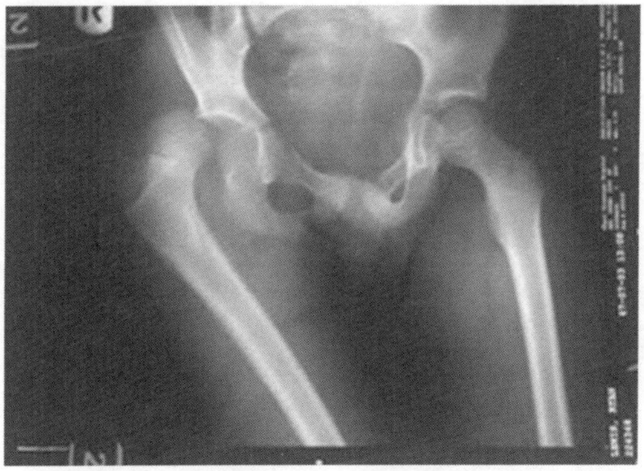

Fig. 5.3: Radiograph showing posterior dislocation of hip

Treatment

The treatment of posterior hip diclocation can either be conservative or surgical.

Conservative management:
The dislocated hip should be reduced under anaesthesia as soon after the injury as possible.
Position of patient: Patient lies supine on the floor with hip and knee flexed to 90^0.
Technique: An assistant grasps the pelvis firmly while the surgeon exerts an axial pull by holding the knee. Reduction is confirmed by a 'click' sound after which the patient is able to move the hip in all directions. The hip is immobilized for a period of 3-6 weeks.

Surgical Management:
The decision of open reduction and internal fixation is taken in following cases:
- Where closed reduction fails.
- Late and neglected cases.
- Presence of intra-articular loose fragment.
- Fracture of weight bearing part of acetabulum.

The immobilization period is slightly longer, i.e., of 6-8 weeks.
Immobilization Techniques:
- Thomas splint with skin traction.
- Hip spica plaster of paris cast.

Complications

- Injury to sciatic nerve.
- Avascular necrosis of femoral head.
- Osteoarthritis.
- Post traumatic ossification.

Anterior Dislocation (Fig. 5.4)

It is not a common injury to occur.

Mode of Injury

Forcible abduction and external rotation.

Attitude of Limb

The limb rests in attitude of external rotation.

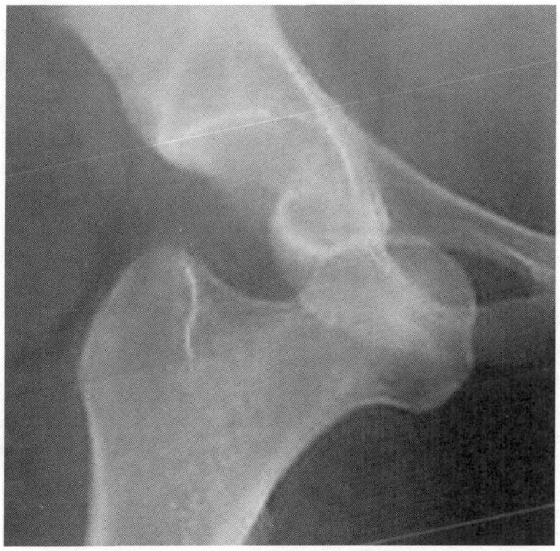

Fig. 5.4: Anteriorly dislocated hip

Clinical Features

- Clinical deformity.
- Lengthening of the limb.
- *On palpation:* Head of the femur is palpable in groin.

Treatment

Manipulative reduction under anaesthesia is effected by strong traction upon the limb combined with medial rotation. The limb is immobilized in Thomas splint or hip spica for 6–8 weeks.

Complications

- Avascular necrosis of femoral head.
- Osteoarthritis.

Central Fracture Dislocation

In this case head of femur is driven through the medial wall of acetabulum towards the pelvic cavity, associated with fracture of acetabular floor (Fig. 5.5).

Mode of Injury

- Heavy lateral blow on femur.
- Fall on the side.

Treatment

The main aim of treatment in cases of central fracture dislocation is to attain as much maximum congruence of articular surface.

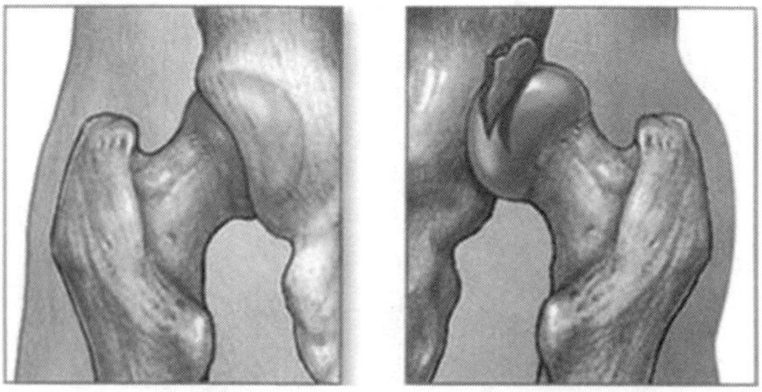

Fig. 5.5: Central fracture dislocation

Conservative Management:
The central fracture dislocation of hip is conservatively managed by skeletal traction. The traction is applied in two directions – longitudinally along the line of leg and laterally through the greater trochanter. The hip is immobilized for 8–12 weeks.

Surgical Management:
Surgical intervention in form of acetabular floor reconstruction is done in cases where the fractured fragment do not fall back to place by conservative means and in young demanding patients.

Complications

- Hip joint stiffness.
- Myositis ossificans.
- Osteoarthritis.

Physiotherapy Management

During immobilization:

- Strong isometrics to glutei, hip flexors, quadriceps and hamstrings are ensured.
- Small range movements to be begun in cases treated with skeletal traction.
- Care must be taken in cases treated with skeletal traction while performing adduction and internal rotation in posterior dislocation; adduction and external rotation in anterior dislocation.

During mobilization

- Vigorous range of motion exercises to the involved hip joint to be initiated at an early stage of mobilization.
- Strengthening of the muscles crossing the hip joint.
- Knee mobilization exercises are necessary in patients treated with hip spica.
- *Regaining control of hip movements:* It could be done by initializing assisted SLR.
- Assisted ambulation is started once the hip movements are controlled by 12 weeks. The patient becomes independent in ambulation by 15-16 weeks.

DISLOCATION OF PATELLA

The patella always dislocates laterally (Fig. 5.6). The dislocations of patella can be categorised into three categories:
- Acute dislocation.
- Recurrent dislocation.
- Habitual dislocation.

Acute Dislocation of Patella

Cause

Sudden strong contraction of quadriceps while the knee is flexed or semi-flexed.

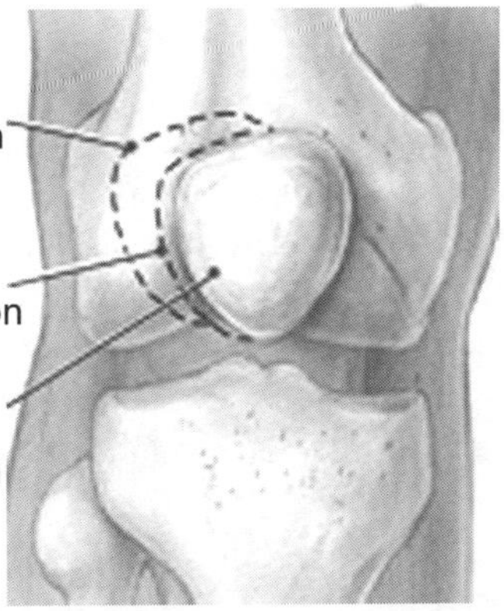

Fig. 5.6: Dislocation of patella

Clinical Features

- The patella lies on the lateral aspect of the knee over the lateral femoral condyle.
- Patient is not able to extend the affected knee actively.
- Swelling may occur eventually due to fluid effusion.
- Local tenderness over antero-medial aspect of the knee joint due to rupture of capsule.
- Medial femoral condyle appears to be more prominent.

Even after the reduction of dislocation and proper healing patient complains of repeated episodes of pain, swelling and sensation of loose body due to tearing of piece of bone covered with articular cartilage from the patella or femoral condyle at the time of dislocation.

Treatment

- Reduction of dislocation.
- Immobilization.

Reduction of dislocation may sometimes occur spontaneously or can easily be done by applying a medial ward pressure upon the patella while the knee is gradually straightened. Immobilization is done with the aid of above knce cylinder cast for three weeks.

Physiotherapy Management

During immobilization

- Gentle isometrics to the quadriceps and hamstrings are initiated at an early stage so as to maintain good muscular strength.
- Passive SLR includes:
  - Isometrics to the quadriceps.
  - Improving hip control.
- As soon as the pain reduces, partial weight bearing (PWB) crutch walking is initiated.

During mobilization

- Knee ROM exercises are initiated as soon as the cast is removed. Procedures of both tibio-femoral and patellofemoral joint mobilization are started simultaneously.
- Quadriceps strengthening exercises are progressed from static isometrics to concentric to eccentric. Resisted exercises should be done regularly so as to avoid any future recurrence of the dislocation.

Recurrent Dislocation of Patella

In recurrent dislocation of patella, the patella dislocates laterally. The ease of dislocation increases after the occurrence of first episode.

Age of onset: Adoloscence

Gender

Girls are generally more susceptible to the dislocation than the boys.

Causes

- Excessive joint laxity.
- Small patella.
- Patella alta.
- Shallow femoral intercondylar groove.
- Genu valgum.
- Underdeveloped lateral femoral condyle.
- Weak knee musculature.

Clinical Features

- The lateral dislocation of patella is associated with severe pain.
- *Apprehension test positive:* When the patella is pushed laterally and the knee is flexed, the patient resists the manoeuvre.
- In between the episodes of dislocations, the patient is usually asymptomatic.

Treatment

Surgical management of the condition is only the effective measure to prevent recurring patellar dislocation.

Principle of surgical treatment:
Realignment of quadriceps mechanism so that the patella is prevented from dislocating laterally when knee is flexed.

Commonly performed surgical procedures:

- *Campbell's operation:* The tight structures on the lateral side of the joint are released and a thin strip of joint capsule on the medial side is mobilized with its base proximally. The strip is then passed under the ligamentum patellae and brought out on the lateral side, and then folded on itself to be stitched back on the medial side. It pulls the ligamentum patellae on the medial side and prevents it from dislocating laterally.
- *Hauser's operation:* The bony insertion of the patellar tendon is detatched and transpose into new bed on tibia, medial and distal to original insertion. In this way patella is drawn lower into the intercondylar groove of femur and line of pull of quadriceps is transferred more to medial side.

Habitual Dislocation

Habitual dislocation of patella does not occur commonly. The patella dislocates every time the knee is flexed.

Causes

- Shortened vastus lateralis component of quadriceps muscle results in abnormal lateral pull on patella when the knee is flexed.
- Abnormal fibrous band tethering the vastus lateralis to iliotibial tract due to which the patella is pulled laterally out of its groove every time the knee is flexed.

Treatment

Surgical treatment aims at releasing the tight structures on the lateral side and repairing of lax structures on the medial side.

Post-Surgical Physiotherapy Management

During immobilization: Post-surgically the knee is immobilized in above knee POP cast for 4 weeks.

- Active movements to all the free joints.
  - Strong toe movements.
  - Active hip movements.
- Non-weight bearing crutch walking is initiated on the second post-operative day.
- Quadriceps strengthening exercises:
  - Indirect isometric quadriceps during passive SLR.

- Direct weak isometrics inside the cast within limits of discomfort should begin.

During mobilization

- To reduce pain
  - Paraffin wax bath.
  - Short wave diathermy.
  - Interferential therapy.

All above mentioned modalities reduces pain and also aids in mobilization.

- Hydrotherapy in the form of whirlpool is extremely useful at this stage.
- Improving range of motion of the knee joint:
  - Gradual knee mobilization is to begin in small range by CPM.
  - Passive movements to the knee joint.
  - Self assisted knee swinging.
  - Passive knee mobilization should begin and progressed very gradually.
- Knee musculature strengthening exercises:
  Both hamstrings and quadriceps has to be strengthened so as to achieve good control of movements. The strengthening exercises should begin with isometrics as they do help in pain relief and reducing swelling. The exercises should be progressed gradually.
- Endurance training:
  - Endurance training in the position of maximum extension.
  - Quadriceps and hamstrings co-contraction.
  - Isokinetic exercises.
- Use of knee orthosis:
  Knee orthosis should be used as a protective measure for 8-10 weeks. Weaning off the orthoses to be done only when:
  - Patient regains full active extension.
  - 70-90° of knee flexion.
- After 10–12 weeks following measures could be initiated:
  - Body resistive squats.
  - Light sports activity.
  - Brief periods of jogging and running.

DISLOCATION OF KNEE

The dislocation of knee is a rare injury caused by severely violent trauma to the knee affecting all its supporting ligaments (Fig. 5.7). The knee joint attains a greater amount of stability by cruciate and collateral ligaments thus the damage to the ligamentous support will result in instability of the knee joint.

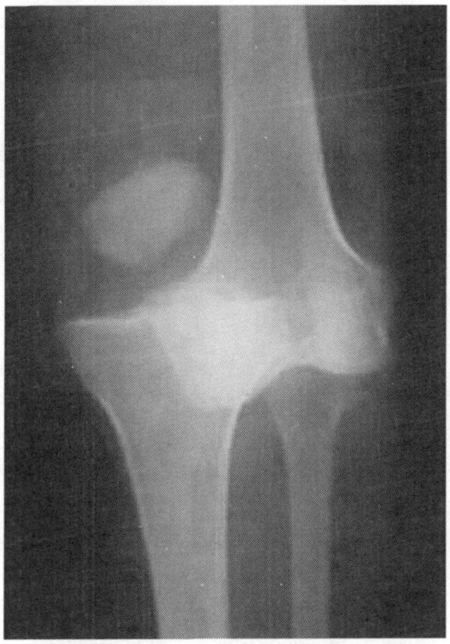

Fig. 5.7: Dislocation of knee

Clinical Features

- Pain.
- Swelling.
- Inability to bear weight on the affected limb.

Treatment

The treatment of a dislocated knee will depend upon the damage to the ligaments. It could either follow a conservative or a surgical pathway.

Conservative Treatment

The conservative management for a dislocated knee includes closed reduction by traction and manipulation. The limb is then immobilized in cylindrical cast for two months.

Surgical Treatment

If conservative treatment fails or there is serious damage to the ligaments then surgery must be done. The surgical procedure aims at repair and reconstruction of torn ligaments. The limb is immobilised for a period of 12 weeks.

Physiotherapy Management

During Immobilization

- Check for proper circulation to the foot to exclude any damage to the popliteal vessels.
- Keep the immobilised limb in an elevated position.
- Vigorous ankle and toe movements are initiated.
- Isometric exercises for the following muscle groups are initiated from first day.
  - Quadriceps.
  - Hamstrings.
  - Glutei.
- After 1 week, begin with assisted SLR which is then progressed to voluntary SLR by the patient.
- Ambulation:
  - Non-weight bearing crutch walking is initiated on the second or third day.
  - As soon as the patient is able to perform voluntary SLR,gradual weight bearing can be initiated which is progressed to full weight bearing.

During Mobilization

There are many problems encountered during the period of mobilization due to the nature of injury and long period of immobilization. Specifically encountered problems are:

- Stiff and painful knee.
- Instability of knee.

Intervention

- Knee mobilization exercises.
- Controlled stabilization of the knee.
- Endurance training.
- Muscle strengthening exercises.

COMPLICATIONS

- Injury to popliteal artery and nerve.
- Persistent knee instability.
- Restriction of knee movement.
- Late osteoarthritis.

UNIT TWO

DEFORMITIES

CHAPTER 6

CONGENITAL DEFORMITIES

SPRENGEL'S SHOULDER

It is also known as congenital high scapula (Fig. 6.1). It is characterized by abnormally high scapula. It may be unilateral or bilateral.

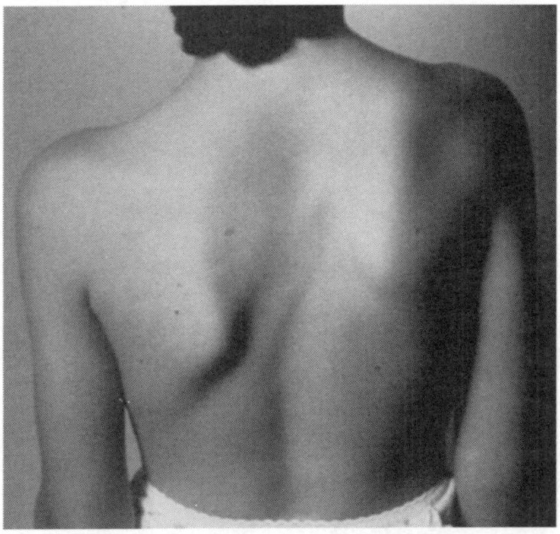

Fig. 6.1: Congenital high scapula

Causes

The condition is caused by failure of descent of the scapula, which is developmentally a cervical appendage.

Clinical Features

- Poorly developed scapular muscles represented by fibrous bands.
- Scoliosis (thoracic curve) with convexity on involved side.
- Markedly limited scapular movements.
- Limitation of shoulder abduction and elevation.

Surgical Management

It consists of excision of the fibrous band or bony bar and bringing the scapula back to its normal position.

Postsurgical Physiotherapy Management

- Suitable pain reducing modalities like TENS and hydrocollateral packs may be used to induce relaxation.
- Gradual relaxed passive mobilization of scapula and shoulder, with special attention to shoulder abduction and elevation.
- Strengthening of scapular and shoulder muscles.
- Maximum possible correction of posture and its maintenance.

RADIOULNAR SYNOSTOSIS

Radius and ulna are fused at proximal radioulnar joint (Fig. 6.2) causing restriction of forearm movements. There is restricted rotation of radius over ulna.

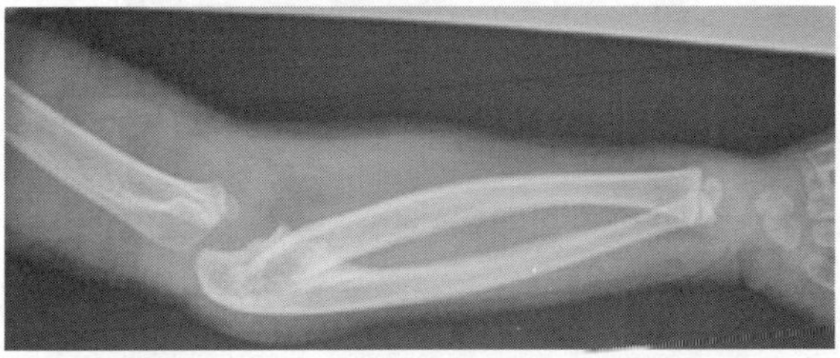

Fig. 6.2: Fused proximal radioulnar joint

Management

Conservative Management

When forearm is fixed in the near range to mid position of forearm or pronation, arm can be effectively used for functional activities by maneuvering movement at shoulder, elbow and wrist joint.

Physiotherapeutic Intervention

Strengthening of compensatory muscle groups.

Surgical Management: When forearm is fixed in an abnormal position, osteotomy becomes necessary.

Physiotherapeutic Intervention

Post surgical emphasis on rotational movements at forearm.

MADELUNG'S DEFORMITY

It is a congenital anomaly associated with defective development of medial part of distal radial epiphysis. Consequently, the radial shaft bows backwards and the lower end of ulna subluxate backwards (Fig. 6.3).

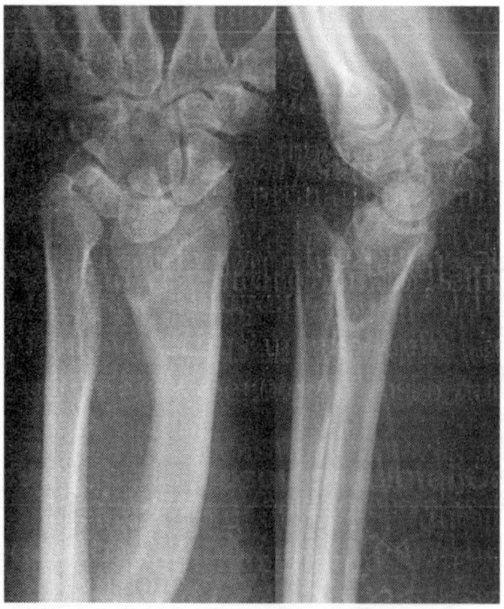

Fig. 6.3: Madelung's deformity

Management

Surgical Treatment

Excision of lower end of ulna is the most commonly performed surgery in this condition. It improves deformity and range of motion.

Physiotherapeutic Intervention

Mobilization is to be initiated as soon as pain permits as there is no plaster post-surgically.

CLUB HAND

This is characterized by distortion of the hand at the wrist from long axis of forearm due to congenital absence of radius (Fig. 6.4) or ulna causing either excessive radial deviation or ulnar deviation.

More commonly, radius is absent along with the thumb.

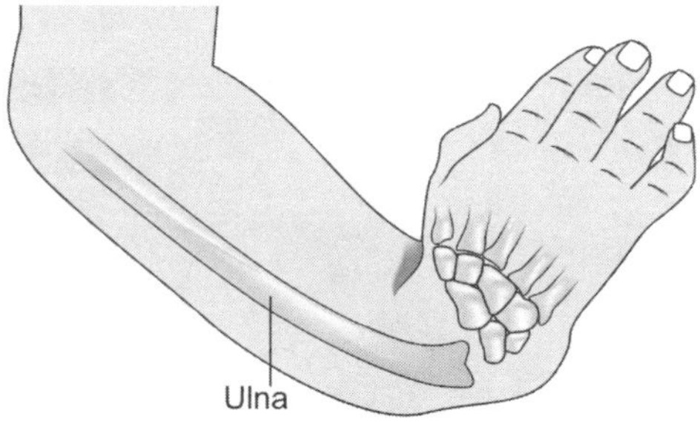

Fig. 6.4: Radial club hand

Deformity

Wrist is in flexion along with radial or ulnar deviation.

Clinical Features

- Weakness of grasp (due to mechanical disadvantage imposed upon the line of action of flexor group of muscles).
- Marked soft tissue tightness or contracture on side of deformity.

Management

Mild Cases

- Passive stretching of contracted soft tissues followed by immobilization in a specially fabricated splint which keeps the hand in overcorrected position.

Moderate Cases

- Forcible manipulation under general anesthesia.
- Premanipulative regime: Splint and regular sessions of passive stretching.

Severe Cases

- *Preoperative regime:* Stretching and splinting sessions.
- *Surgical regime:* Centralization of ulna i.e., alignment of ulna with third metacarpal. This alignment is maintained with an internal fixation and plaster cast for period of six weeks.
- *Postoperative regime:*
  - Maintenance of proper positioning of wrist in overcorrected position with the help of splints.
  - Sessions of gentle relaxed passive movements towards overcorrection as well as wrist extension should be concentrated.
  - Strengthening procedures for muscle groups antagonistic to side of deformity needs special attention.
  - Functional use of hand is emphasized.
  - Gradual weaning of splint to be done.

TORTICOLLIS

It is characterised by malposition of neck due to muscular shortening.

Causes

- Malposition of neck in uterus.
- Shortening of sternocleidomastoid muscle (Fig. 6.5).

Associated Shortened Muscles

- Scaleni.
- Platysma.
- Splenius.
- Trapezius.

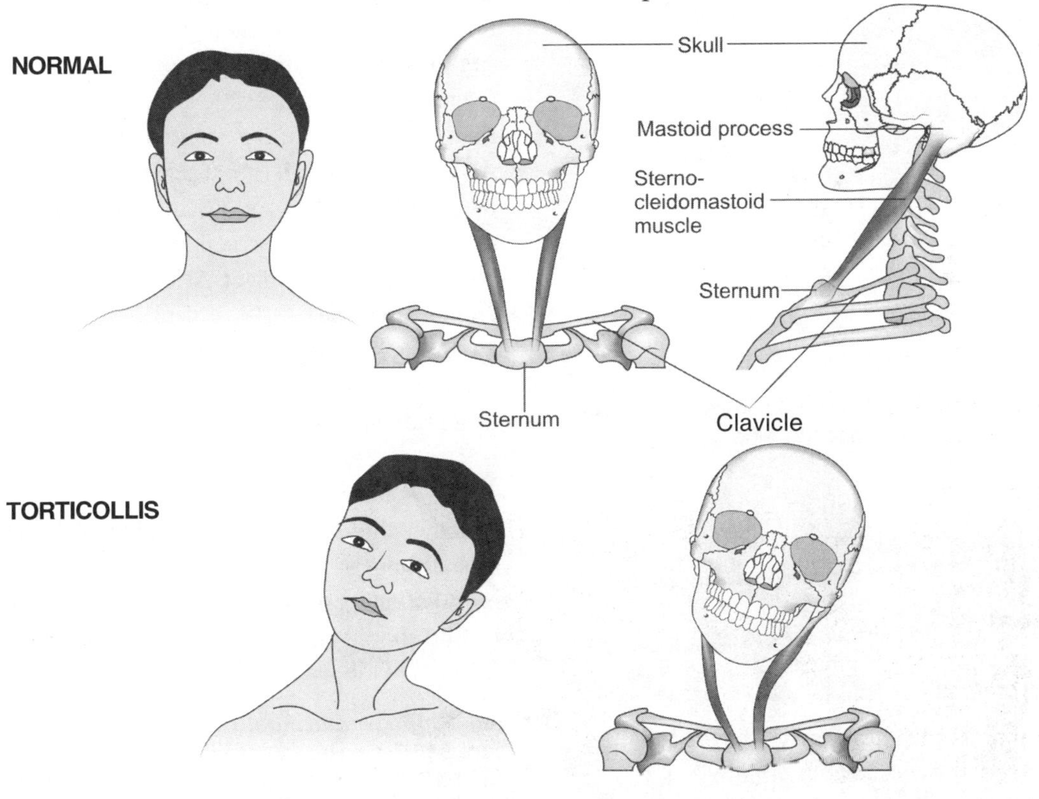

Fig. 6.5: Shortening of sternocleidomastoid muscle

Aetiology

It is more common in girls, side usually affected is left.

Nature of Deformity

In Unilateral Cases

- Head is fixed in side flexion to same side, while it is rotated to opposite side (Fig. 6.6).
- Affected shoulder is raised.
- Scoliosis with convexity to sound side may be present in cervical region.
- Facial asymmetry with smaller eye and lowering of corners of mouth and eye.
- Deviation of nose on affected side.

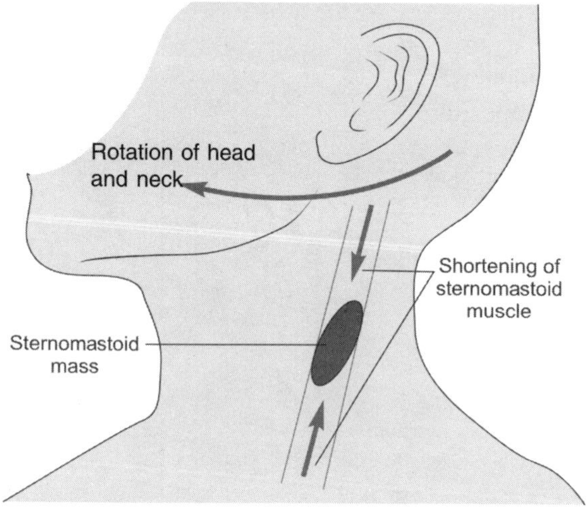

Fig. 6.6: Shortening of SCM resulting in rotation of head to opposite side

In Bilateral Cases

- Head is protruded forward with associated kyphosis.

Treatment

Aims of Treatment

- To correct the deformity by release of contracted soft tissues.
- To maintain correction by suitable exercise regime.

Early Mild Cases

Physiotherapy procedures employed are:

- Careful evaluation of range of motion and degree of deformity.
- Massage can relax the affected muscle preceding the stretching maneuvers.
- Relaxation of the affected muscle by adequate thermotherapy modality.
- Passive movements:
  - Child is placed in supine position with head beyond edge of table with neck in extension by positioning a pillow under thoracic region. Shoulders are stabilized by an assistant.
  - To attain relaxation, all movements of cervical spine are performed in form of slow relaxed passive movements.
- *Passive stretching of sternocleidomastoid:* Head should be gradually bend in side flexion to the unaffected side and then gradually rotated to the affected side. Try to gain as much overcorrection as possible by applying gradual traction to gain further stretching.
- *Active correction:* It is best achieved by assisting the child's head to follow an object moved in the proper arc of correction. Bright coloured sound producing object is ideal to attract the child's attention.
- *Proprioceptive neuromuscular facilitation (PNF):* Patterns of neck extension can be used at an advantage with emphasis on stretch and traction.
- *Home Treatment Programme*

The mother should be properly taught manipulation to repeat them at home.

Exact positioning of head during sleep is important. The child should be made to sleep on opposite side of lesion.

Older Children and Adults

Surgical treatment: The sternal and clavicular heads of sternocleidomastoid are divided close to origin along with release of tight fascia. The head is then immobilized in plaster cast in overcorrected position for 2 to 4 weeks.

Postsurgical Physiotherapy Regime

- *Control of pain:* Pain relieving modality like hot pack or infra red should be given before exercises because pain at surgical incision may persist particularly during exercises.
- *Active movements:* The sternocleidomastoid muscle will become weak after surgery so active movements should be emphasized. Initially free active movements are encouraged. Then specific exercises for sternocleidomastoid in a correct groove to attain lateral flexion to opposite side and rotation to same side is encouraged.
- *Resistive movements:* The affected SCM should be strengthened resistively.
- *Self correction:* Methods of self correction in front of mirror and its maintenance by active efforts should be well educated.
- Specially moulded cervical collar should be used.
- *Postural guidance:* Proper posture should be maintained especially during sleep.

Guidance on proper posture while working or during activities of daily life forms an important part of treatment to avoid recurrence.

CERVICAL RIB

The presence of extra rib is the extension of costal process of seventh cervical vertebra. It may compress neurological and vascular structures (Fig. 6.7) i.e. brachial plexus (lower part) and axillary artery.

Clinical Features

- Paraesthesia in hand.
- Hypothenar wasting.
- Atonia in shoulder girdle muscles.
- Drooping of shoulder.
- Lower trunk paresis.
- Sympathetic disturbance with increased sweating in hand.

Management

Medical Treatment

- Anti-inflammatory drugs.
- Analgesics.

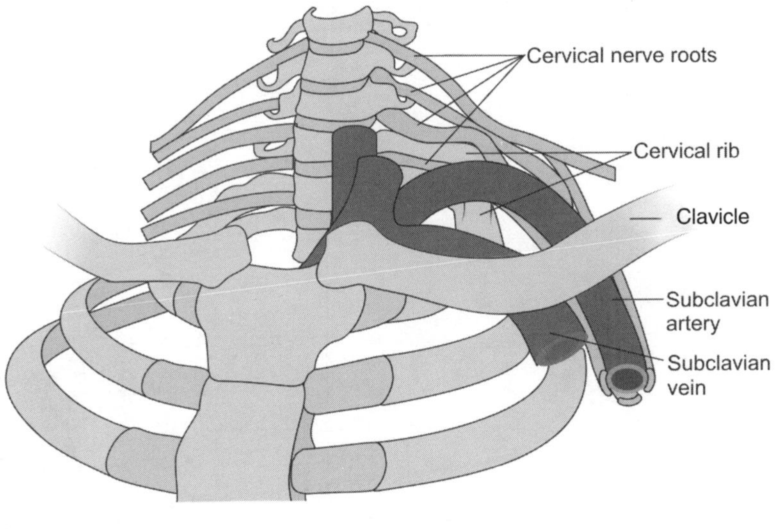

Fig. 6.7: Cervical rib compressing the neurological and vascular structures

Surgical Treatment

- Excision of cervical rib.

Physiotherapy Treatment

- Strengthening of shoulder girdle muscles: Elevators and retractors.

Specific interventions are as follows:
– Self resistive exercise.
– Progressive resistive exercises.
– Scapular PNF patterns.

CONGENITAL DISLOCATION OF HIP (CDH)

This is spontaneous dislocation of hip occurring before, during or shortly after birth.

Incidence

It is 3-5 per 1000 live births.

Gender

Girls are affected three times more than boys.

Causes

- Genetically determined joint laxity.
- Hormonal joint laxity.
- Genetically determined dysplasia of hip.
- Breech malposition.

Pathology (Fig. 6.8)

Bony Changes

- The femoral head is dislocated upwards and laterally; its epiphysis is small and ossifies late.
- The femoral neck is excessively anteverted.
- The acetabulum is shallow, with steep sloping.

Ligaments

- The ligamentum teres is hypertrophied.
- The fibrocartilaginous labrum of acetabulum (limbus) may be folded into the cavity of acetabulum (inverted limbus).
- The capsule of hip joint is stretched.

Muscles

- The long muscles passing from pelvis to femur or to tibia or fibula will tend to become shortened and thus will offer resistance to reduction. These muscles are hamstrings, sartorius, rectus femoris, adductors.
- The short muscles attached between pelvis and femur are altered in direction and this alter their function. Gluteus medius and minimus become more horizontal in direction and this makes their angle of pull largely ineffective, not only as abductors of hip but in their important function

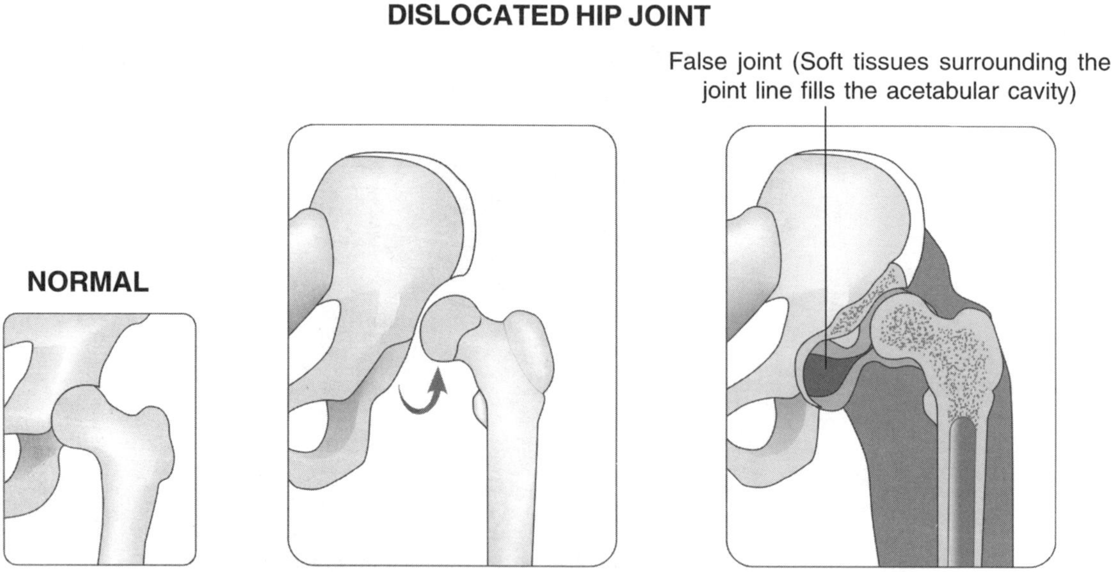

Fig. 6.8: Pathology of congenital hip dislocation

of keeping the pelvis level during weight transference.

- The tendon of psoas major is displaced so it compresses the capsule of hip joint producing an 'hour-glass shape' in posterior dislocations. It thus stretches between the origin and insertion like a sling, and the pelvis is supported on it, and on the capsule.

Clinical Features

The clinical features are not very obvious until the child begins to walk but the observer should look for following specific signs and symptoms in neonates:

Gait

- In unilateral cases, there is marked limp, the patient droops the pelvis towards the sound limb every time the weight is placed on the affected limb. In order to counteract this, trunk is jerked in opposite direction i.e. towards affected side (Fig. 6.9).
- In bilateral cases the gait is an exaggerated waddle, the pelvis being dropped alternately on both sides, and the trunk jerked correspondingly from side to side.

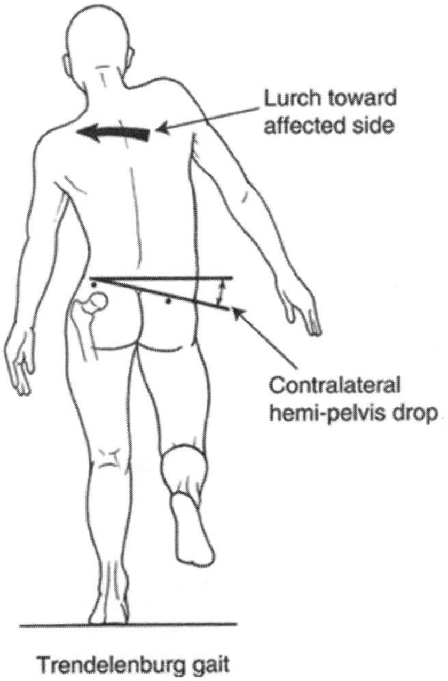

Fig. 6.9: Trendelenburg gait

Lordosis

This is usually exaggerated in posterior dislocation because the back gets hollow to compensate for anterior pelvis tilt. It disappears on hip flexion. It is more marked in bilateral cases as compared to unilateral cases.

Scoliosis

It develops in unilateral cases with convexity of curve towards the sound limb as the pelvis is dropped on this side.

Apparent Shortening

The affected leg appears to be shortened than the other because of upward dislocation of head of femur (Fig. 6.10).

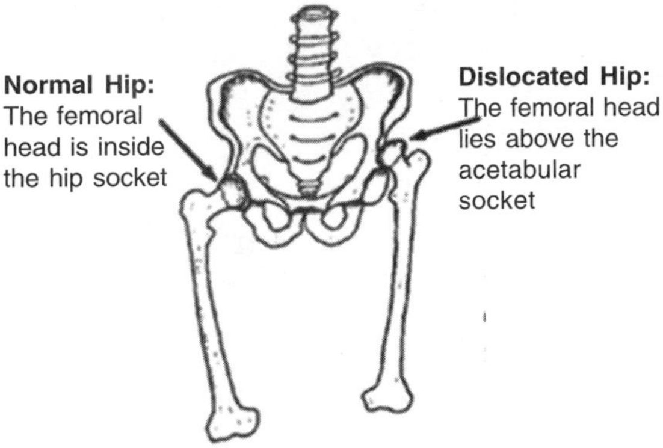

Fig. 6.10: Affected limb appears shortened

Position of Greater Trochanter

This lies above Nelton's line instead of on the line. Since it protrudes above the upper border of gluteus maximus it is prominent, though this is more noticeable in adults than in children.

Buttocks

In bilateral cases the buttocks are broad, flat and somewhat triangular in shape, owing to altered position of gluteus maximus. Also, in bilateral cases, the perineum is wider than normal.

Pain

As a rule children do not suffer any pain, but as they grow older there is fatigue on exertion, especially in bilateral cases. Spasm of muscles may also cause considerable pain.

Range of Motion

Abduction is limited on the affected side (Fig. 6.11).

Thigh Folds

In a child with congenital dislocation of hip thigh folds are asymmetrical with increased number of folds on affected side (Fig. 6.12).

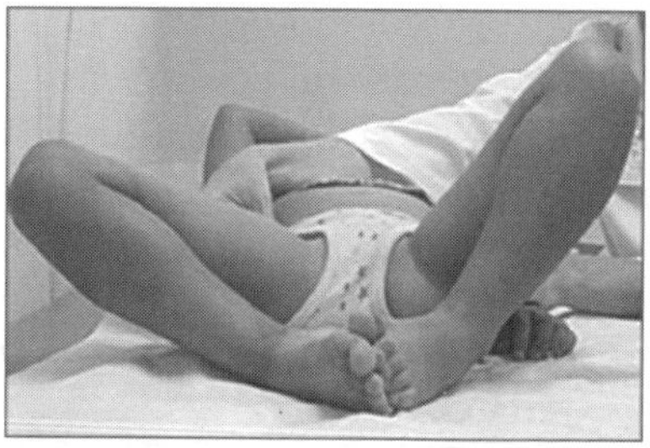

Fig. 6.11: Limited hip abduction on affected side

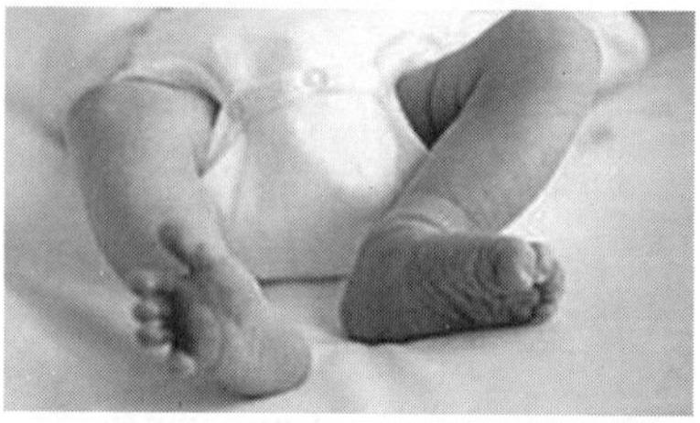

Fig. 6.12: Increased number of thigh folds on affected side

Diagnosis

Clinical Signs

- *Barlow's Test:* The test has two parts. In first part examiner faces the child's perineum. He/she grasps the upper part of each thigh, with fingers behind greater trochanter and thumb in front. The child's knee is fully flexed and hips flexed to right angle. The hip is now gently adducted (Fig. 6.13). As this is being done, gentle pressure is exerted by examiner in proximal direction while the thumb tries to push out the hip. As femoral head rolls over posterior lip of acetabulum, it may if dislocatable slip out of acetabulum. One feels an abnormal posterior movement, appreciated by finger behind the greater trochanter. There may be a distinct 'clunk'.

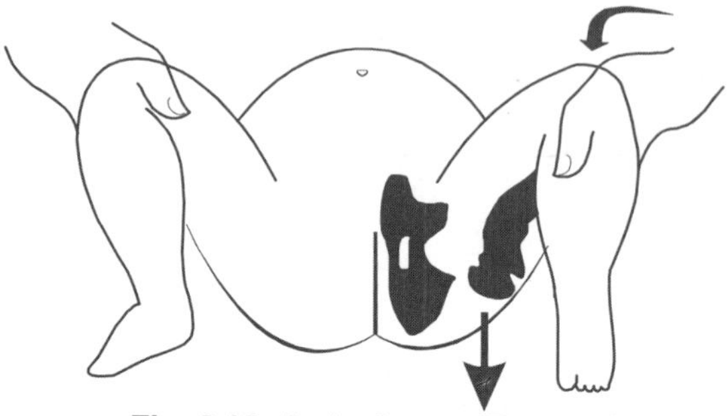

Fig. 6.13: Barlow's test (First part)

In the second part of the test, with the hips in 90° flexion and fully adducted, thighs are gently abducted (Fig. 6.14). The examiner's hand tries to pull the hips while the fingers on greater trochanter exert pressure in forward direction, as if one is trying to put back dislocated hip. If the hip is dislocated either due to first part of test or if it was dislocated to start with, a clunk will be heard and felt indicating reduction of dislocated hip.

- *Ortolani's Test:* The test is similar to second part of Barlow's test. The hips and knees are held in a flexed position and gradually abducted (Fig. 6.14); a 'click' of entrance will be felt as femoral head slips into acetabulum from the position of dislocation.

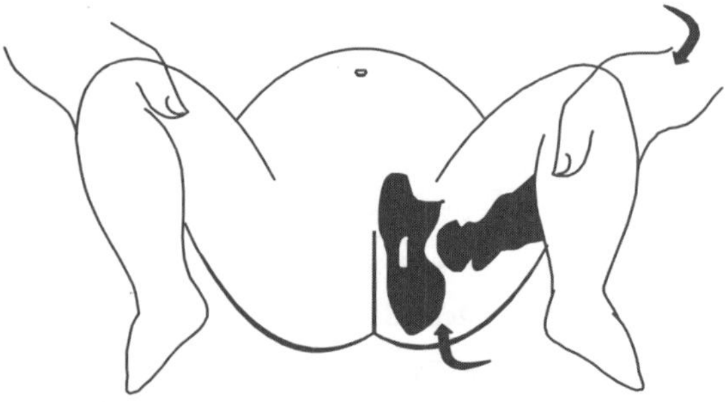

Fig. 6.14: Barlow's test (Second part); Ortolani's test

- *Trendelenburg's Test:* The test is performed in an older child. The child is asked to stand on the affected side. The opposite anterior superior iliac spine (ASIS) (unaffected side) dips down (Fig. 6.15).
- *Galeazzi's Sign:* The levels of knees are compared in a child lying with hip flexed to 70° and knee flexed. There is lowering of knee on the affected side (Fig. 6.16).
- *Telescopy Test:* In case of dislocated hip, it will be possible to produce an up and down piston like movement at affected hip. This can be appreciated by feeling the movement of greater trochanter, under the fingers.

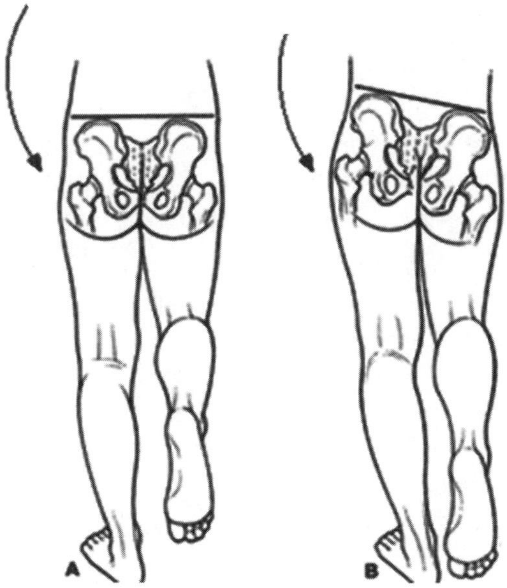

Fig. 6.15: Trendelenburg's test

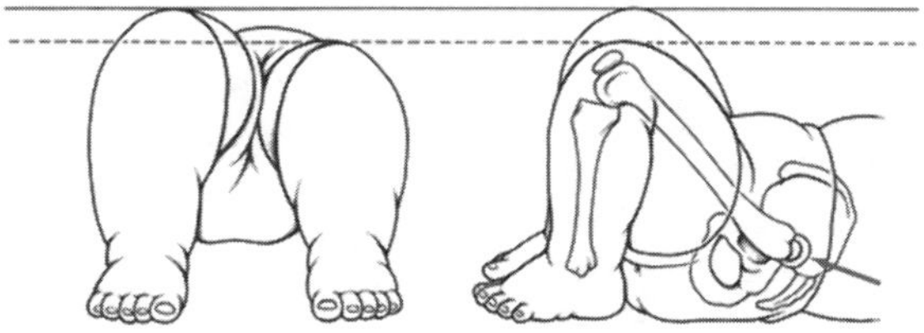

Fig. 6.16: Galeazzi's sign

Radiological Features (Fig. 6.17)

- In a child below the age of 1 year, since the epiphysis of femoral head is not ossified, it is difficult to diagnose a dislocated hip on plain radiograph. Von Rosen's view may be helpful in diagnosis.
- In an older child, following are important X-ray findings:
  - Delayed appearance of ossific centre of head of femur.
  - Retarted development of ossific centre of head of femur.
  - Sloping of acetabulum.
  - Lateral and upward displacement of ossific centre of femoral head.
  - A break in Shenton's line.

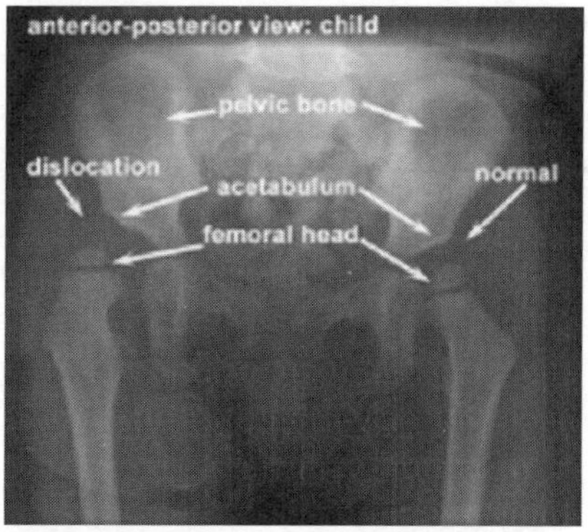

Fig. 6.17: Radiograph of congenitally dislocated hip

Management

Principles of Treatment

- To achieve reduction of head into acetabulum.
- Maintenance of reduction until hip becomes clinically stable.

Methods of Reduction

- *Closed manipulation:* It is sometimes possible in younger children to reduce hip by gentle closed manipulation under general anaesthesia.
- *Traction followed by closed manipulation:* In cases where manipulative reduction requires a great deal of force or if it fails, the hip is kept in

traction for some time, and is progressively abducted. As this is done, it may be possible to reduce the femoral head easily, under general anaesthesia. An adductor tenotomy is often necessary in some cases to allow the hip to be fully abducted.

- *Open reduction:* This is indicated if closed reduction fails. The reasons of failure of closed reduction could be:
  - Fibrofatty tissue in the acetabulum.
  - Fold of capsule and acetabular labrum between femoral head and superior part of acetabulum.

In such situations, the hip is exposed, the soft tissues obstructing the head are excised or released, and the head repositioned in acetabulum.

Maintenance of Reduction

Once the hip has been reduced by open or closed reduction, the following methods may be used for maintaining the head inside the acetabulum.

- *Plaster Cast*
  - Frog leg or Lorenz cast (Fig. 6.18A).
  - Bachelor cast (Fig. 6.18B).

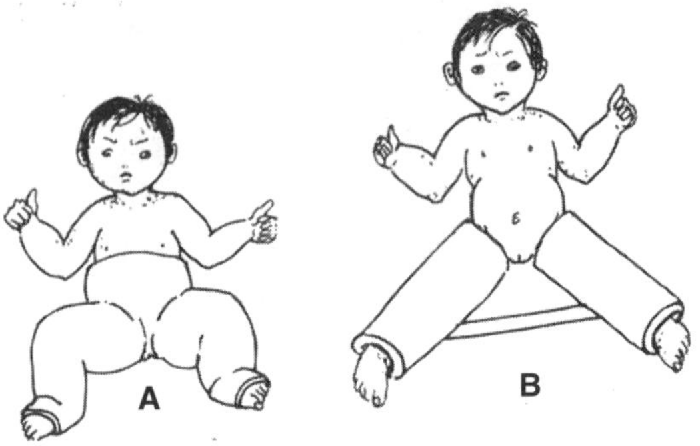

Fig. 6.18A: Frog leg or Lorenz's cast

Fig. 6.18B: Bachelor's cast

- *Splint*
  - Von Rosen splint (Fig.6.19).

Procedures for Acetabular Reconstruction

- Salter's osteotomy.
- Chiari's pelvic displacement osteotomy.
- Pemberton's pericapsular osteotomy.
- Varus derotation osteotomy.

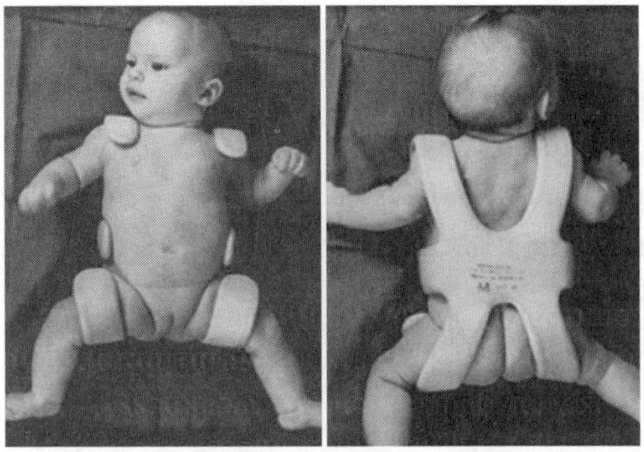

Fig. 6.19: Von Rosen's splint

Treatment Plan

The treatment plan in case of congenital dislocation of hip varies according to the age of the patient. It can be divided into four categories:

- Upto 6 months of age.
- Six months to 2 years of age.
- Two years to 8 years of age.
- Above 8 years.

Upto Six Months of Age

When diagnosed and treated in an early age, the prognosis of the deformity is excellent. In this age group the application of splint is the preferred treatment. The splints applied maintains hip in position of flexion and abduction. Various types of splints available are as follows:

- Craig nappy splint.
- Von Rosen splint.
- Pavlik harness (Fig. 6.20).

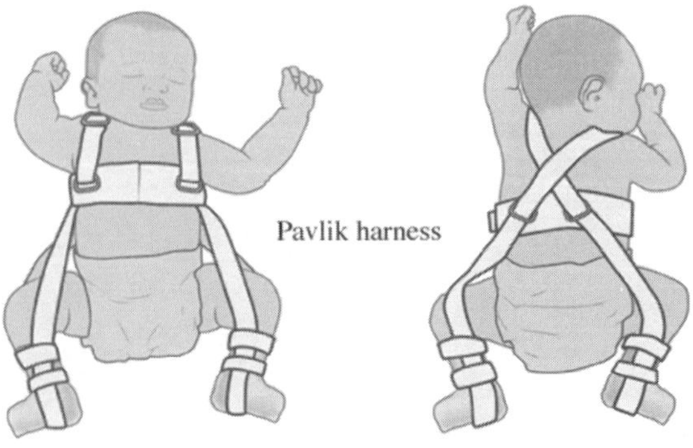

Fig. 6.20: Pavlik harness

Six Months to Two Years of Age

Conservative treatment: The dislocation is reduced by manipulation under general anaesthesia and maintained in plaster of Paris hip spica. The spica is removed after three months to check the stability of joint.

Surgical treatment: Open reduction is indicated when conservative method fails in case of soft tissue contractures, particularly hip adductors. The adduction contractures prevent the reduction of hip joint of closed manipulation. Therefore, adductor tenotomy is done followed by reduction of hip by skin traction. Skin traction may be applied using Wingfield frame and pelvic traction or by overhead Gallows traction. The reduction can also be maintained in POP hip spica for 3-6 months.

Two Years to Eight Years of Age

In this age group, the conservative management usually fails and the dislocation is reduced following surgical reconstruction of acetabulum. Plaster immobilization is continued till the osteotomy/ reconstruction is united. After removal of plaster cast, the mobilization of the hip joint has to be emphasized.

Above Eight Years of Age

The prognosis of any form of treatment is poor in this age group. The patient is therefore left untreated and is considered for total joint replacement at a later age when secondary osteoarthritis develops.

Physiotherapy Management

During Immobilization

- Active movements to all the free joints.
- Active movements of the affected hip within available range in cases where splints are harnessed.
- Isometric exercises to the gluteal muscles and quadriceps.

During Mobilization

- *Range of motion exercises:* As the limb is immobilized in abduction for a prolonged period of time, the maximum limited movement is of adduction. Therefore, relaxed passive adduction in a very small range should be initiated and progressed. Care to be taken to stabilize the pelvis to avoid tilting during adduction.
  Other hip movements should also be given to improve range of motion. Hip rolling can be started with stabilization of the pelvis.
- *Strengthening exercises:* Strengthening exercises for the glutei are well planned and progressed. Initially it should be started as quadruped knee standing progressed to kneeling i.e. standing on knees.
- *Gait:* Walking should be initiated with enough support so that proper weight bearing and weight transfers without drooping of the pelvis are achieved. It may be necessary to initiate ambulation with wide base.
  Assisted ambulation should be progressed to independent ambulation as the muscle power, stability and range of motion improves.

CHAPTER 7

ACQUIRED DEFORMITIES

DUPUYTREN'S CONTRACTURE

It is gradually progressing flexion deformity of the digits especially ring and little fingers (Fig. 7.1). It is initiated at metacarpophalangeal joint which later on progresses to first and second interphalangeal joints. It results from thickening and shortening of palmar aponeurosis.

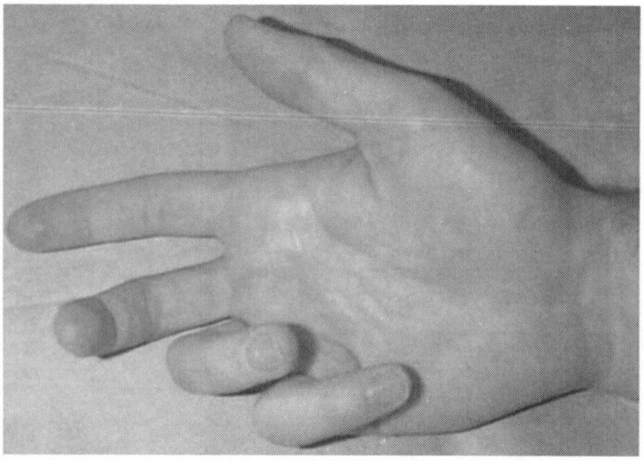

Fig. 7.1: Dupuytren's contracture

Predisposing Factors

- Injury to palmar soft tissue.
- Gout.
- Rheumatism.
- Metabolic diseases.
- Occupational hazard where hands are exposed to pressure, overuse or friction.

Aetiology

Men are affected more than women with bilateral involvement.

Pathology

The palmar aponeurosis (palmar fascia) is normally a thin tough membrane whose fibres radiate from the termination of the palmaris longus tendon at front of the wrist to gain insertion into proximal and middle phalanges of the fingers. Chronic inflammatory reaction sets in whereby the palmar fascia gets thickened and nodular. The skin also gets contracted along with palmar fascia and draws the fingers into the palm producing flexion at metacarpophalangeal joint.

The joint capsules get contracted producing shortening of flexor tendons. The deformity gradually progresses to the proximal and then to distal interphalangeal joints. The skin gets adherent and the tendons stand out like cords (Fig. 7.2) with muscular thickenings.

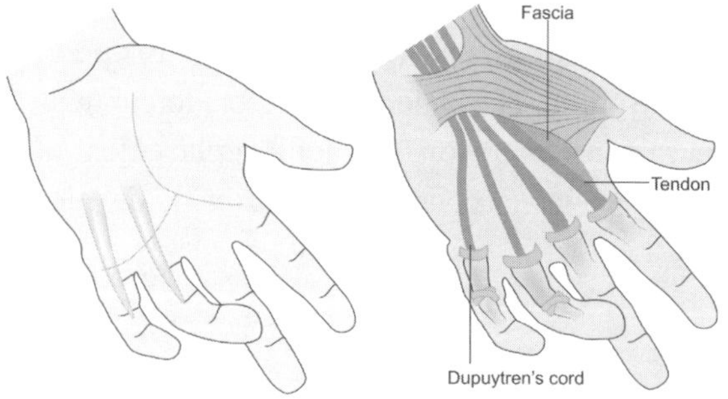

Fig. 7.2: Flexor tendons standing out like cords

Clinical Features

The earliest sign is a small thickened nodule in the mid-palm opposite to base of ring finger. The area of thickening gradually spreads from this point, giving rise eventually to firm cord like bands that extend into ring finger or little finger or both. It prevents full extension of metacarpophalangeal and proximal interphalangeal joints. The skin is closely adherent to fascial bands, and is often puckered. The flexion deformity becomes progressively worse in the course of months or years.

In some cases these changes in the palm are accompanied by thickening over the dorsum of the interphalangeal joints (knuckle pads). The feet may also show nodules in the sole.

Physiotherapy Management

In Early and Mild Cases

- Paraffin wax bath followed by deep friction massage to the palm especially over the tendons and thickened fascia.
- *Stretching*
  - *Passive stretching:* Relaxed passive stretching of the fingers in stages and holding the stretched position.
  - *Active assisted stretching:* This can be done by the patient himself extending metacarpophalangeal joints to the maximum and holding the stretch.
  - *Self stretching:* This can be done by putting the affected hand inverted on the table and pushing the joints to normal by the normal palm.

In Severe Cases

Surgical management: Surgical excision of the contracted fascia is done when the contracture is not relieved by conservative treatment.

Post-Surgical Physiotherapy Management

- Post-surgically pain relieving modalities like hot pack, ultrasound can be used.
- *Splinting:* Serial dynamic splintage may be necessary in severe contractures even after the surgery.
- *Stretching:* The stretching exercises should be continued even after full correction to avoid recurrence.

COXA VARA

The term coxa vara includes any condition in which the neck-shaft angle of femur is less than normal of about 120-135 degrees (Fig. 7.3). The angle is sometimes reduced to 90 degrees or less.

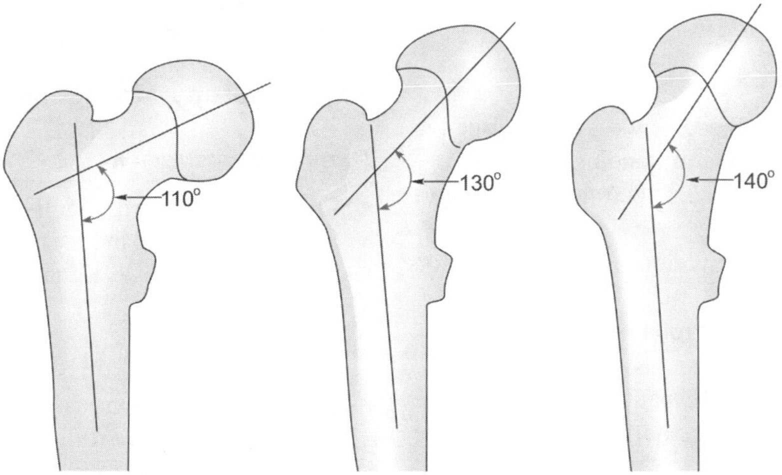

Fig. 7.3: Reduced femoral neck shaft angle (Coxa vara)

Causes

It occurs as a result of increased strain to the growing bone or sudden injury to the bone that is not sufficiently hardened.

Effect

This leads to the epiphyseal slipping. The slipped epiphysis may unite in an abnormal position if not properly treated.

Precipitating Factors

- Fracture neck femur.
- Rickets.
- Osteomyelitis.
- Osteochondritis.
- Tuberculosis.
- Arthritis.

Pathology

There is depression of neck of femur thereby reducing its normal angle with shaft from normal 120°-135° to more or less to a right angle. The neck may be distorted backwards and head may get deformed and subluxated from the acetabulum. The greater trochanter is raised producing shortening and making the action of abductors ineffective.

Clinical Features

- Abductor muscles become weak and ineffective especially in single limb standing.
- Adductor muscle groups tend to become short and contracted.
- There is marked limitation of range of motion of flexion and abduction.
- External and internal rotations are excessively free.
- *Standing posture:* The patient stands with the hips in adduction and external rotation and the foot in eversion.
- *Gait:*
  - *In bilateral cases:* There is waddling gait with occasional scissoring. It is also associated with bilateral swaying of the trunk.
  - *In unilateral cases:* There is marked limp. The patient drops the pelvis towards the sound side, everytime the weight is borne on affected limb. To counteract this, the trunk is jerked to opposite side. There may be associated compensatory lordosis and scoliosis with apparent limb shortening.

Management

Conservative Treatment

- Bed rest to relieve strain on epiphysis for 4 to 6 weeks.
- Traction to femur in abduction if slipping of epiphysis is confirmed, for a period of 4 to 6 weeks.
- Weight relieving orthosis or plaster is given for 12-18 months.

Surgical Treatment

- After reduction, some surgeons pin the epiphysis in position.
- In long standing cases, wedge osteotomy may be necessary which will need 8 weeks of immobilization in abduction. The angle of abduction has to be brought to neutral position by corrective serial plasters.

Physiotherapy Management

During Immobilization

- Strong and vigorous active movements are initiated for ankle and toes.
- Isometeric exercises to quadriceps and glutei.

During Mobilization

- Initiation of relaxed passive range of motion exercises with emphasis on hip abduction and internal rotation. Abduction in suspension apparatus is useful to improve ROM.
- Gradual sitting up and partial weight transfers on the affected hip joint.

- Standing balance on ischial weight relieving orthosis, with emphasis on maintaining the level of pelvis.
- Re-education in walking eliminates pelvis drop and waddling gait.
- Other ambulatory activities like back walking, side walks, negotiating stairs and ramps should be taught.
- Limb length disparity should be compensated by shoe raise. The shoe raise has to be checked and corrected with growth.

GENU VALGUM

The inward or medial angulation of the leg over thigh at the knee joint is termed as genu valgum (Fig. 7.4). The condition is also known as knock knees. In this condition both the knees come close together with feet lying apart (Fig. 7.5). A line drawn from the head of femur to the middle of ankle joint passes lateral to knee joint (Fig. 7.6) instead of passing through the centre of the knee.

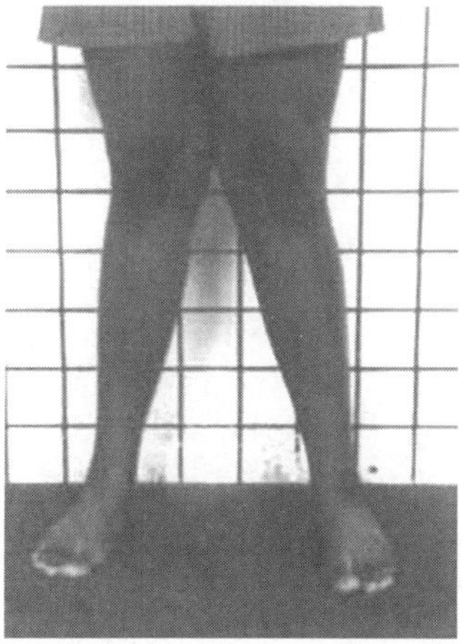

Fig. 7.5: Feet lie apart in genu valgum

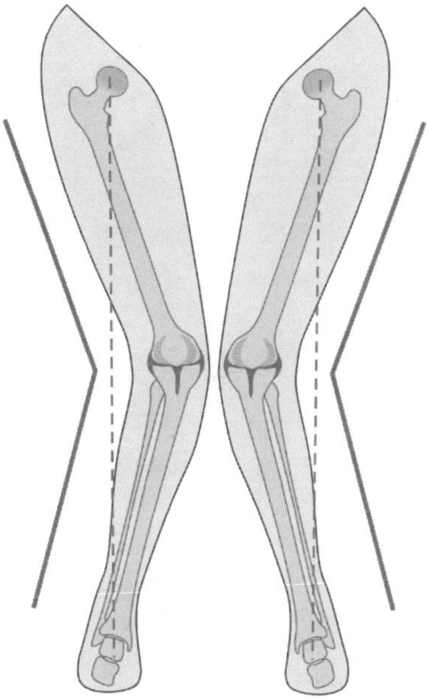

Fig. 7.6: In genu valgum a straight line from head of femur to ankle joint passes lateral to knee joint

Causes

- Rickets producing curvatures of femur or tibia.
- Growth imbalance between the medial and lateral femoral condyles. Rapid overgrowth of medial condyle leads to knock knees.
- Muscular or ligamentous weakness.
- Muscular paralysis of semimembranous, semitendinosus.

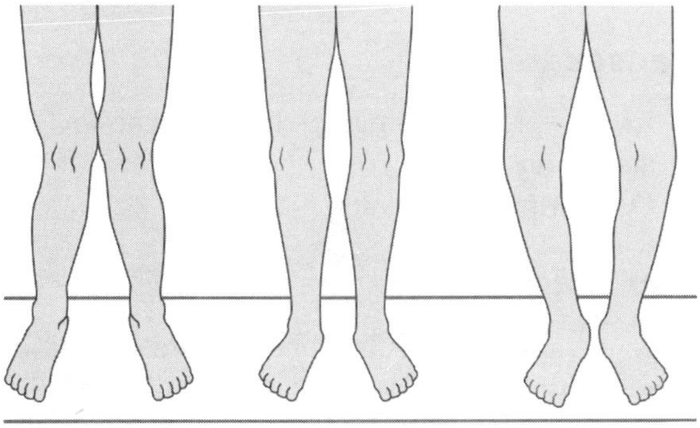

Fig. 7.4: Genu valgum (Knocked knees)

- Fractures and injuries involving knee joint.
- Secondary to coxa vara, flat foot, OA knees or spinal curvatures.

Effect

There is increased rotational or posterior mobility at knee joint.

Assessment

- Intermalleolar distance is noted which could vary from 2 to 20 inches (Fig. 7.7).
- Degree of deformity in the weight bearing position is noted.
- Angle of genu valgum is measured with goniometer or on weight bearing radiographs.
- Muscular strength of all the muscles around the knee joint, should be assessed.
- Range of motion of the knee joints should be recorded carefully.
- Functional status of the patient should be recorded.

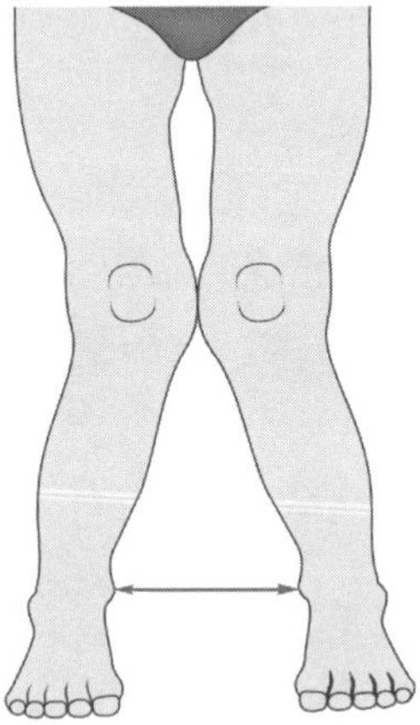

Fig. 7.7: Increased intermalleolar distance in knock knees

Treatment

Cases with Negligible Bony Changes

- Correct method of applying the accurate orthosis: Specially designed orthosis with lateral uprights and broad knee strap to pull the knee joint laterally is given.
- Weight transfers.
- Proper ambulation techniques.
- Stretching of lateral structures of knee joint.
- Strengthening of medial structures of the knee joint.

Cases with Marked Bony Changes

The patients are treated by corrective osteotomy.

Post-surgical Physiotherapy:

- Thermotherapy adjunct should be used as pain controlling measure.
- Graded and gradual knee mobilization should be initiated as relaxed free movement.
- Strengthening exercises for quadriceps, hamstrings and glutei.
- When the patient starts walking, weight transfer should be done in all stages till independent ambulation is achieved.
- Orthosis are used to avoid any recurrence.

GENU VARUM

In this condition there is lateral angulation of tibia in relation to the knee (Fig. 7.4). Thus in standing with the feet together the knees remains wide apart (Fig. 7.8). It is usually bilateral. It is also known as bow legs.

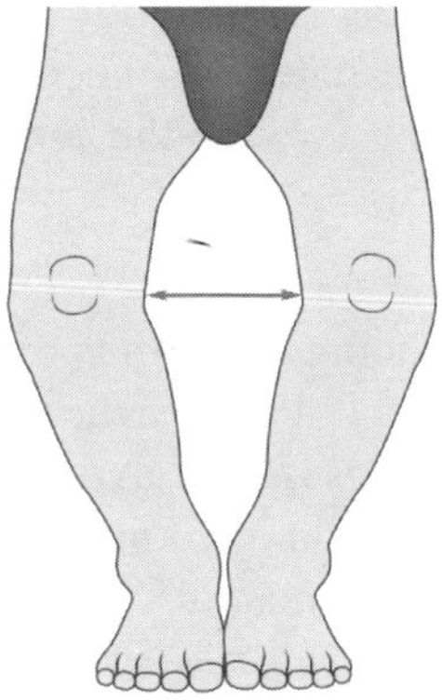

Fig. 7.8: Knees remain apart in bow legs

Causes

- Early weight bearing in children who are fat and heavy.
- Osteoarthritis in adults.

Pathology

In genu varum there is lateral curvature of shaft of femur, tibia as well as fibula, the maximum convexity being at the knee. In bow legs, only the shafts of tibia and fibula are bent with lateral convexities. Internal rotation may be present at the hip joints with knee in hyperextension. The muscles and ligaments on the lateral aspect of limb are stretched, whereas those of medial aspects are shortened. The child adopts waddling pattern of gait with toes turned in and weight bearing is on lateral border of the feet.

Treatment

In Mild Cases

There occurs spontaneous improvement or full correction as the child grows upto age of five years.

In Moderate Cases

If the deformity persists, orthosis to pull the knee joint medially is given.

In Severe Cases

Corrective osteotomy is recommended.

Physiotherapy Treatment

On same lines as for genu valgum.

PES CAVUS

There is marked accentuation of longitudinal arch of foot with drooping of the tarsus (Fig. 7.9). It is also known as contracted foot or hollow foot.

Causes

- Muscle weakness: Intrinsic foot muscles, lumbricals, interossei.
- Muscle paralysis: Plantar flexors.

Fig. 7.9: Pes cavus deformity

Pathology (Fig. 7.10)

The metatarsal heads are lowered in relation to the hind part of foot, with consequent exaggeration of longitudinal arch. The soft tissues in the sole are abnormally short, and eventually the bones themselves alter shape, perpetuating the deformity. There is always associated clawing of toes which are hyperextended at metatarsophalangeal joints. This clawing seems to result from defective action of intrinsic muscles—lumbricals and interossei.

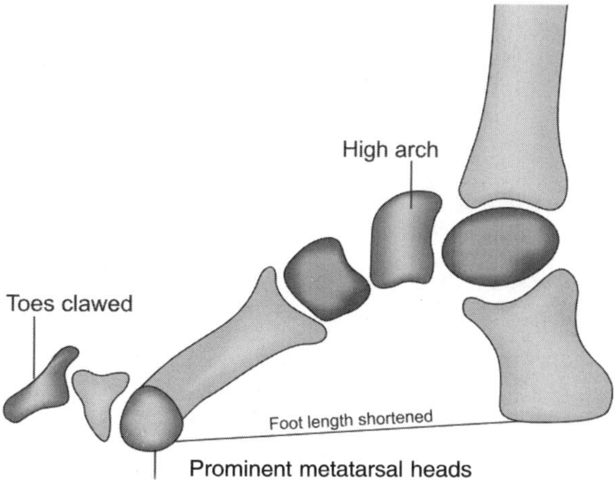

Fig. 7.10: Pathology of pes cavus

In case of paralysis of intrinsic muscles, their stabilizing action is lost resulting in uncontrolled action of long toe flexors, which cause clawing of toes. When the long toe flexors are paralysed, the anterior tibial muscles exert excessive pull, resulting in raising of the anterior part of calcaneum and depression of the anterior transverse arch along with hyperextension of the toes producing clawing.

The effect is that the toes are almost functionless, and unable to take their normal share in weight bearing. Due to which, the excessive weight falls upon metatarsal heads on walking or standing, and hard callosities form in the underlying skin. The malalignment of the tarsal joints predisposes to the later development of osteoarthritis.

Clinical Features

- Painful callosities beneath the metatarsal heads.
- Tenderness over the deformed toes from pressure against the shoe.
- Pain in tarsal region from osteoarthritis of tarsal joints.

On Examination

- Characteristic and easily recognized deformity.
- High longitudinal arch.
- Thick and splayed forefoot.
- Callosities beneath metatarsal heads.
- The toes cannot be straightened at will by the patient, nor can they be pressed firmly upon the ground to take a share in weight bearing.

Management

In Early and Mild Cases

Conservative management can help the patient in mild cases. Physiotherapy and special shoes can control the deformity in early stage.

Physiotherapy Management

- Pain to be controlled by suitable pain relieving modality.
- A small sand bag is placed over the dorsum of the foot in contact with the ground or by offering self-stretching by placing the heel of normal foot over dorsum of deformed one. The weight of the sand bag or pressure of normal foot offers relaxed passive stretch to contracted plantar fascia.
- Movements of dorsiflexion combined with toe extension have a stretching effect on longitudinal arch. Resisted toe extension is useful in preventing clawing of the toes.
- Corrective shoes with soft padding are given to encourage weight bearing over the arch.

In Severe Cases

In neglected and severe cases, surgical intervention is needed.

Surgical Management

- *Steindler's management:* All the muscles on under surface of calcaneum along with plantar fascia are divided. The divided muscles slide forward and get attached to bone distally. The cavus position is thus corrected. A below knee POP cast is applied in correct position for 3-4 weeks.
- *Lambrinudi's operation:* This consists of arthrodesis of interphalangeal joints to correct the clawing, also long toe flexors act at the metatarsophalangeal joints supporting the metatarsal heads. Thus the muscle power is re-distributed in the foot.
- Fasciotomy: Plantar fascia is divided along with tendons of extensor digitorum longus. The foot is then stretched; the deformity is corrected and immobilized in plaster cast for 3-4 weeks.

Post-Surgical Physiotherapeutic Intervention:

During Immobilization:

- Exercises to the joints free from immobilization.

During Mobilization:

- Active exercises to metatarsophalangeal joints, ankle and foot.
- Stretching sessions to flatten the longitudinal arch by weight bearing and weight transfers to it.
- Friction massage is helpful on painful surgical scar.
- Re-education in ambulation.

HALLUX VALGUS

The deformity is characterized by abnormal abduction of first metatarsal with adduction of phalanges (Fig. 7.11).

Aetiology

Females of any age group are more commonly affected as compared to males.

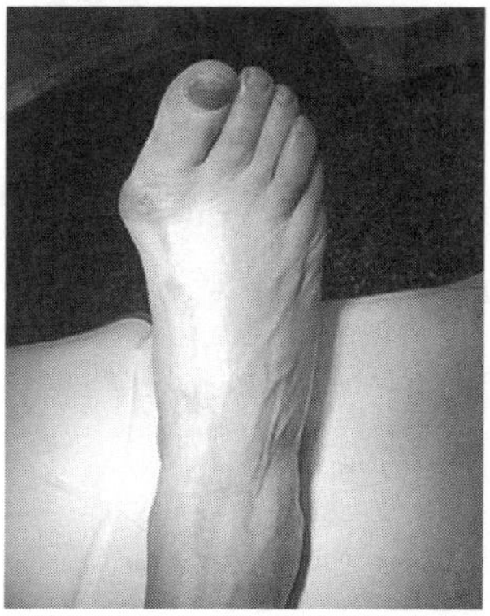

Fig. 7.11: Hallux valgus deformity

Precipitating Factors

- Gout.
- Arthritis.
- Bad footwear.

Pathology

A false bursa may form over first metatarsal head, which may get thickened and enlarged (Fig. 7.12), known as bunion (Fig. 7.13). The articular cartilage may get inflammed, eroded and atrophied. New bone formation may take place on medial side of metatarsal head, known as exostosis or spur. Tendon of extensor hallucis longus is shortened and displaced laterally. It acts with a mechanical disadvantage increasing the deformity. Intrinsic muscles, too, cannot act effectively. These inadequacies result in drooping of arch and eversion of foot.

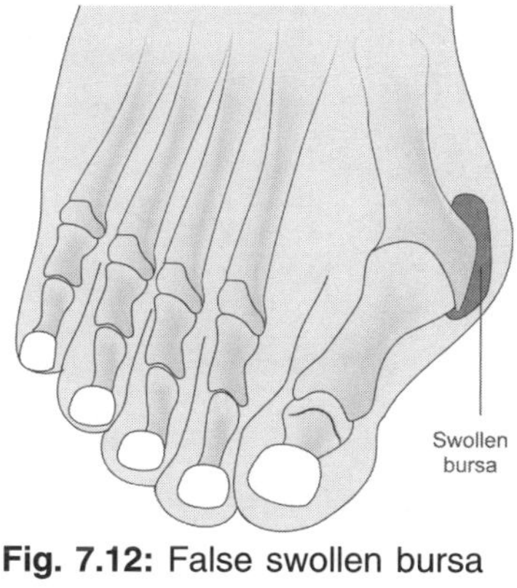

Fig. 7.12: False swollen bursa

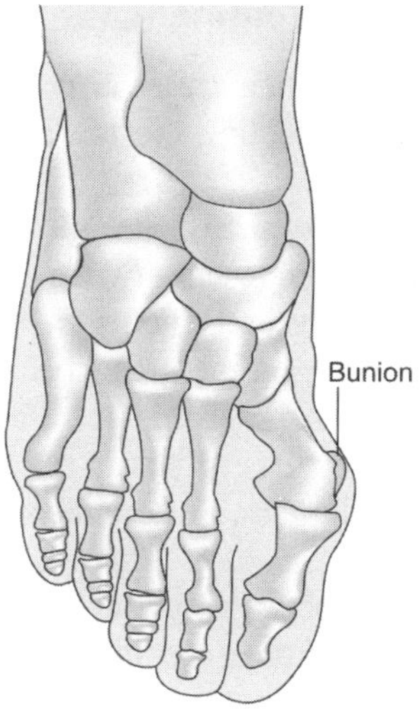

Fig. 7.13: Bunion

Clinical Features

- Tenderness over bunion from pressure against the shoe.
- Difficulty in getting comfortable footwear.
- Flattening of transverse arch.

On Examination

- Obvious deformity.
- Hard, reddened and tender skin over prominent joint.
- Thick walled bursa occasionally fluid filled can be felt.
- *In early cases*: Joint movements are free and painless.
- *In severe cases*: Joint movements are limited and painful.
- Forefoot is often flat and splayed in late cases.

Management

In Mild Cases:

- Physiotherapy.
- Proper foot wear.

In Severe Cases

Surgery is indicated.

Physiotherapy Treatment

- The patient is taught to carry out relaxed passive stretching by abducting the toe many times a day.
- *Specially designed shoes:* Straight inner border footwear with wedge in between the great toe and second toe greatly helps in maintaining abduction stretch on the great toe.
- Night splints may be given.
- Strong active exercises are given for strengthening lumbricals and interossei.
- *Proper weight bearing:* The weight bearing which tends to be more on the lateral aspect of the foot to avoid pressure and pain, should be discouraged.
- Faradic foot bath may be necessary to relieve pain, improve circulation and induce contraction of intrinsic muscles.

Surgical Treatment

- *Arthroplasty:* The bunion and exostoses are removed, shortened soft tissues are divided. The joint is aligned in the maximally corrected position.
- *Keller's operation:* Proximal two thirds of proximal phalanx is removed with bunion and medial portion of head of metatarsal.
- *Mayo's operation:* The head of metatarsal is excised. Firm dressings or plasters cast are given for 2-3 weeks following surgery. Traction may be applied through pulp of toe.
- Arthrodesis of metatarsophalangeal joint of big toe.

Post-Surgical Physiotherapy

During Mobilization:

- The patient is trained in relaxed passive stretching of toe. It is advised to put soft cotton or foam wedge between great toe and second toe.
- Strong exercises are given to intrinsic foot muscles.
- Active fanning of toes in warm water with assisted abduction of great toe.
- Faradic foot bath is useful in assisting active efforts.
- Weight transfers, gait training and ambulatory activities to be gradually added avoiding limp.

HALLUX RIGIDUS

This deformity results in stiffness of the great toe at metatarsophalangeal joint.

Cause

It is caused by wear and tear of small joint.

Predisposing Factors

- Focal sepsis.
- Direct injury to great toe.
- Tight footwear.

Pathology

The changes are seen in articular cartilage and bone surface. The articular cartilage is gradually worn away from both surfaces of the joint until eventually the subchondral bone is exposed. The exposed bone becomes hard and glossy i.e. eburnation. The marginal bone hypertrophies to form osteophyte (Fig. 7.14), which often cause obvious thickening, especially at dorsum of toe known as dorsal bunion (Fig. 7.15).

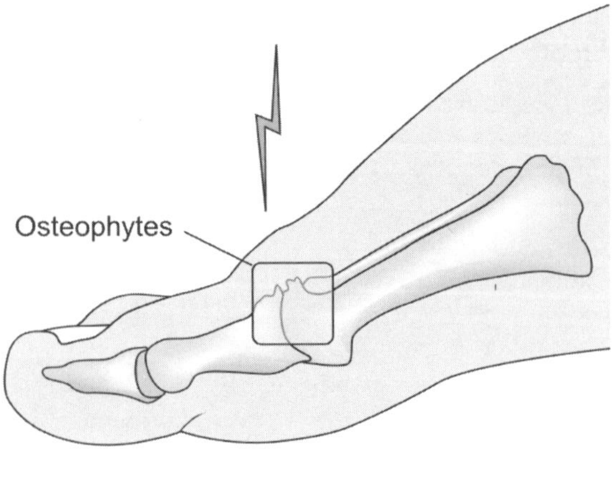

Fig. 7.14: Osteophyte formation

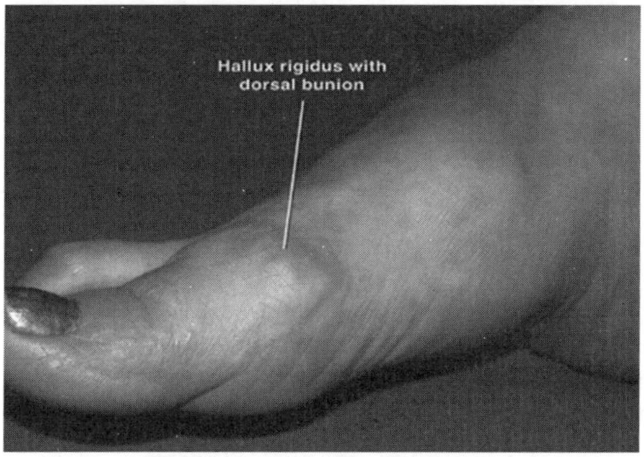

Fig. 7.15: Dorsal bunion

Clinical Features

- Pain in base of great toe on walking.
- Metatarsophalangeal joint is palpably thickened from osteophyte formation.
- Flexion and extension at metatarsophalangeal joint are restricted (Fig. 7.16).
- The first phalanx may even be fixed in flexion (hallus flexus).
- Interphalangeal movement is not affected.

Radiological Examination

- Cartilage space is narrowed.
- Sclerosis of subchondral bone.
- Osteophytic spurring of joint margins.

Management

Physiotherapy Treatment

- Thermotherapy modality with other measures should be used to relieve inflammation.
- Pressure relieving measures like metatarsal bar, soft sole and modified foot wear should be used.
- Stress on the toe to be reduced by guiding modified gait with minimum toe extension during push off phase of gait.

Surgical Treatment

Excision arthroplasty of proximal half of first phalanx.

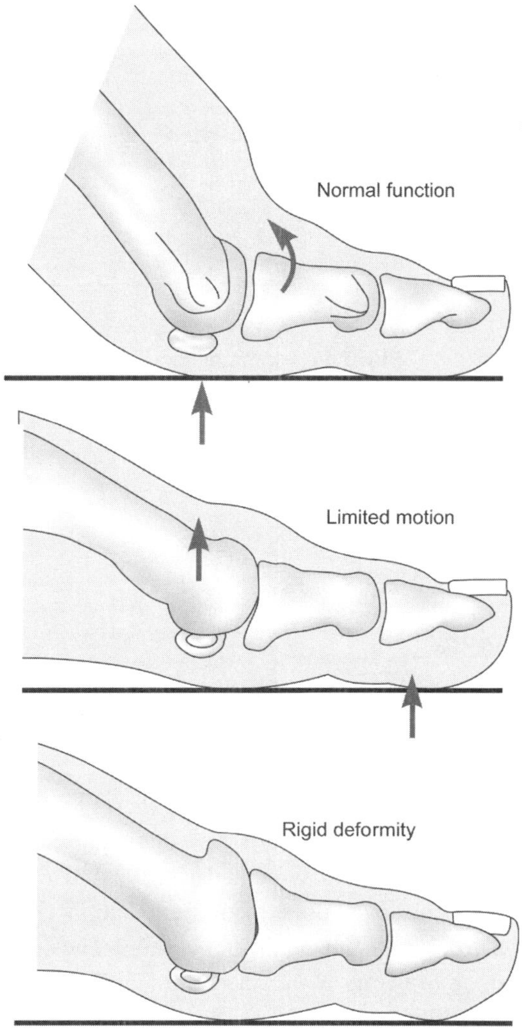

Fig. 7.16: Reduced motion at metatarsophalangeal joint

Post-Surgical Physiotherapy

- Repeated active flexion—extension exercise in warm water restores range of motion early.
- Intrinsic muscles exercises.
- Gait training.

HAMMER TOE

The term hammer toe denotes fixed flexion deformity of interphalangeal joint of toes (Fig. 7.17).

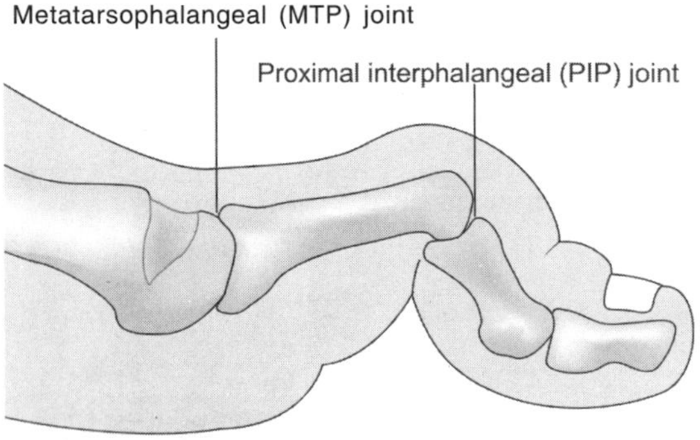

Fig. 7.17: Hammer toe

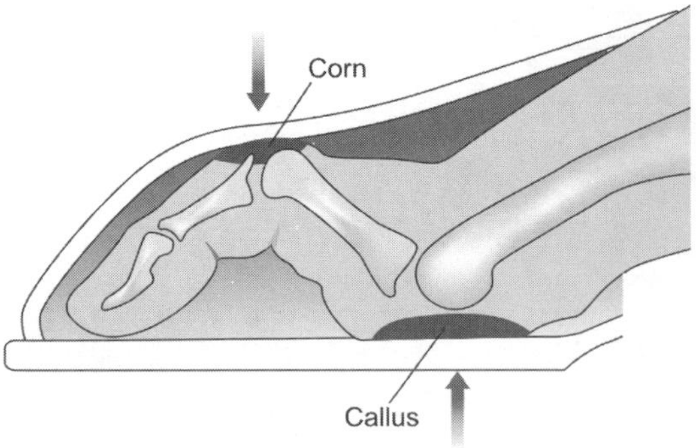

Fig. 7.18: Corn over dorsum of the flexed joint

Causes

- Imbalance of delicate arrangement of flexor and extensor tendon.
- Associated with hallux valgus.
- Tight shoes.

Aetiology

It could be congenital or familial in origin.

Pathology

The proximal interphalangeal joint is sharply angled into flexion. Secondary contracture of plantar aspect of joint capsule fixes the deformity, and corn usually forms over dorsum of flexed joint (Fig. 7.18), from pressure against the shoe. The long extensor tendons are contracted along with overlying skin.

Deformity

In the characteristic deformity the proximal interphalangeal joint is in fixed flexion, and the distal interphalangeal joint, though still mobile, rests in compensatory hyperextension.

Management

Physiotherapy Treatment

- The toe is strapped to neighboring toes in corrective position with adhesive plaster (Fig. 7.19).
- Corrective splint during rest is necessary to maintain small constant stretch.
- Relaxed passive stretching with axial traction and its retention stretches the short muscles.

Surgical Treatment

It is needed in the severe cases:
- Excision of proximal interphalangeal joint.
- Arthrodesis of first interphalangeal joint.
- Immobilization period is 4-6 weeks.

Post-Surgical Physiotherapy

- Mobilization and stretching of metatarso-phalangeal and interphalangeal joints are encouraged.

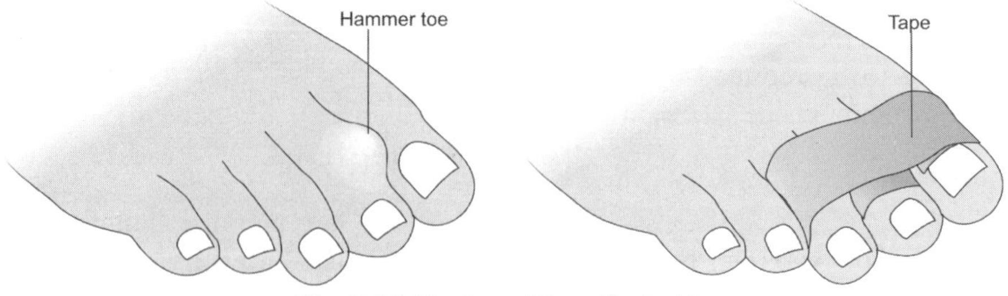

Fig. 7.19: Taping of the affected toe

CHAPTER 8

SPINAL DEFORMITIES

KYPHOSIS

This is a general term used for excessive backward convexity of the spine. It is the exaggeration of the posterior spinal curve (Fig. 8.1) localized to dorsal spine. It is also known as kyphosis—arcuata or round back.

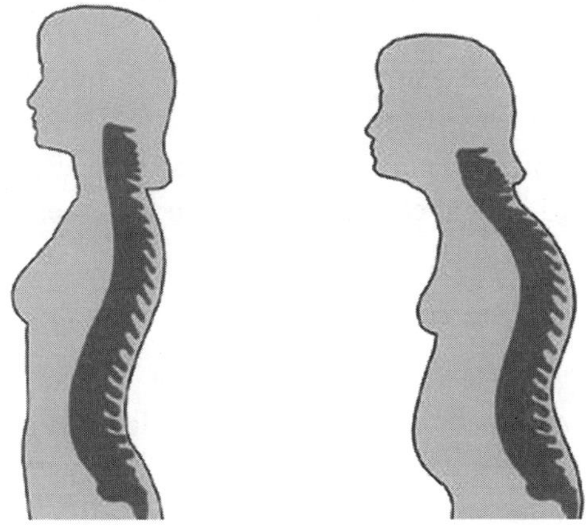

Fig. 8.1: Kyphotic deformity

Causes

- Habitual bad posture.
- Arthritis.
- Rheumatism.
- Lung affections.
- Muscular weakness.
- Degeneration of vertebral bodies and discs.
- Tuberculosis.
- Ankylosing spondylitis.
- Scheuermann's disease.
- Congenital anomalies.

Types of Kyphosis

Round Kyphosis

It means gentle backward curvature of spinal column (Fig. 8.2). It is caused by diseases affecting number of vertebrae as for example senile kyphosis. It may be localized to a spinal segment or may be diffuse.

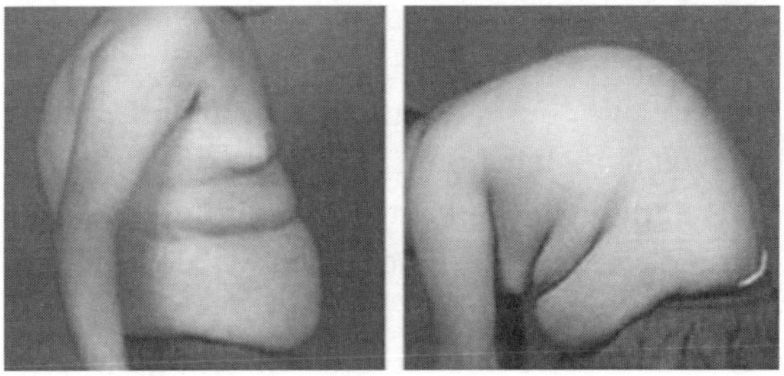

Fig. 8.2: Round kyphosis

Angular Kyphosis

It means a sharp backward prominence of spinal column. It may be prominence of only one spinous process because of collapse of only one vertebral body as may occur in compression fracture of vertebra. This is called knuckle. There may be kyphosis localized to a few vertebrae, and is known as gibbus (Fig. 8.3). It is seen commonly in tuberculosis.

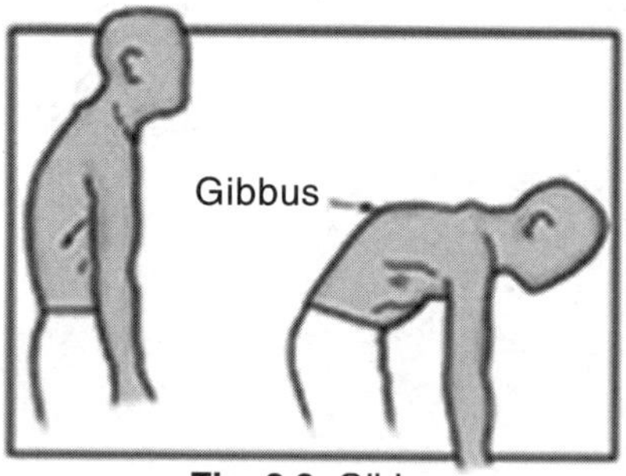

Fig. 8.3: Gibbus

Classification of Deformity According to Severity

- First degree kyphosis.
- Second degree kyphosis.
- Third degree kyphosis.

First Degree Kyphosis

A habitual bad posture is the precipitating factor. There is no imbalance between the muscles. If the treatment is not adequate it progresses to the further stages.

Second Degree Kyphosis

- The pectoral muscles become short, thereby restricting chest expansion resulting in reduced respiratory function.
- Longitudinal back muscles, rhomboids and middle trapezius are weakened with loss of tone and are in a stretched position.
- Posterior ligaments are lengthened with corresponding shortening of anterior structures. This results in increased posterior laxity.

Third Degree Kyphosis

During the adolescent stage of growth period, wedging of the vertebral body may occur. The deformity gets organized which is a difficult syndrome.

Postural Adaptation in Kyphosis

- Rounded back.
- Forward head.
- Flattened chest.
- Rounded shoulders.
- Excessive protrusion of scapulae.

Management

First Degree Kyphosis

It is best managed by physiotherapy.
- Relaxation of body especially upper back.
- Repeated stretching sessions of shortened anterior structures by bracing shoulders and maintaining the position.
- *Postural training:* Posture of head, neck and shoulder during activity or rest in optimal position should be trained and checked.
- Mobilization of spine, scapula and shoulders.
- Diaphragmatic and costal breathing exercises with emphasis on inspiration.
- Resistive exercises to weak longitudinal and transverse back muscles.
- Controlled pelvic tilt associated with abdominal and gluteal contractions and pelvic rocking are useful.

Second Degree Kyphosis

Active correction and maintenance is difficult. The milwaukee brace is prescribed with pads applied to posterior uprights. The patient is encouraged to apply maximum pressure on posterior pads. It stretches the shoulder, scapula and kyphotic curve. It is difficult to achieve enough correction, but it prevents further deterioration of curve. Exercises to improve mobility and respiration reduce overall impact of deformity.

Third Degree Kyphosis

Surgical treatment is recommended. Surgical procedures undertaken are:
- Bone graft.
- Spinal cord decompression.
- Spinal stabilization.

Post-Surgical Physiotherapy

- Gradual progression of corrective mobilization.
- Muscle strengthening techniques.
- Prevention of post-surgical complications especially respiratory ones.

LORDOSIS

It can be described as the exaggeration of the anterior curve of the spine (Fig. 8.4). The commonly involved sites are cervical and lumbar spine where the spinal curvature is of anterior convexity in normal. The condition is also known as hollow back.

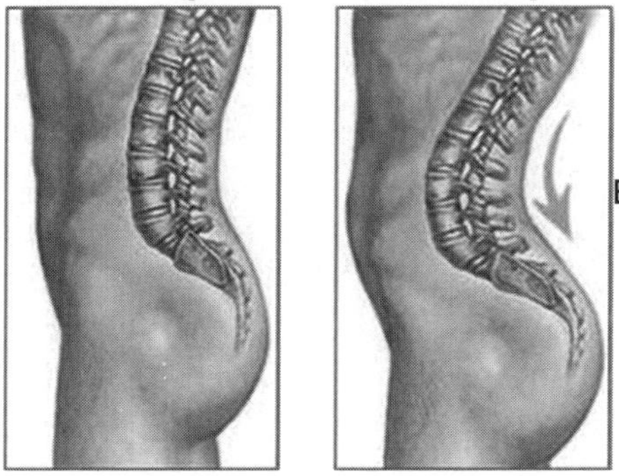

Fig. 8.4: Exaggerated lumbar lordosis

Causes

- Hip flexion contracture due to:
  - Congenital dislocation of hip.
  - Tuberculosis.
- Positional or habitual tightness of hip flexors.
- Paralysis of abdominal muscles or spinal flexors.
- Congenital or acquired spinal deformities like spondylolisthesis.
- Obesity with protruding abdomen.
- Associated with other diseases like:
  - Pseudohypertrophic muscular deformity.
  - Ankylosing spondylitis.
  - Fixed flexion deformity at hip or knee.

Pathology

The forward tilting of pelvis produces compensatory exaggerated lumbar lordosis. This leads to stretching of abdominal muscles and anterior spinal ligaments. There is reciprocal shortening of posterior ligaments and muscles. It may be associated with weakness of glutei and lengthening of hamstrings.

Physiotherapy Treatment

- Lumbar spine mobilization.
- Strengthening of abdominals, glutei and hamstrings.
- Active backward or posterior pelvic tilting by contracting abdominals and glutei in supine lying. It is progressed to sitting and standing.
- *Postural guidance:* Postures like "make yourself as tall as you can" or toe touching in long sitting or forward bending are simple procedures.

Precaution

Attitudes involving spinal extension or hyper-extension should be strictly avoided.

KYPHOLORDOSIS

The condition can be described as the exaggeration of the normal spinal curves including both kyphosis and lordosis (Fig. 8.5). The lordosis is the primary curve. Kyphosis occurs as a compensatory attitude to the exaggerated curves.

Management

The approach to the patient of kypholordosis is very individualized to exact segment. The exercises should be well localized for each of the individual involved segment.

- Thoracic spine must remain extended while exercising abdominal muscles.
- Flexion of lumbar spine should not produce flexion of thoracic spine as well.

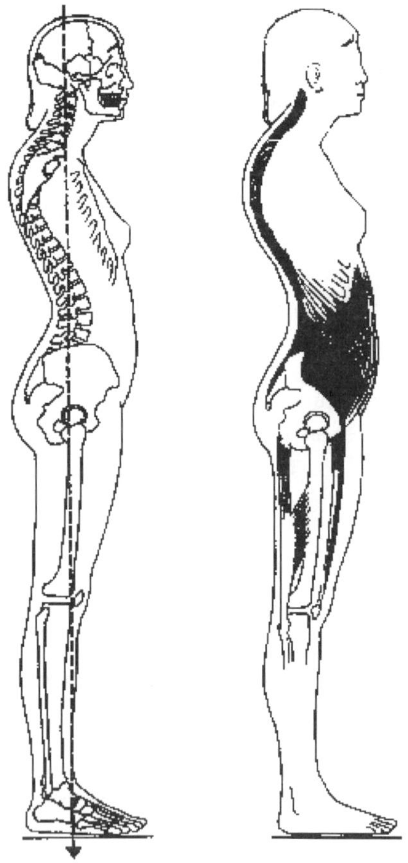

Fig. 8.5: Kypholordosis posture

- Corrective braces should be applied if required.
- Breathing capacity needs careful monitoring in thoracic curves.

SCOLIOSIS

Scoliosis can be described as the lateral curvature of spine (Fig. 8.6) which exceeds by 10 degrees from normal.

Pathology

The main pathology is lateral curvature of part of spine. This is called *primary curve*. The spine above or below the primary curve undergoes compensatory curvatures in opposite direction known as *compensatory or secondary curves* thus assuming an S-shape (Fig. 8.7). The lateral curvature is constantly accompanied by rotation of vertebrae on vertical axis, the body of vertebra rotating towards convexity of curve and spinous

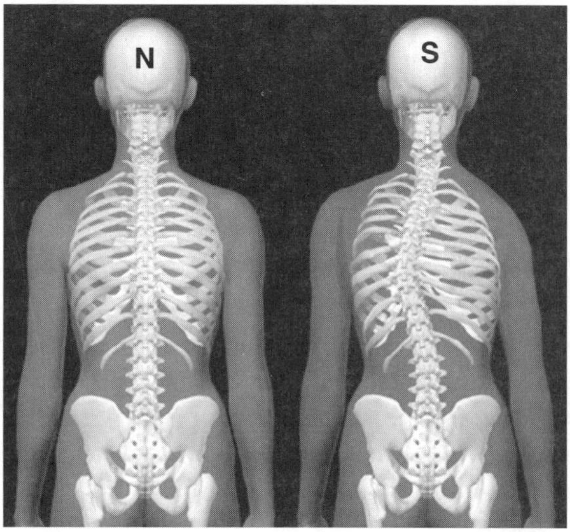

N: Normal spine **S:** Scoliotic spine

Fig. 8.6: Scoliotic spine

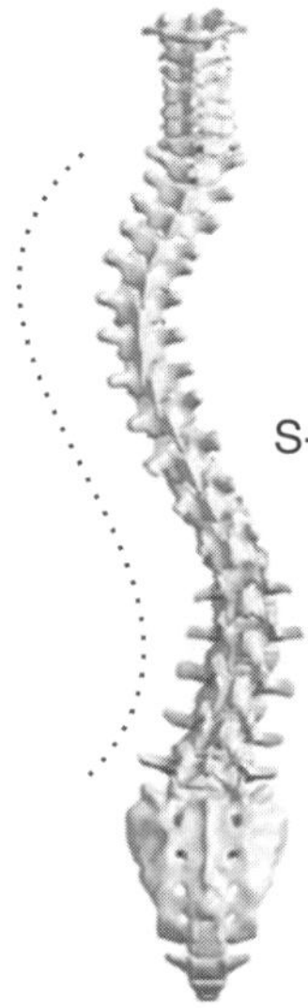

Fig. 8.7: S-shape spine in scoliosis (Primary thoracic and secondary lumbar lateral curvatures)

process away from convexity (Fig. 8.8). By thrusting the ribs backwards on the convex side this rotation increases ugliness of the deformity giving rise to *rib hump*.

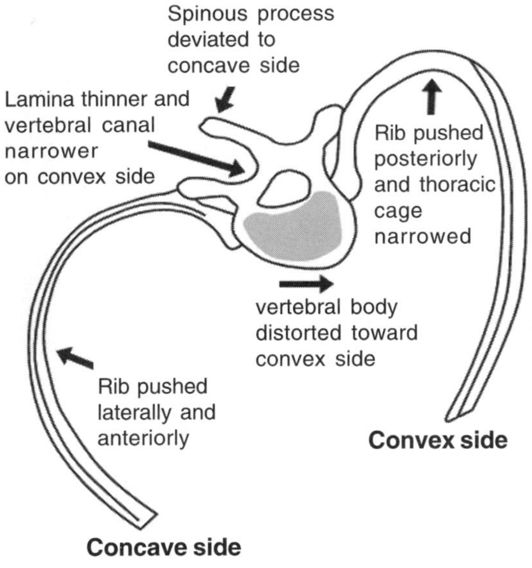

Fig. 8.8: Rotation of vertebra on vertical axis

Types of Scoliosis

Scoliosis is basically classified into following two categories:

- Structural scoliosis.
- Non-structural scoliosis.

Structural Scoliosis

It is grade II and grade III scoliosis. In this type of scoliosis there is defect in bone which results in contractures of soft tissues on concave side of curve and reciprocal stretching on convex side. It is a scoliosis with component of permanent deformity.

Types of Structural Scoliosis

Idiopathic Scoliosis

It is the most common type affecting girls more than boys. It may begin during infancy, childhood or adolescence and tends to increase progressively until the cessation of skeletal growth. Infantile scoliosis begins in first year of life and can be resolving or progressive type. Scoliosis which begin later in life progresses at variable rate, and leads to ugly deformity. The deformity is most obvious in thoracic scoliosis because of formation of rib hump.

Congenital Scoliosis

This is always associated with some form of radiologically demonstrable anomaly of vertebral bodies like hemivertebra, block vertebra or bar of bone. These curves grow often at a very fast rate. Sometimes there are associated anomalies in growth of neural structures, leading to neurological deficit in lower limbs. Its complications render the brace ineffective and surgery may be required.

Paralytic Scoliosis

An unbalanced paralysis of the trunk muscles along with greater degree of muscular imbalance causes paralysis. It may occur due to poliomyelitis, cerebral palsy, spina bifida and muscular dystrophies. In the growing age, the condition is worst with rapidly deteriorating curve. Surgery becomes necessary when the progression of curve is rapid.

Non-Structural Scoliosis

It is grade I scoliosis. This is mobile or transient scoliosis. This type is without any bony changes or muscular weakness. It may get organized to structural one due to secondary soft tissue contractures (muscles and ligaments) on concave side of curve.

Types of Non-Structural Scoliosis

Postural Scoliosis

It is most common overall type seen in adolescent girls. The curve is mild, and convex usually to left. The causative factor may be the impairment of postural reflex, wrong postural habits, e.g., standing with stress on one leg or psychological factors. The main diagnostic feature is that the curve straightens completely when the patient bends forwards.

Compensatory Scoliosis

In this type scoliosis, there is a compensatory phenomenon occurring in order to compensate for pelvic tilt; hip disease; short leg; deformities of neck, arm, trunk or leg. These may be due to post-paralytic, congenital, rachitic or static causes. Unilateral organ diseases like pleurisy, empyema or disc lesion may also act as a causative factor. There is no intrinsic abnormality of spine. The curve disappears with correction of primary factor.

Sciatic Scoliosis

This is a temporary deformity which occurs as result of unilateral painful spasm of paraspinal muscles, in certain painful conditions of spine such as prolapsed intervertebral disk, impinging upon the nerve or acute lumbago. The curve is usually in the lumbar region. The abnormal posture is assumed involuntarily in an attempt to reduce as far as possible the painful pressure over nerve or joint. The treatment is that of underlying condition.

Clinical Features

- Visible deformity.
- In long standing cases; pain is the symptom manifested by adults.
- In severe cases, the sharp angulation of spinal cord over the apex of curve may result in interference with cord functions, leading to neurological deficit.

Radiological Features

Full antero-posterior radiograph of spine in supine and erect position along with a lateral view are necessary.

- *Cobb's Angle*: It is an angle between the lines passing through margins of vertebrae at the ends of curve (Fig. 8.9). It measures the severity of the curve.

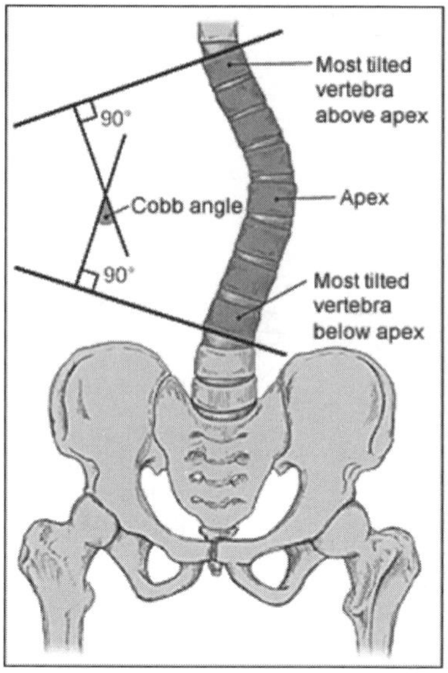

Fig. 8.9: Cobb's angle

- *Reisser's Sign:* It assesses the likelihood of progression of curve by looking at iliac apophysis. Iliac apophysis fuses with iliac bones at maturity and indicates completion of growth and thus no further possibility of the curve worsening.
- *Rotation of Vertebra:* It is appreciated by looking at the position of spinous process and pedicles on AP view. Normally a spinous process is in the centre of vertebral body. In case where there is rotation of vertebra, the spinous process is shifted to one side. There will be asymmetry in the position of pedicles on two sides.

Assessment

Inspection (Fig. 8.10):

- *Level of Ears and Contour of Neck:* Disparity in the level of ears indicates the presence of cervical curve.

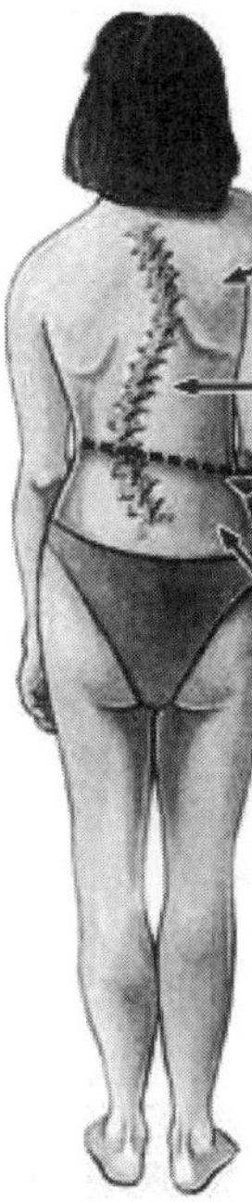

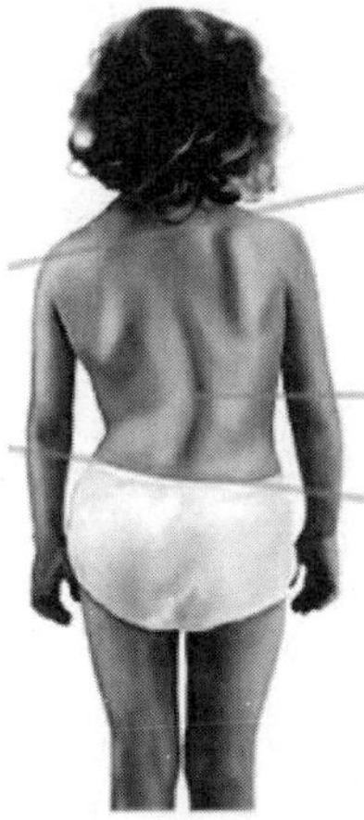

Fig. 8.10: Postural deviations in scoliosis

- *Shoulder Level:* Disparity in shoulder level indicates high dorsal or cervicodorsal curve. Shoulder will be higher on convex side of curve.
- *Scapular level:* Level of inferior angle and vertebral border of scapula is examined in relation to midline of spine. Shifting of vertebral border away from midline with higher scapula and eversion of inferior angle indicates a dorsal curve.
- *Position of Arms and Waist Line:* The arm on the side of higher shoulder hangs close to the body and waist line may be more on opposite side. The width of back appears unequal. Back appears wider on convex side due to bulging of ribs.
- *Thorax:* The ribs appear to be crowded on concave side, and further apart on convex side of curve. When the dorsal curve is more pronounced there is rotation of thorax. The ribs bulge backward on convex side and appear flattened on concave side.
- *Hips:* The hips and posterior superior iliac spine are higher on concave side.
- *Pelvis:* Forward rotation of pelvis occurs on the concave side of lumbar curve. Iliac crest will be prominent on concave side. The gluteal fold on side of raised pelvis appears higher.

ROM Assessment

Range of motion is measured and recorded for all spinal movements that are flexion, extension, lateral flexion and rotation.

Forward Bending Test

The patient in stride standing bends forwards with relaxed arms. The spine is observed for any obliteration of curve. The curve is reduced by this test in case of non-structural scoliosis but remains the same in case of structural scoliosis.

Measurement of Curve by Cobb's Method

A postero-anterior radiograph of the spine is taken for measurements. The vertebra at either end of curve, which is tilting towards concavity of curve, is taken as end-vertebra. A straight line is drawn which passes through the upper border of upper end vertebra and another that passes through lower border of lower end vertebra. The angle formed by the lines drawn perpendicular to these lines at the side of concavity represents the angle of scoliosis (Fig. 8.9).

The curve measuring 60° or more with respiratory insufficiency is an absolute indication for surgery.

Respiratory Status

In scoliosis of thoracic spine, the vital capacity and chest expansion are reduced. These should be measured and recorded.

Rib Hump

In a thoracic curve the rib hump is measured with a gauge (Fig. 8.11). The depth of the valley is measured in the low thoracic or lumbar curve either in forward flexion or prone position by scoliometer. The outline of hump can be traced and transferred onto graph paper. Distortion also occurs in ribs and vertebral in thoracic curve.

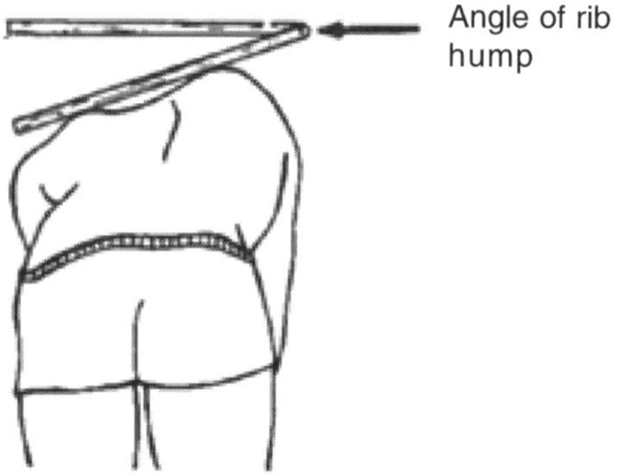

Fig. 8.11: Angle of rib hump

Pain Assessment

The whole spine is palpated with finger tips over spinous process from occiput to sacrum. Tenderness or pain indicates the presence of inflammatory lesion. This focus of pain and tenderness may occasionally be confirmed by exerting vertical compressive force from top of head with patient in stable standing.

Monitoring of Curve Progression

Scoliosis in growing children or adolescents needs to be monitored till cessation of spinal growth. This coincides with cessation of growth in iliac apophysis known as Risser's sign. It first appears about one year before its completion. It gradually progresses from Risser's 1, 2, 3, 4 beginning at front of iliac crest and progresses to Risser 5 indicating complete fusion of iliac apophysis, thus indicating the end of further deterioration of the curve.

Types of Scoliotic Curves

The scoliotic curves (Fig. 8.12) are termed by the apex of curvature.

- *Cervical Scoliosis:* The apex of curvature is between C_1 and C_6.
- *Cervicothoracic Scoliosis:* The apex of curvature is at cervicothoracic junction.
- *Thoracic Scoliosis:* The apex of the curve is in between T_2 and T_{11}.
- *Thoracolumbar Scoliosis:* The apex of the curve is at thoracolumbar junction.
- *Lumbar Scoliosis:* The apex of the curve is in between L_2 and L_4.
- *Lumbosacral Scoliosis:* The apex of the curve is at lumbosacral junction.

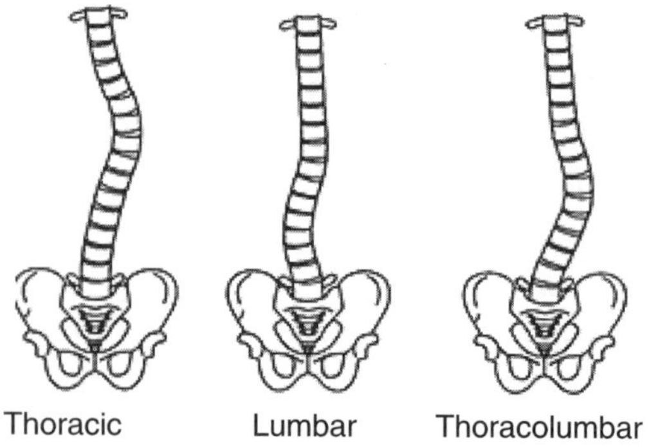

Fig. 8.12: Type of scoliotic curves

Management

Mild Postural Curves: Curve less than 40°

- *Active correction:* As these curves are correctable the most important aspect is to detect self corrective postural attitude. The physiotherapist identifies the postural adaptation by asking the patient to move and place the legs or trunk in such a position that optimal self correction of curve is attained.
- *Passive Correction:*
  - Hanging provides the best method of passive correction. Unequal hanging or hanging with one arm is useful method of correction. Hanging in head suspension apparatus gives satisfactory results.
  - Axial traction is also a mode of passive correction. One physiotherapist grasps the pelvis and gives traction towards the legs while the other grasps the chin and occiput and stretches the spine in opposite direction in supine lying position.

Management of Grade I Scoliosis

- General body relaxation.
- *Postural re-education:* The patient is trained to feel and hold the corrected posture. The posture can be passively corrected by the physiotherapists. Its maintenance is important.
- Free mobility exercises to the whole spine.
- Strengthening exercises to spinal extensors and abdominals.
- Deep breathing exercises.
- Balance exercises.

Stretching of Tight Soft Tissue Structures

Correction of contractures and shortening of soft tissues can be achieved by guiding the correct posture in lying.

Precaution

Avoid the positions and activities prone to produce and reproduce the deformity.

Management of Grade II Scoliosis

The structural curve of less than 40° is treated conservatively. Active self correction is not possible therefore bracing is advised. Exercise programme is progressed on same lines as for grade I scoliosis. Both are continued uninterrupted for a long time period. The brace needs repeated adjustments as the child grows. It is continued till the child attains skeletal maturity. It can be weaned off gradually thereafter. The brace needs to be worn day and night except during sessions of spinal mobilization and deep breathing exercises. The following braces are commonly used:

- Milwaukee brace (Fig. 8.13).
- Boston brace (Fig. 8.14).
- Reisser's turn buckle cast (Fig. 8.15).
- Localiser cast.

Exercise Regime

- Spinal stabilization and mobility exercises.
- Pelvic tilt with knees flexed.

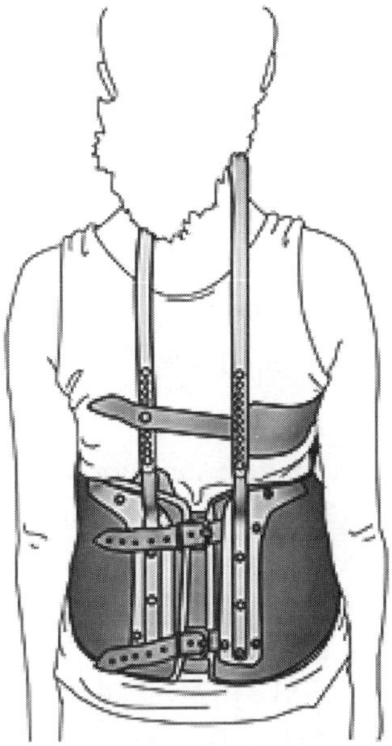

Fig. 8.13: Milwaukee brace

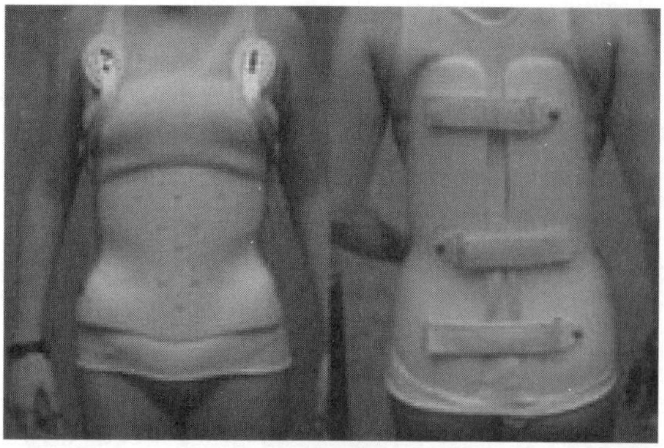

Fig. 8.14: Boston's brace

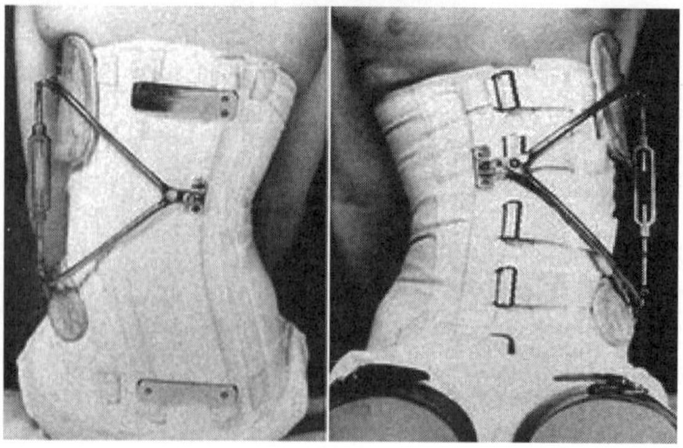

Fig. 8.15: Reisser's turnbuckle cast

- Pelvic tilt with extended knees.
- Sit ups with pelvic tilt, stabilizing the feet initially, progressing to partial sit up with unsupported feet.
- Modified bicycle exercises: Legs should not be raised over the hips.
- Pelvic tilt in standing position.
- Push ups with pelvic tilt.
- Deep breathing exercises.
- Exercises to reduce and correct the anterior pelvic tilt due to associated lumbar lordosis.
- Correction of major curve is also achieved by putting a pad over rib hump in the brace on convex side of curve.
- This thoracic pad will prers against the rib hump and helps to derotate the spine. Derotation should be performed many times throughout the day be inhaling deeply expanding backward against the posterior uprights with chest wall that is arch like a cat.
- Stretching of hip flexors and hamstrings.

Management of Grade III Scoliosis

The curves which are greater than 40° need surgical intervention.

Indications for Surgery

- Cord compression.
- Rapid progression of curve.
- Excruciating pain.
- Respiratory impairment.
- Cosmetic reasons.

Principles of Surgical Intervention

- Correction of curve.
- Maintenance of correction.

Aims of Surgical Intervention

- To restore the symmetry of trunk as much as possible by correction of curve.
- To straighten the thoracic curves to stop the deterioration in the pulmonary functions.

Correction of Curve

Any of the following methods are employed to achieve maximal correction of curve.

Turnbuckle Cast Technique (Reisser's)

The patient is put on Reisser's table. The head and pelvis are pulled by traction in opposite direction. A POP localiser cast is then applied over the trunk with scoliotic curve in corrected position. A few days later, a window is made in the cast through which surgery of spinal fusion is performed. The cast is maintained postoperatively for about 6 months till fusion consolidates.

Distraction Techniques

Certain distraction techniques are employed to correct the spinal deformity.

- *Skeletal traction*
  - Halo-femoral traction.
  - Halo-pelvic traction.
  - Halo-wheelchair traction.
- *Non-skeletal traction*
  - Intermittent traction followed by sustained traction.
  - Cotrel traction
  - Gravitational traction.

Contraindication to Distraction Techniques

- Arterial hyperextension.
- Congenital spinal malformation.
- Neurological disease.
- Flaccidity of cervical spine ligaments.

Loosening of curve: In rigid scoliotic curves, the operation of loosening of curve is performed as first stage procedure. In this operation the intervertebral discs of affected vertebra are removed so that spine gets loosened. After that distraction technique is applied in order to straighten the spine. It is followed by spinal fusion with instrumentation after 4-6 weeks.

Methods to Maintain the Curve Correction

- Spinal fusion.
- Spinal instrumentation
  - Harrington instrumentation.
  - Segmental spinal instrumentation (Luque).
  - Dwyer's instrumentation.
  - Zielke instrumentation.

Pre-Surgical Physiotherapy Assessment

- Measurement of rib hump.
- Assessment of pulmonary function.
- Muscle charting of whole body.
- Detailed neurological examination.
- Gait analysis.
- Functional status.

Pre-Surgical Physiotherapy Training

- Vigorous and strong ankle toe movements.
- Isometric exercises to quadriceps and glutei.
- *Postural guidance:* Techniques of postural correction and its maintenance.
- Intervertebral spinal mobility exercises.
- *Spinal stretching:* Stretching of whole spine to maximum. This stretches the contracted soft tissues in preparation for surgery.

Postsurgical Physiotherapeutic Intervention

First Two Days

- *Respiratory exercises.*
  - Deep breathing.
  - Vibrations.
  - Assisted coughing.
- Ankle toe movements.
- Upper extremity movements to the maximum painless range.
- Slow relaxed passive movements to lower limbs helps in increasing circulation, relieving pain and stiffness.
- Changing the position of patient every 2 hourly is important.

Third and Fourth Day

Active movements to hip and knee joints alternated with relaxed passive movements may provide pain relief.

After Five Days

- Reverse climb down technique is taught for getting out of bed. The procedure is rolling to prone, coming to prone kneeling and getting down by slowly sliding down from foot end of the bed.

- Assisted sitting over the side of bed with legs hanging for not more than 15 minutes.
- Chair sitting with lumbar roll or support progressing to unsupported sitting as the patient learns to actively support the spine.
- Assisted standing is initiated. It should be functional. As the balance and proprioception returns to normal assistance is decreased.
- *Walking:* Walking is initiated with correct gait pattern once the standing balance is acceptable. The patient should be made to walk in the parallel bars with height of hand rail raised and adjusted to avoid forward flexion thus avoiding the stress on lumbar spine.

  During ambulation elbow crutch or cane can be used as assistive devices.

UNIT THREE

DEGENERATIVE ARTHROPATHIES

CHAPTER 9

OSTEOARTHRITIS

Definition

Osteoarthritis is a chronic, non-inflammatory degenerative disorder of joints with exacerbation of acute inflammation characterized by progressive deterioration of the articular cartilage and formation of new bone (osteophytes).

Synonyms

- Degenerative arthritis.
- Degenerative joint disease.
- Arthritis deformans.

Aetiology

Osteoarthritis is seen commonly in weight bearing joints, predominantly in the middle age and older age groups. It is equally common in men and women but under the age of 50 there are more men, and over the age of 50, more women are affected. But the joint distribution pattern is different for both the sexes.

In men, the order of affected joints is hip (most common), knee, spine, ankle, shoulders and fingers. In women the order is knee, finger, spine, hip, ankle and shoulder (Fig. 9.1).

Cause

The concept of wear and tear is generally attributed as a cause of osteoarthritis. If a joint would never put under stress, it would never become osteoarthritic. Hence the relatively less stressed joints of upper limb are in general, less prone to osteoarthritic changes than the heavily stressed joints of lower limb.

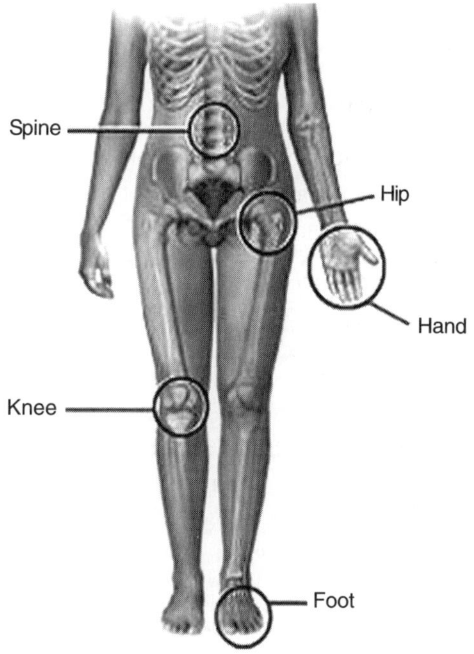

Fig. 9.1: Affected joints in osteoarthritis

Nearly always, there is a predisposing factor that accelerates the wear and tear process. Almost any deformity of a joint may be responsible, indirectly for the development of osteoarthritis, often many years later.

Predisposing Factors

- Hereditary.
- Poor posture.

- The ageing process in joint cartilage.
- Defective lubricating mechanism and uneven nutrition of the articular cartilage.
- Crystals (calcium pyrophosphate and hydroxyapetite) have been associated with synovitis in osteoarthritic joints.
- Obesity and overweight.
- Congenital ill-development.
- Irregularity of joint surfaces.
- Internal derangements, such as loose body or torn meniscus.
- Malalignment of a joint.

Classification

Osteoarthritis can be classified into two categories:

- Primary osteoarthritis.
- Secondary osteoarthritis.

Primary Osteoarthritis:

In primary osteoarthritis, there is no obvious cause of the diseased process. It is always idiopathic.

Secondary Osteoarthritis:

Secondary osteoarthritis arises as a consequence of other conditions. There is always an obvious cause for the disease process. Some of the causes may be categorized as:

- Trauma.
- Dislocation.
- Repeated minor trauma.
- Occupational
  - In miners, knees are at risk.
  - In tailors, first carpometacarpal and metacarpophalangeal joints.
  - In pneumatic drillers, elbows and shoulders.
- Infection
  - Tracking into a joint from open wound.
  - Tuberculosis of a joint.
- Deformity.
- Obesity.
- Haemophilia.
- Acromegaly.
- Hyperthyroidism.
- Tabes dorsalis, syringomyelia: Charcot's joints.

Pathology

This will be considered in relation to each joint structure as follows:

- Articular cartilage.
- Bone.
- Synovial membrane.
- Capsule.
- Ligaments.
- Muscles.

Articular Cartilage

Cartilage is usually the first structure to be affected (Fig. 9.2). Fibrillation which causes softening, splitting and fragmentation of cartilage occur in both weight bearing and non-weight bearing areas. Flakes of cartilage break off and may be impacted between the joint surfaces causing locking and inflammation. Proliferation occurs at the periphery of joint cartilage.

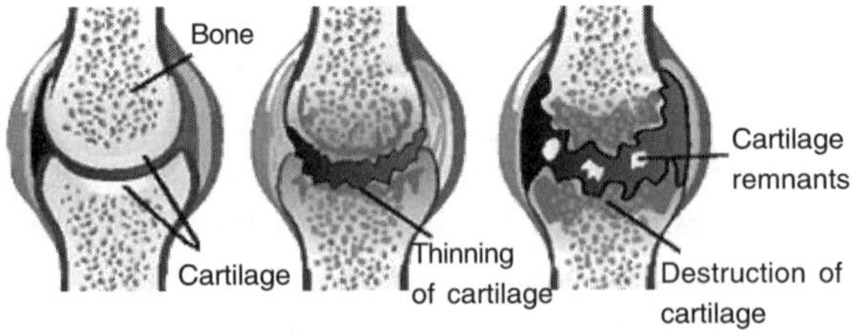

Fig. 9.2: Evolution of osteoarthritis

Bone

The bone surfaces become hard and polished as there is loss of protection from the cartilage.
Cystic cavities form in the subchondral bone (Fig. 9.3) because eburnated bone is brittle and microfractures occur allowing the passage of synovial fluid into the bone tissue. There can also be venous congestion in the subchondral bone.

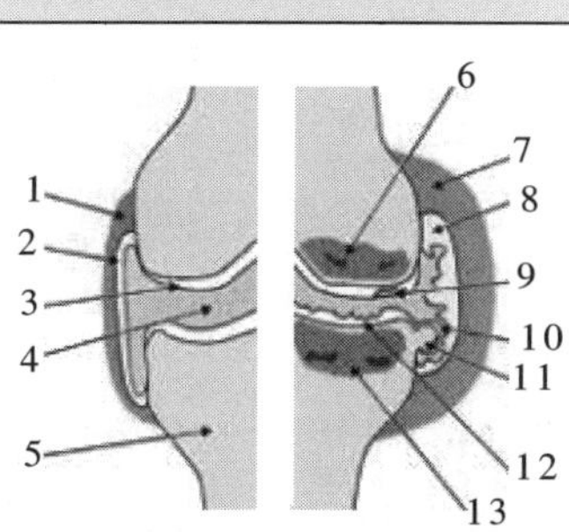

1. Joint capsule, 2. Synovium membrane, 3. Articular cartilage, 4. Joint cavity, 5. Bone, 6. Subchondral bone cyst, 7. Thickened joint, 8. Inflammation of the synovitis membrane, 9. Early degeneration of articular cartilage, 10. Cartilage cap of osteophyte, 11. Osteophyte, 12. Fibrillated cartilage, 13. Altered bone turnover, "sclerosis" on radiograph

Fig. 9.3: Osteoarthritic changes

Osteophytes form at the margin of the articular surfaces where they may project into the joint or into the capsule and ligaments. Bone of the weight bearing joints alter in shape.

Synovial Membrane

This undergoes hypertrophy and become oedematous. Later there is fibrous degeneration. Reduction of synovial fluid secretion results in loss of nutrition and lubrication of the articular cartilage.

Capsule

This undergoes fibrous degeneration and there are low-grade chronic inflammatory changes.

Ligaments

According to the aspect of joint, they become either elongated or contracted.

Muscles

These undergo fibrous atrophy which may be related to disuse because pain limits movement and function.

Clinical Features

The signs and symptoms related to osteoarthritis may be generalized as follows:

- Pain.
- Muscle spasm.
- Stiffness.
- Loss of movement.
- Muscle wasting and weakness.
- Joint enlargement.
- Deformity.
- Crepitus.
- Loss of function.

During active inflammation, the appearance of joint is characterized by the characteristic features of inflammation, which are as follows:

- Heat.
- Redness.
- Swelling.
- Pain.

Pain

Onset of Pain

The onset of pain is of low intensity and can be described as of three types:

- Pain on weight bearing, severe aching, due to stress on synovial membrane and later due to contact of bone surfaces, which are rich in nerve endings.
- During and after exercise there is pain described as being around the joint.
- At night, especially after a very active day there is severe aching. This is thought to be due to venous congestion in bone ends. It is worse in patients with varicose veins and can be reduced if the end of bed is elevated.

Nature of Pain

- Aching is dominant, at first fleeting and then becoming more constant.
- Referred pain is described as passing down a limb distally from the affected joint.
- Sharp stabbing pain is associated with a loose body becoming impacted in the joint.
- Throbbing is related to an episode of inflammation and is worse at night.

Muscle Spasm

This occurs over one aspect of joint and is initially protective but when it remains beyond the active episode it must be treated to prevent contractures.

Stiffness

This is present after rest and takes little time to wear off with movement. It may be due to:

- Loss of joint lubrication.
- Chronic oedema in periarticular structures.
- Swelling of articular cartilage.

Loss of Joint Movement

This may occur due to:

- Articular cartilage destruction.
- Muscle spasm.
- Soft tissue contracture.

Muscle Wasting and Weakness

Muscles become weak often on the aspect of joint which is opposite to contractures.

Joint Enlargement

Chronic oedema of the synovial membrane and capsule together with muscle wasting makes the joint appear large.

Deformity

Each joint tends to adapt a characteristic deformity.

Crepitus

The flaked cartilage and eburnated bone ends grate with characteristic sound on movement.

Loss of Function:

Pain, muscle weakness, giving way lead to inability to use the limb normally and can be severely disabling.

Radiographic Features (Fig. 9.4)

In the initial stages the radiological appearance may be normal. Subsequently the changes which are seen include:

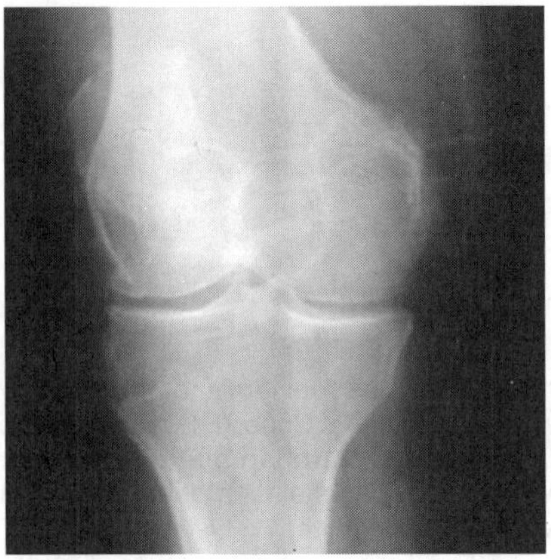

Fig. 9.4: Radiographic appearance of an osteoarthritic knee joint

- Joint space narrowing. This reflects the gradual disappearance of cartilage.
- Sclerosis (increased density) of bone beneath the cartilage as the process of eburnation takes place.
- Osteophyte formation at the joint margin.
- Cystic changes in the peri-articular bone. These are seen as translucent areas of varying size in close proximity to the joint. They can result in local collapse of bone.
- Deformity resulting from subluxation.
- The presence of loose bodies.
- Irregularity of bone surfaces.

Diagnosis

This is usually clear by the history, clinical findings, and radiographic features. Osteoarthritis is not easily confused with inflammatory form of arthritis, because there is no synovial thickening, no increased local warmth, and the erythrocyte sedimentation rate is not increased. The radiographs show sclerosis rather than rarefaction.

Course

Osteoarthritis usually increases slowly year by year. In many cases the disability never reaches the stage at which treatment is required. In others increasing pain, stiffness, or deformity drives the patient to demand measures for its relief.

Treatment

Principles of Treatment

The disease once started progresses gradually and there is no way to stop it. Hence efforts are directed, wherever possible, to the following:

- To delay the occurrence of the disease, if the disease has not begun yet.
- To stall progress of the disease and relieve symptoms, if the disease is in early stages.
- To rehabilitate the patient, with or without surgery, if his disabilities can be partially or completely alleviated.

Methods of Treatment

To achieve the above objectives, the following therapeutic measures may be taken:

- *Drugs*: Analgesics are used mainly to suppress pain.
- *Chondroprotective agents:* Agents such as glucosamine and chondroirtin sulphate have been introduced, claiming to be the agents which result in repair of the damaged cartilage.
- *Viscosupplementation:* Sodium hylarunon has been introduced. It is injected in the joint 3-5 times over weekly interval. It is supposed to improve cartilage functions, and is claimed to be chondroprotective.
- *Supportive therapy:* This is useful and harmless method of treatment and often gives gratifying results.
- *Surgical treatment:* In selected cases, surgery can provide significant relief. The following are some of the surgical procedures performed:
  - *Osteotomy:* Osteotomy near a joint has been known to bring about relief in symptoms, especially in arthritic joints with deformities.
  - *Joint replacement:* For cases crippled with advanced damage to the joint, total joint replacement operation has provided remarkable rehabilitation. These are now commonly performed for hip and knee. An artificial joint serves for about 10-15 years.
  - *Joint debridement:* This operation is not so popular now. In this, the affected joint is opened, degenerated cartilage smoothened and osteophytes and the hypertrophied synovium excised. The results are unpredictable.
  - *Arthroscopic procedures:* Arthroscopic removal of loose bodies, degenerated meniscus and other such procedures have become popular because of their less invasive nature. In arthroscopic chondroplasty, the degenerated fibrillated cartilage is excised using a power-driven shaver under arthrosporic vision. Results are unpredictable.

Physiotherapy Management

Osteoarthritis is neither a condition of relentless progression, nor a disease. It is the result of imbalance between the mechanical stresses on joint and the ability of the tissue to withstand them. Patient present to physiotherapy department with varying distribution and degree of deterioration in the affected joints and are treated according to the stage of degenerative process.

Assessment

Pain: The level of pain experienced by the patient indicates the degree of joint irritability but not necessarily the amount of joint deterioration. Information concerning the pain can be elicited by careful questioning of the following points:

- Site and distribution of pain.
- *Quality of pain:* Burning, aching, throbbing, searing.
- *Duration:* Permanent, persistent or intermittent.
- *Triggering factors:* Weight bearing, jarring, sustained stress, specific movement, rest, posture, weather, emotional state, no recognizable trigger.

- *Relieving factors:* Rest, movement, postural adjustment, temporal adjustment, physiotherapeutic procedures.

Loss of Function: Damage to a single joint such as hip or knee will have significant effect on the patient's function. The patient will be able to identify specific problems and treatment should be oriented towards their relief.

Joint Stiffness: All affected joints display restriction of movement, and careful examination is required of the active and passive ranges so that deficiencies may be noted. The quality of movement, point of pain limitation or muscle guarding should be noted and recorded. Movement must be localized to the joint under examination and care must be taken to prevent movement in adjacent joints.

When examining joint movement, the physiotherapist must also check accessory movements at the joints involved. These movements are an essential part of the normal movement and cannot be performed voluntarily in isolation. Restriction of accessory movement due to mechanical disruption to the joint surfaces will give rise to pain on movement and will preclude normal range or smooth quality of movement within the existing range.

Assessment is completed by noting the posture, identifying any deformity or asymmetry of limb lengths and testing the strength of muscles around the affected joints using MRC scale.

Assessment of tenderness: The degree and area of tenderness, effusion and crepitus are carefully examined by palpation, volumetric measures or measuring tape and relaxed passive ROM respectively.

Assessment of deformity: It is extremely important to measure the degree of deformity accurately. The deformity may be fixed or dynamic when exposed to compression. The assessment should, therefore be done in the position of maximum compression, e.g., weight bearing on the affected limb alone.

General Principles of Physiotherapeutic Management

- Prevention.
- To control pain.
- To improve range of motion.
- To prevent further damage.
- To improve strength, endurance and muscle function.
- To improve functional status of the involved joint and the whole body with correct ergonomic control.

Prevention

Physiotherapy can play a vital role in the prevention of painful symptoms of osteoarthritis.

Measures of Prevention

- Early identification of the individuals at risk, e.g., with history of trauma to the joint, those with obesity and deformities at the related joints.
- Critical examination of the joint kinematics in weight bearing and non-weight bearing positions.
- Guided measures are to be taken depending upon the findings of the examination to prevent deterioration of degeneration which could be:
  - Strengthening, improving flexibility and endurance of concerned muscle groups.
  - Corrective measures to compensate the influence of altered stresses on the joints by using viscoelastic inserts, avoiding undue strain.
  - Exercises should be directed to lower the impact of excessive force across the joint. This is achieved either by decreasing the contractile force on the muscles, or by making the muscles more efficient so that they do not have to contract as strongly to produce the same effect. Thus, controlled activity of the muscle group can prevent compression of the joint due to excessive contraction.

- Guidance on avoiding various postures and activities causing excessive compression of the susceptible joints, e.g., repetitive sitting and standing.
- Nutritional guidance for obese individual.
- Inhibition of degenerative changes during immobilization by providing safe and limited ROM devices like non-weight bearing functional orthosis. Traction or continuous passive motion (CMP) is also useful.
- Early management of congenital anomalies, infective condition of joints and intra-articular fractures.
- Graduate resistance to the full arc of movement or controlled loading through full ROM. It is necessary to expose the maximum area of cartilage to the stimulus of weight bearing.

Public awareness of these facts can prevent progression of osteoarthritis.

Intervention

The treatment is planned by giving due considerations to the patient's lifestyle, physical requirements, body weight, and the reports of evaluation. It is difficult to generalize the treatment for all the patients of osteoarthritis. Only basic approaches can be enumerated as follows:

- *Pain Control:* To control pain, suitable electrotherapy modality should be used. In the acute phase pain relief is achieved better by the superficial heat modalities or cryotherapy. Ultrasound, TENS, diapulse, pulsed diathermy and stimulation are also effective. Short wave diathermy may be used in the later phase when the tissue oedema is less.
  - *Traction:* Distraction of joint surfaces, either manually or mechanically; either intermittently or prolonged, will reduce pain by relieving pressure on sensitive intra-articular structures. Protective muscle guarding is reduced and this will also ease the pain.
  - *Heat:* Superficial or deep heat will relieve discomfort by reducing the protective muscle spasm. Hot packs, radiant heat, paraffin wax bath, short save diathermy are all beneficial.
  - *Cold:* The application of cold is often more effective than heat. Ice packs or ice toweling techniques are useful.
  - *Ultrasound:* This is indicated when pain is centered on peri-articular soft tissues.
  - *Interferential therapy:* This is used for its analgesics and circulatory effects.
  - *Hydrotherapy:* The warmth of the water and its buoyancy are helpful in relieving pain particularly when weight-bearing joints are effective.

- *To prevent further strain or damage to affected joints:* The identification of activities which produce strain followed by reduction or elimination of them is obviously the best method. Improvement of posture, the selection of appropriate walking aid or correction of leg length inequality by a shoe raise may also be required. A period of rest in the corrected position during the day will ease strain and should be encouraged.

- *To improve range of motion:* As there is no systemic involvement in osteoarthritis, vigorous techniques can be used to improve joint movement once the protective muscle spasm has been reduced. Mobilization may be active or passive.
  - *Active:* Active free relaxed rhythmic movements improve the range as well as promote relaxation of the joint. Methods include the use of suspension therapy for the larger limb joints and lumbar spine. Pool therapy is beneficial for the lower limb joints as are PNF techniques such as hold-relax and slow reversal hold-relax used in appropriate patterns.
  - *Passive:* Passive techniques are used where mechanical dysfunction or alteration of length

of peri-articular soft tissues are limiting movement. Relaxed passive movements should be started first to mobilize stiff joints. Hydrotherapy and PNF techniques are useful in improving ROM. When mechanical dysfunction blocks the movement, manipulation and mobilization techniques are effective.

- *To improve muscle power, endurance and tone:* Muscle power can only be improved by active exercise. There should be selection of appropriate standing positions, type and quality of resistance so that the patient works to the limit of his capabilities in order to hypertrophy muscle. Endurance will be increased by working muscles for a longer time against a sub-maximal resistance.
  Graduated exercise programme is initiated which consists of progressive resistance (PRE), strong and sustained repeated sessions of isometrics holding or sustaining muscle contractions in static and mid range position of isotonics.

- *To improve functional independence:* Function of the whole body in relation to the degenerated joint can be improved by:
  - Proper guidance to relieve compression over the affected joints.
  - Providing assistive aids, modified supports, orthoses, adaptations and ergonomic advice on the performance of ADLs.

By relieving pain and muscle guarding the patient's level of functional independence may improve. If problem remains the solution may lie in the use of an alternative method by supplying an aid, for example a stocking gutter, elasticated shoe laces or a half-step.

CHAPTER 10

SPONDYLOSIS

DEFINITION

Spondylosis is a condition in which there are degenerative changes in the intervertebral joints between the vertebral bodies and the discs.

Osteoarthritis results in degenerative changes in synovial joints and therefore can occur in the apophyseal joints of the spine. Clinically the two conditions often occur together.

Aetiology

The age range is 30 years onwards and is most common around 45. Women are more commonly affected than men.

Predisposing Factors

- Poor posture associated with anxiety, habit.
- Occupational stress, e.g., typists at poorly positioned desks, coal miners, drivers, people whose work involve lifting, twisting and carrying.
- Body type, neck that is thickest with a 'Dowager's hump' and long backs are prone to spondylosis.

Affected Sites

The sites commonly affected are:

- Cervical – C_4 to T_1
- Lumbar – L_2 to L_4
- Thoracic – T_4 to T_6

Pathology

The pathological changes that occur are the same regardless of site but the difference in anatomy gives rise to different signs and symptoms.

Intervertebral Discs

- The annulus fibrosis becomes coarser, the collagen fibres tend to separate and cracks appear at various sites.
- The nucleus pulposus loses fluid and becomes more fibrous.
- The disc overall loses height.
- These changes occur as part of the ageing process of the discs and can be present without causing any signs or symptoms.

Vertebral Bodies

'Lipping' of vertebral body occurs. This is due to alteration of disc mechanics producing traction to the periosteum by attachment of the annulus fibrosis. There can be decalcification within the bodies which predisposes to crush fractures.

Ligaments

The intervertebral ligaments may become contracted and thickened especially at the sites where there are gross changes.

Meningeal Sleeves

The dura mater of the spinal cord forms a sleeve around the nerve root and this undergoes inflammatory changes because as the disc space narrows there is diminished lumen of the intervertebral canal. The inflammation is low grade and chronic in nature resulting in adhesions around the nerve root.

Apophyseal Joints

These undergo the changes of osteoarthritis. Osteophytes form at the margins of the articular surfaces and these together with the capsular thickening can cause pressure on the nerve root and reduce the lumen of intervertebral foramen.

CERVICAL SPONDYLOSIS

Degenerative changes are common in the cervical spine. Indeed, they are found almost universally in some degree in persons over 50 years of age. Beginning in the intervertebral discs, they affect the posterior intervertebral (facet) joints secondarily, causing pain and stiffness of the neck, sometimes with referred symptoms in an upper limb.

Synonyms

- Cervical spondylarthritis.
- Cervical spondylarthrosis.
- Cervical osteoarthritis.
- Cervical osteoarthrosis.

Causes

The primary degenerative changes may be initiated by injury, but usually the condition is simply a manifestation of normal wear and tear.

Pathology

Degenerative arthritis occurs most commonly in the lowest three cervical joints. The changes affect first the central intervertebral joints (between the vertebral bodies) and later the posterior intervertebral (facet) joints. In the central joints there is degenerative narrowing of intervertebral disc, and bone reaction at the joint margins leads to formation of osteophytes. In the posterior intervertebral joints the changes are those of osteoarthritis in any diarthrodial joint–namely wearing away of articular cartilage and the formation of osteophytes (spurs) at the joint margin.

Secondary Effects (Fig. 10.1)

Osteophytes commonly encroach upon the intervertebral foramina, reducing the space for transmission of the cervical nerves. If the restricted space in a foramen is reduced still further by traumatic oedema of the contained soft tisses, manifestations of nerve pressure are likely to occur.

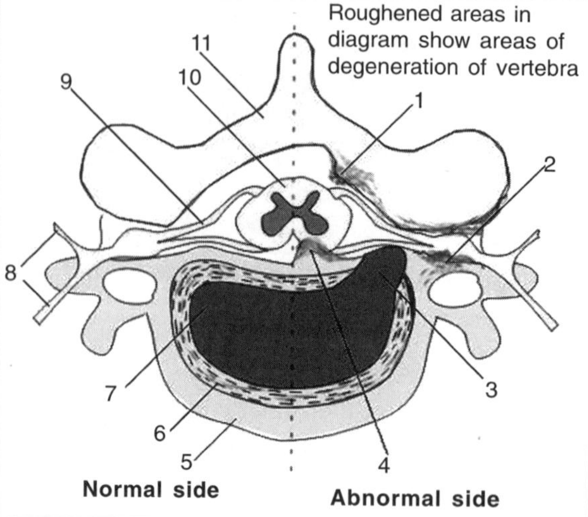

1. Degeneration (osteophyte) not causing any problems
2. Degeneration (osteophyte) irritating or pressing on nerve root coming out from spinal cord. This is one cause of cervical radiculopathy
3. Prolapsed disc pressing on a nerve root coming from the spinal cord. This is one cause of cervical radiculopathy
4. Degeneration (osteophyte) pressing on spinal cord. This is one cause of a cervical myelopathy
5. Anterior part of vertebra
6. Annulus fibrosus
7. Nucleus pulposus
8. Nerves coming and going to spinal cord to take messages to and from arms and neck
9. Nerve root emerging from the spinal cord
10. Spinal cord
11. Posterior part of vertebra

Fig. 10.1: Changes in a degenerated vertebra

Exceptionally, the spinal cord itself may suffer from damage from encroachment of osteophytes within the spinal canal.

Clinical Features

The symptoms are in the neck or in the upper limb or both.

Neck symptoms consist mainly of:

- Aching pain in the back of neck or in the trapezius area.
- Feeling of stiffness.
- Grating on movement.
- Occipital headaches are due to upper cervical pathology.
- Neck ache usually due to mid-cervical pathology.

They are liable to periodic exacerbations, probably from unremembered strains or repetitive movements.

In the upper limb, there may be vague, ill-defined and ill-localized referred pain spreading over the shoulder region. The main feature of nerve root irritation is radiating pain along the course of the affected nerve or nerves, often reaching the digits. There may also be paraesthesia in the hand, in the form of tingling or 'pins and needles'.

Examination

Patient's Lifestyle

A meticulous examination is essential to identify precipitating factors in the patient's lifestyle:

- Working condition that demand concentration resulting in 'poking chin and round shoulders'.
- Habit of holding the telephone on one shoulder.
- Sitting or standing still for long times.
- Driving for long time, especially in traffic jams.
- Sleeping in awkward positions.

Referred Pain

- There may be no pain perceived in neck but pain is in the arm (Fig. 10.2).
- Pain down to the elbow—C5 (Fig. 10.3).

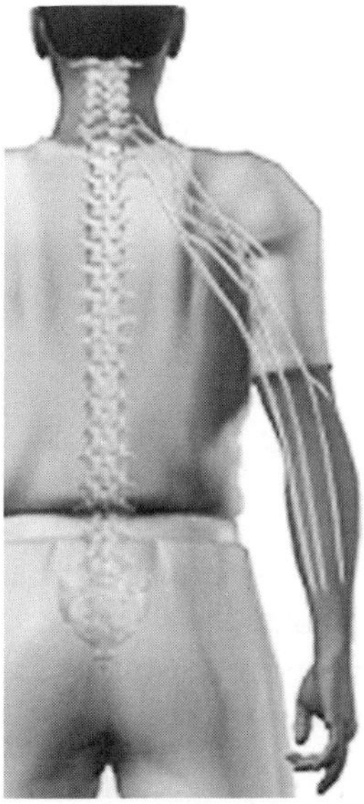

Fig. 10.2: Cervical radiculopathy

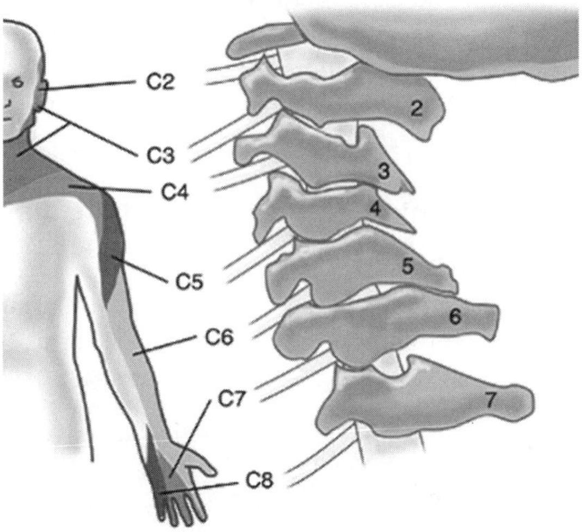

Fig. 10.3: Pattern of referred pain in upper extremity

- Pain to thumb and index finger—C6.
- Pain on middle three fingers and forearm—C7.
- Pain on inside the forearm, little finger and possibly chest—C8/T1.
- In addition pain may be referred down to thoracic area, for example the medial border of scapula.

Nature of Pain

The pain is described as dull aching superimposed by sharp stabbing pain and from time to time as cramp-type throbbing.

Paraesthesia

Pins and needles or altered sensation may be present in the area supplied by an impinged nerve root (dermatome).

Limitation of Movement

- Neck movements are all limited often bilaterally but during an acute episode of pain one side is more affected than the other. It is important to note that the upper cervical flexion is often very limited together with lower cervical spine extension.
- Muscle spasm and muscle tightness.
- Limitation of movements, including limiting factors and exact vertebral levels affected.
- Loss of accessory intervertebral movements detected by palpation.
- Loss of soft tissue mobility also detected by palpation.

Radiographic Features (Fig. 10.4)

- Narrowing of the intervertebral disc space.
- Formation of osteophytes at vertebral margins. Encroachment of osteophytes upon the intervertebral foramen is demonstrated best in oblique projection.

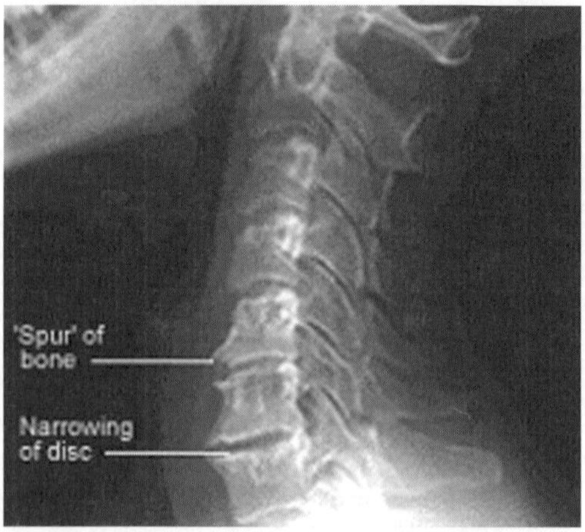

Fig. 10.4: X-ray of the cervical spine (lateral view) showing cervical spondylosis

Differential Diagnosis

Distinction has to be made from other causes of neck pain and upper limb pain.

Other Causes of Neck Pain

- Prolapsed cervical disc.
- Tuberculous or pyogenic infection.
- Tumours involving the vertebral canal.
- Fibrositis.

Other Causes of Upper Limb Pain

1. Central lesions
   - Tumours involving spinal cord or its roots
   - Cervical spondylolisthesis
2. Plexus lesions
   - Tumours at thoracic inlet
   - Cervical rib
   - Prolapsed intervertebral disc
3. Shoulder lesions with radiating pain in upper arm.
4. Skeletal lesions
   - Tumours
   - Infection
   - Paget's disease of bone of upper extremity
5. Elbow lesions
   - Tennis elbow
   - Arthritis
6. Distal nerve lesions
   - Friction neuritis of ulnar nerve at elbow
   - Compression of median nerve in the carpal tunnel

Complications

If the spinal canal is markedly narrowed by osteophytes the spinal cord may be damaged, with progressive upper motor neurone disturbances affecting all four limbs and possibly the bladder.

This complication is serious but fortunately rare.

Treatment

There is strong tendency for the symptoms of cervical spondylosis to subside spontaneously, though they may persist for many weeks and the structural changes are clearly permanent. There are chances of remissions of the symptoms.

Aim of Treatment

Treatment is aimed towards assisting natural resolution of temporarily inflammed or oedematous soft tissues.

During the period of remission, the prevention of any further attacks is of utmost importance and is done by advising the patient regarding the following:

- *Proper neck posture:* The patient must avoid situations where he has to keep his neck in one position for a long time.
- *Neck muscle exercises:* These help in improving the neck posture, cervical range of motion and muscular strength.

During an acute episode, the following treatment is required:

- Analgesics.
- Hot fomentation.
- Rest to the neck in cervical collar.
- Traction to the neck if there is stiffness.
- Anti-emetics if there is giddiness.

In *mild cases*, measures include analgesic drugs.

In the *more severe cases* it is wise to provide rest and support for the neck by a closely-fitting protective cervical collar, which should be worn for one to three months according to progress.

In the *exceptional cases* in which the spinal cord is constricted, decompression either from in front or by laminectomy may be required, and thereafter it may be advisable to fuse the affected segments of the spinal column by a bone grafting operation.

Physiotherapy Management

- *Heat:* A heat pad applied with the patient in lying or half-lying so that the neck is supported can reduce muscle spasm and increase the circulation which brings nutrition to the neck structures and remove metabolites.
- *Relaxation:* Tension in the neck and shoulder girdle muscles is nearly always present in a patient who presents with pain from cervical spondylosis, and education of relaxation is therefore an essential component of the total management.

Physiological relaxation *(Laura Mitchell Method)* is the best approach as it can be applied in various positions and at rest, work or play. To encourage relaxed sleeping the patient and physiotherapist work out a position of comfort and support. Prone lying should be strongly discouraged. In side-lying there should be sufficient pillows to fill in the space between shoulder and the head so that the neck is straight. A pillow between the legs or under the top knee plus another folded up and positioned to support the top arm are important so that the patient can truly relax in a position of support. The patient is instructed to push the legs down into the bed, feel the support and stop pushing. This is then repeated with the trunk, arms, and head until the whole body is fully supported and muscular tension is reduced to minimum. The mouth is stretched open as in yawning and allowed to close gently. The eyes are closed and the eyebrows raised with a feeling of 'smoothing' the scalp back over the top of the head. The patient should then be encouraged to think of something pleasant, e.g., a piece of music, lying on warm sunny beach, making a floral display, playing a sport. This promotes refreshing sleep making the patient feel better and breaking the cycle of pain. While sleeping in supine one pillow under the head (not shoulders) is best and another pillow under the knees to flatten the lumbar spine is helpful. If a patient has a problem that precludes lying flat, the upper thoracic spine may be supported on pillows but there must be a pillow for the head alone—possibly 'butterflied', i.e., flattened in the middle so that the ends support the head on either side.

In sitting, relaxation can also be practised. The position depends on activity being pursued. Where the patient is relaxing, e.g., watching television, the head, neck and shoulders should be supported by high-backed chair with a small pillow in the lumbar region, the feet supported and the arms resting either on the arms of the chair or on a pillow on the lap. The same principles are followed of pushing the parts of the body into the supporting structure. The fingers should rest in extension, the elbows in slight flexion and the shoulders slightly abducted. This is opposite to the position of tension. The shoulder girdles are positioned by pushing them down and back, holding and then releasing. If the patient practices this and checks for relaxation every half hour the reduction in muscle tension is of great benefit. Sitting at work should also include components of relaxation, especially pushing the shoulders down and back and stretching the head up 'out of neck' at regular intervals. The same principles are applied to walking with shoulder girdles relaxed.

- *Posture Education:* This is closely associated with teaching of relaxation. The classical postural abnormality is much the same as the position of tension. This in the extreme is:
  - Head thrust forwards (stressing C5/6/7 level and resulting in shortening of upper cervical spine extensors).
  - Shoulders held up and forward (causing excess tension in upper fibers of trapezius muscles).
  - Thoracic spine flexed and rounded (causing shortening of the pectorals and lengthening of shoulder girdle retractors).
  - Lumbar spine flexed, pelvis tilted backwards, hips flexed, knees flexed, ankles dorsiflexed, feet pronated.
  - Correction of only one component will not succeed which is why it is essential to examine the posture of patient from head to toe, identify abnormalities and teach alignment in total. It is very important to impress upon the patient that it is perfectly possible to reduce the pain and discomfort associated with spondylosis by paying attention to posture.
  - Position sense needs to be developed so that the patient can think of correction during daily activities.
- *Collar (Fig. 10.5):* During a phase of acute pain, a firm collar will help to steady the neck and relieve pain especially during travelling or work. It is important to remind the patient that it is very unwise to drive or operate intricate machinery whilst wearing a collar because the altered input from the nerve receptors in the facet joint capsules results in impairment of coordination of upper limb activities. When the

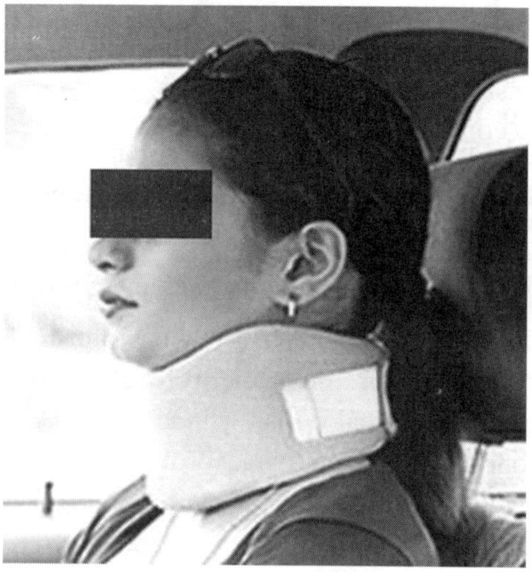

Fig. 10.5: Cervical collar

pain subsides the collar should be taken off when the patient is resting. The periods without the collar should be gradually extended. Generally it is wise to keep the collar on for travelling until there is no pain at rest and neck movements are pain free for atleast a third of full range. A soft collar is often helpful at night to prevent awkward positions of the neck during sleep. If the patient cannot tolerate a collar in bed then it is useful to put a rolled-up thick towel round the back of neck crossed over in front and if necessary tied with pin. A 'butterfly' pillow may be used for the patient who likes sleeping supine. The pillows may be tied in the middle and this part supports the neck whilst the sides prevent the head and the neck from rolling over.

- *Manipulative Therapy*
  - *Mobilizations:* These are undoubtedly essential in treatment of patients suffering from pain related to spondylosis. Restoration of intersegmental mobility by accessory pressure and physiological techniques enables the patient to regain full functional pain free movements. Scrupulous palpation is required to identify stiff segment. When there is acute pain and muscle spasm at $C_{4,5}$ there is often stiffness at C_7,T_1. These segments are not contributing the percentage they should to total spinal movement and therefore stress occurs above ($C_{4,\ 5}$). Grade I and II techniques will settle the pain and spasm of $C_{4,5}$ and grade III techniques will mobilize C_7,T_1. The ribs often need mobilization. This is effectively and comfortably achieved by alternate flat hand pressure on the thoracic cage.
  - *Soft tissue techniques:* Kneading to mobilize tethered fascia is required especially around the dowager's hump C_7-T_2. Kneading also helps to release tightness in the upper fibers of trapezius. Finger kneading helps to mobilize the occipital attachment of the trapezius and scalene muscles on the transverse process of the vertebrae. Picking up, wringing and skin rolling achieve similar effects.
  - Finger kneading or frictions are often necessary to stretch interspinous ligament (C^7-T^1 and T^1-T^2) or localize thickenings in the paravertebral muscles. The benefit of soft tissue techniques are underrated but can be objectively demonstrated in terms of increased pain-free range of movement in neck, thoracic spine and shoulder girdle immediately after treatment.
- *Traction*: Oscillatory traction is considered to be mobilizing therefore is appropriate where the neck is generally stiff. Continuous traction is used to relieve nerve root pressure but if target segment is stiff then it must be mobilized first otherwise the traction force is distributed between the other mobile segments. Also it is essential to ensure that the paravertebral muscles are relaxed and lengthened (e.g., by heat, hold-relax, passive stretching) prior to the application of traction.
- *Hydrotherapy:* Total relaxation in float support lying, together with the warmth of the water gains relief of muscle spasm. Head, neck and trunk side-flexion (legs fixed) performed slowly through full range gains mobility and ensures that the muscles lengthen and shorten fully. To stretch tight paravertebral muscles the patient practices tucking the chin in and pushing the $C_{4,5}$ level into the neck float. Float support lying pushing one hand then the other towards the feet helps to relax the upper fibers of trapezius. Sitting, holding floats down with both hands works the lower fibers of trapezius and serratus anterior and trains the neck and shoulder joint receptors and muscles to hold a good position.

Swimming is not advisable—except possibly for backstroke or if the patient is very accomplished swimmer. Breast stroke with the head held out of water is the worst possible thing for the well-being of cervical spine.

- *Movement:* Hold-relax are necessary to lengthen the muscles especially the side flexors and upper cervical spine extensors. Lengthening the shoulder girdle elevators is achieved by the physiotherapist holding the head steady and applying hold-relax to gain shoulder girdle depression. Lengthening the upper cervical extensors is achieved by deep longitudinal stroking and by teaching the patient to lift the head out of shoulders pushing the back of the head backwards and upwards. Generally these techniques are applied with the patient in lying but half-lying or sitting can also be used. Stabilizations are helpful to retain correct muscle balance so that the upper cervical spine flexors and lower cervical extensors work to counteract the hypertonia in their antagonists. Free active exercises should be practised everyday particularly oblique patterns (flexion, side flexion rotation right to extension, side-flexion rotation left and repeat opposite way).
- *Advice:* During the day, every half hour or so, the neck should be stretched and moved through full range especially in sitting, reading, writing, car driving and similar activities. If the neck starts to feel stiff it is advisable to see a physiotherapist soon so that movement can be restored before a severe acute episode of pain ensues.

LUMBAR SPONDYLOSIS

This is a degenerative disorder of lumbar spine characterized clinically by an insidious onset of pain and stiffness and radiologically by osteophyte formation. The lumbar complex has always been a seat of degenerative changes due to excessive mobility over this area of spine.

Causes

- Bad posture.
- Chronic back strain.
- Previous injury to spinal joints.
- Previous disease involving the joints.
- Birth defects.
- Intervertebral disc prolapse.
- Increasing age – wear and tear of joints.

Pathology

The annulus fibers undergo fibrillation, which predisposes annulus tears. Dehydration sets in the intervertebral disc resulting in reduction of the disc space. The reduced disc space brings about approximation of the zygoapophyseal and facet joints resulting in slackening in the posterior longitudinal ligament (PLL). The stretching of PLL detaches it from the periosteum due to increased intradiscal pressure and disc extrusion results. The extruded disc material becomes fibrous and eventually gets calcified into a spur.

The changes affect the central intervertebral (body to body) joints and the posterior intervertebral (facet) joints. One segment or several segments may be affected. In the central joints, which are affected first, there is degeneration with consequent narrowing of intervertebral disc, and hypertrophy of bone at the joint margins leads to formation of osteophytes. In the posterior intervertebral (facet) joints the changes are those of osteoarthritis in any diarthrodial joint—namely, attrition of the articular cartilage and osteophyte formation (spurring) at the joint margins. These changes in the facet joints are probably more important from a clinical point of view.

Secondary Effects

Rarely, osteophytes encroach upon an intervertebral foramen sufficiently to interfere with the function of the issuing nerve. Thinning of the articular cartilage of the posterior intervertebral (facet) joints reduces the stability of the affected segment and predisposes to one type of spondylolisthesis.

Clinical Features

Lumbar spondylosis or spinal osteoarthritis can exist in quite marked degree without causing symptoms but the clinical complaint of the patient often starts with pain.

- *Pain:* There is often a complaint of aching pain in the affected area, worse on activity or after prolonged standing or sitting in one position and especially after stooping or lifting. Pain is often worse first thing in the morning, and there may be a feeling of stiffness when rising from a sitting position.

Referred Pain (Fig. 10.6)

Interference with a nerve in narrowed intervertebral foramen leads to radiating pain in the distribution of the affected nerve. Pain may radiate into a leg because of nerve root irritation. It tends to be dermatomal (Fig. 10.7).

- Groin - L1.
- Anterior aspect of thigh - L2.
- Lower third of anterior aspect of thigh and knee – L3.
- Medial aspect of leg to big toe – L4.
- Lateral aspect of leg to middle three toes – L5.
- Little toe, lateral border of foot, lateral side of posterior aspect of whole leg – S1.
- Heel, medial side of posterior aspect of whole leg – S2.

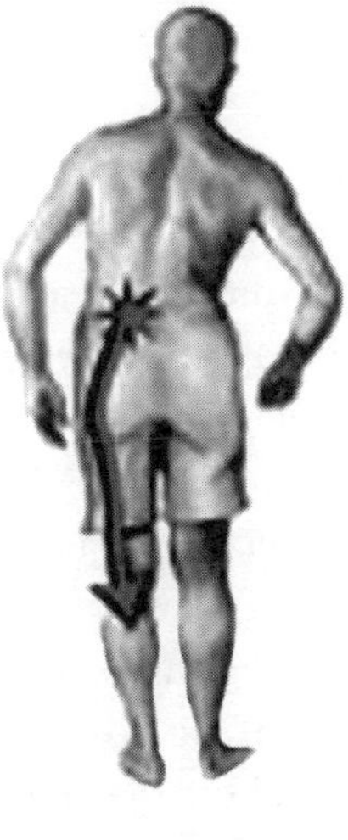

Fig. 10.6: Referred pain

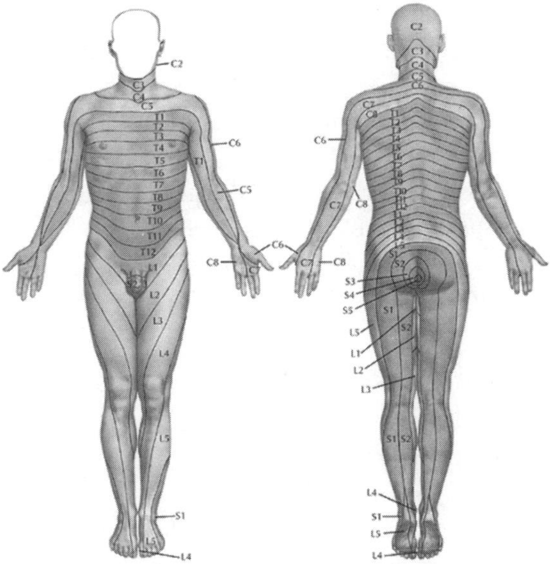

Fig. 10.7: Dermatomal pattern of pain distribution

Nature of Pain

Dull or severe ache superimposed from time to time by sharp stabbing pain.

- *Paresthesia:* This can follow dermatomal distribution and may be pins and needles, a sensation of 'creeping ants' or feeling of numbness.
- *Muscle spasm:* There is usually increased tone in erector spinae and in one or both quadratus lumborum muscles. There is often unequal tone between the hip abductors and also in between

adductors. Sometimes one hamstrings muscle is tighter than other.

- *Limitation of movement:* All lumbar spine movements tend to be limited—on attempted flexion there is no movement between L1 and S1. Hip movements are often limited asymmetrically. Limiting factors are generally soft tissue tightness more than spasm or pain.
- *Muscles weakness:* The abdominal muscles and the glutei may be weak.

Radiographic Features

- Narrowing of intervertebral space.
- Osteophyte formation (spurring) at the joint margins.
- Posterior intervertebral (facet) joints also show changes.
  - There is narrowing of the joint space.
  - Sharpening of margins of the facets.

Examination

This identifies:

- The pain picture.
- Precipitating factors at work or leisure.
- Posture abnormalities.
- Muscle spasm and tightness.
- Limitation of movements and the limiting factors.
- Loss of accessory movement and soft tissue mobility by palpation.

A logical treatment programme can be planned only after these findings are assessed.

Treatment

This depends upon severity of the disability. In mild cases treatment is unnecessary: explanation and reassurance suffice. In lumbar osteoarthritis with moderate disability a well fitted surgical corset (orthotic brace) will usually afford adequate relief. If the pain from a localized lesion is bad enough to cause serious hardship, operative fusion of the affected segments of spine may be required.

Physiotherapy Management

Physiotherapy is directed at:

- Relief of pain.
- Restoration of movement.
- Strengthening of muscles.
- Education of posture.
- Analysis of precipitating factors to reduce recurrence.

The following treatments may be used:

- *Heat:* A heat pad can help to relieve the aching which comes from prolonged muscles spasm. The best position is lying with one pillow under the head and two or three under the knees. Sometimes it is helpful to warm tight muscles in a stretched position. For the lumbar spine extensor pulsed or continuous electromagnetic energy can be applied to the patient, supported in side-lying with the knees, hips and lumbar spine flexed.
- *Ultrasound:* This is very useful for treating the thickenings in the periosteal attachments of erector spinae, quadratus lumborum and the thickened ligaments—sacrotuberous and sacroiliac ligaments.
- *Corsets:* Generally corsets are not indicated in these patients because mobility and good postural tone are the important themes. Short term elasticated strapping may be helpful during an episode of acute pain.
- *Relaxation:* This follows the same principles as described for cervical spondylosis.
- *Posture Education:* As in all postural deformities this includes training the patient in total body alignment. Foot and leg positions affect pelvic balance and can often be the underlying problem

even when patient insists that the pain is in the back and there is nothing wrong with the legs. *For example*, a habit of standing with the right knee slightly bent causes shortening of the hamstrings which pull the ischial tuberosity attachments tending to cause backward rotation of the right hip bone which pulls the quadiatus lumborum and these muscles start to ache. Standing habitually on the right leg with the knee straight causes shortening of the right hip abductors and the left trunk side flexors. Aching can start in both these muscles groups. Breaking these 'habits of lifetime' may not be possible but the patient can certainly be trained in the habit of regular stretching in the opposite direction. Mobility of joints and soft tissues must be gained before posture training is possible. At first correct alignment feels squint to the patient but it is essential to persevere until good alignment feels normal.

- *Manipulative Therapy:*
  - *Mobilizations:* Applied to stiff segments of lumbar spine, sacroiliac and hip joints these techniques gain mobility at a target level which is not possible by exercise. It is important to remember that all of these joints must contribute movement to lumbar pelvic rhythm. Stiffness of one component throws stress on the others.
  - *Soft tissue techniques:* Passive stretching of tight structures is also essential.
    - o The iliotibial tract is stretched by crossing the affected leg over the other together with side flexion of trunk.
    - o Tight side-flexors are stretched with the patient in side lying over a firm roll and the legs lowered over the edge of the bed or table.
    - o The posterior sacroiliac ligament is stretched with the patient prone and the knee on the affected side flexed. The sacrum is fixed by the physiotherapist and the patient's leg carried outwards (medial rotation of hip).

    Kneading, finger kneading and friction are all important in restoring mobility to supraspinous ligaments, quadratus lumborum, erector spinae (especially the sacral attachments) and glutei at their femoral attachment.
  - *Traction:* This is applied under same principle for cervical spine.
  - *Hydrotherapy:* Provided the patient is happy in water, hydrotherapy is very beneficial. It is not sensible to have a patient in the pool that holds the head out of the water in float lying because the back pain is aggravated. Relaxation in float lying followed by the physiotherapist moving the patient through the water and gradually moving the trunk increasingly from side to side gains mobility. This is especially useful for the patient who is afraid to move the spine after an episode of severe pain. The patient joins in the exercise and eventually should be able to swing the legs from side to side adding in trunk extension or flexion. Trunk rotation in sitting gains range in a relatively weight free position. Exercise against buoyancy–pushing both legs into the water in float lying strengthens the lumbar extensors. Swimming is generally beneficial. The freedom of the movement in water gains mobility and strength more quickly than on land. Mobilizations given before hand in water complement the benefits of pool.
  - *Movement:* Hold-relax can be applied to gain flexion. At first the patient is in lying with the knees flexed and crossed. The physiotherapist applies the technique by pushing on the knees. Later, provided there is no danger of disc prolapse, the technique can be applied in long sitting. The side flexors

can be lengthened by hold-relax applied to alternate hip updrawing. Active exercise comprises teaching the patient pelvic tilting forwards, backwards and sideways in crook lying, prone kneeling, sitting and standing. Then smooth pelvic movement needs to be re-educated, i.e., backwards to allow forward flexion, forwards to allow extension and sideways to allow side-flexion. Oblique movements should be taught for daily practice after discharge. Together with mobility, the patient should practice strengthening exercises for all the lumbar and hip muscles.

- *Advice:*
  - Always sleep on firm mattress.
  - Do not bend forwards from waist.
  - Do not lift heavy weights.
  - While getting from supine, always take a side turn.
  - Always bend by flexing the knees.

UNIT FOUR

INFLAMMATORY ARTHROPATHIES

CHAPTER 11

ANKYLOSING SPONDYLOSIS

DEFINITION

It is a chronic perhaps autoimmune seronegative disease characterized by progressive inflammatory stiffening of the joints with a predilection for the joints of axial skeleton, especially the sacro-iliac joints (Fig. 11.1).

The disease is also known as Marie-Strumpell disease.

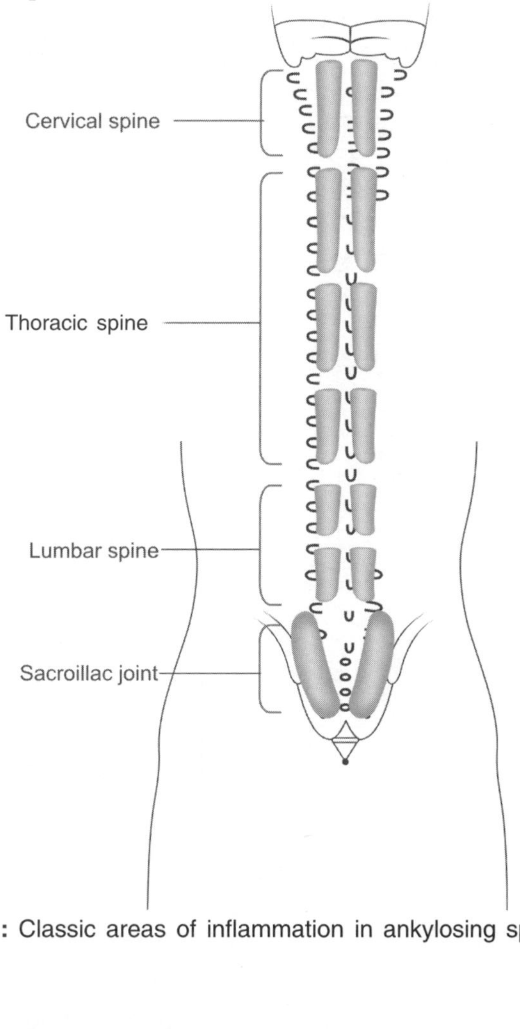

Fig. 11.1: Classic areas of inflammation in ankylosing spondylosis

Aetiology

Age: Onset is most common between 15 and 40 years although it can occur at any age.
Sex: It is most common is men than in women by a ratio of 3:1.
Incidence: 0.6% of adult males are affected.
Heredity: The disease occurs 30 times more commonly in relatives of patients than in general population.
Tissue type: 95% of patients with ankylosing spondylitis are HLA-B27 positive.

Pathology (Fig. 11.2)

There is involvement of synovium, articular capsule and ligaments where attached to bone. There is also cellular infiltration of periosteum to ligament or muscle junctions. Inflammation at the site of attachment of ligaments to bone is known as entheses and enthesopathy is the name given to formation of new bone at these areas. It is the characteristic feature of the disease process. It occurs especially in spine and around pelvis resulting in tufting of bone often along the iliac crests and from the femoral tuberosities as well as spine.

As a result of inflammatory change in spine, reactive bone formation occurs and bridging (Fig. 11.3) takes place between the vertebral bodies, usually from the edge of one body to that of next along the outer layers of the disc: this is known as marginal syndesmophyte formation. Anterior and posterior spinal ligaments are ossified. After bony fusion occurs, the pain may subside, leaving the spine permanently stiff resulting in *bamboo spine*. The disease is thus known as burnt out disease.

The disease can progress to bony ankylosis of sacroilic joints, sympyisis pubis, joints of lumbar, thoracic and cervical spines, costovertebral joints and manubriosternal junction. Sometimes the shoulders and knees also become affected. The changes undergo exacerbations and remissions.

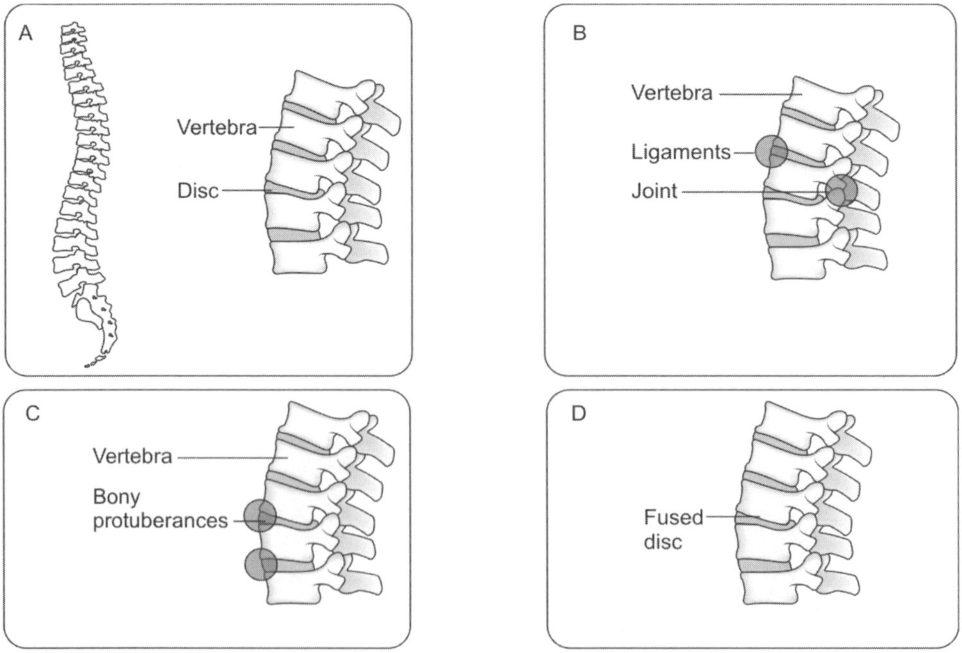

Fig. 11.2: Changes in ankylosing spondylosis

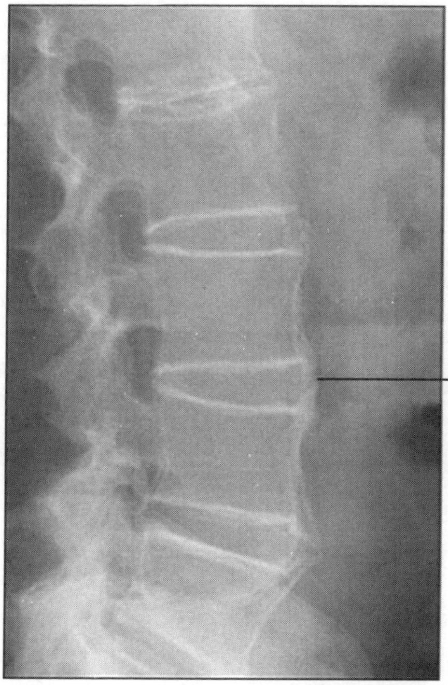

Fig. 11.3: Bony bridges

Clinical Features

Onset

This is often insidious with mild pain and stiffness in the lower lumbar spine. Sometimes the onset is acute with severe pain over sacroiliac joints and lumbar spine.

Clinical Presentations

The following clinical presentations may be seen:

- *Classical Presentation:* The patient is a young adult 15-30 years old male, presenting with gradual onset of pain and stiffness of lower back. Initially, the stiffness may be noticed only after a period of rest, and improves with movement. The pain tends to be worst at night or in early morning, awakening the patient from sleep. He gets better only after he walks about or does some exercises. There may be pain in the heel, pubic symphysis, manubrium sterni and costosternal joints. In later stages, kyphotic deformity of spine and deformity of hips may be prominent features.
- *Unusual Presentation:* The patient may occasionally present with the involvement of the peripheral joints such as shoulders, hips and knees. Smaller joints are rarely involved. Sometimes, a patient with ankylosing spondylitis may present with chronic inflammatory bowel disease; the joint symptoms follow.

Signs and Symptoms

- *Morning stiffness:* This is common in early stages.
- *Fatigue:* This is also common.
- *Spinal features (lumbar spine):*
  - Pain and stiffness in lumbar spine.
  - Radiating pain down the leg.
  - Spasm of lumbar paravertebral muscles.
  - Flattening of lumbar spine.
  - Loss of spinal movements.
- *Thoracic features:*
  - Loss of thoracic expansion.
  - Diminished costovertebral and manubriosternal movements.
  - Reduction in vital capacity.
- *Peripheral joints:* Pain and stiffness may develop in shoulders, hips and knees.

Extra-Articular Manifestations

In addition to articular symptoms, a patient with ankylosing spondylitis may have following extra-articular manifestations:

- *Occular:* About 25% patients with ankylosing spondylitis develop atleast one attack of acute iritis sometimes during the natural history of the disease. Many patients suffer from recurrent episodes which may result in scarring and depigmentation of the iris.
- *Cardiovascular:* Patients with ankylosing spondylitis, especially those with a long standing illness, develop cardiovascular manifestations

in the form of aortic incompetence, cardiomegaly, conduction defects, pericarditis etc.

- *Neurological:* Patients may develop spontaneous dislocation and subluxation of atlantoaxial joints or fractures of cervical spine with trivial trauma, and may present with signs and symptoms of spinal cord compression.
- *Pulmonary:* The involvement of costovertebral joints lead to painless restriction of thoracic cage. This can be detected clinically by diminished chest expansion, or by performing pulmonary function tests. There may also occur bilateral apical lobe fibrosis with cavitation, which remarkably simulates tuberculosis on X-ray.
- *Systemic:* Generalized osteoporosis occurs commonly. Occasionally a patient may develop amyloidosis.
- *Skin:* Associated psoriasis.
- *Colon:* Ulcerative colitis.

General Posture

The patient is observed from anterior, posterior as well as from both the sides to detect the overall postural deviations.

Initially the whole spine assumes a stiff posture. Later on, it may get totally fused. The spinal fusion gives rise to stiff and deformed posture where cervical spine is fixed in flexion with atlantoaxial hyperextension. Thoracic spine is fused in marked kyphosis leading to a rounded back. The hips and knees tend to assume compensatory attitude of flexion. Accurate measurements of the posture are taken at regular intervals with the help of spondylographs and/or clinical photographs.

Assessment

Tests for Detecting Sacroiliac Joint Involvement:

- *Tenderness:* Localised to the posterior superior iliac spine or deep in gluteal region.
- *Sacro-iliac compression (Fig. 11.4):* Direct side to side compression of pelvis may cause pain at sacroiliac joints.

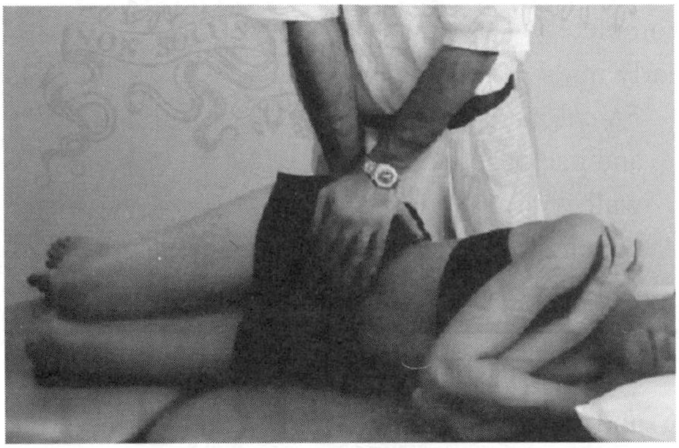

Fig. 11.4: Sacro-iliac compression test

- *Ganslen's test (Fig. 11.5):* The hip and knee of opposite side are flexed to fix the pelvis, and the hip joint of the side under test is hyperextended over the edge of the table. This will exert a rotational strain over sacroiliac joint and will give rise to pain.

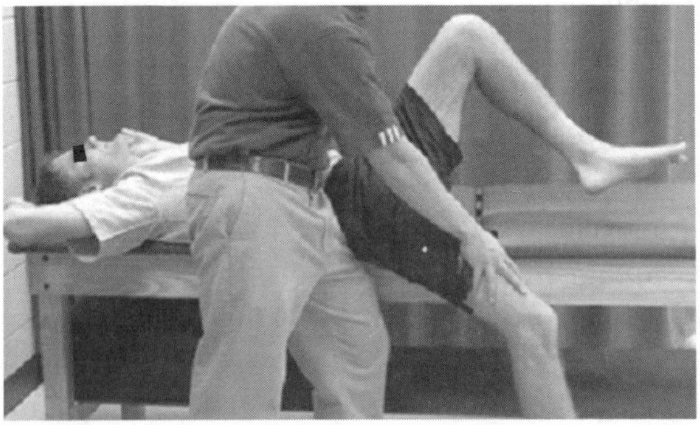

Fig. 11.5: Ganslen's test

- *Straight leg raising test:* The patient is asked to lift the leg up with the knee extended. This will cause pain at the affected sacroiliac joint.
- *Pump handle test:* With the patient lying supine, the examiner flexes hip and knee completely, and forces the affected knee across the chest so as to bring it close to the opposite shoulder.

This will cause pain on the affected side.

Tests for Cervical Spine Involvement

In advanced stages, the cervical spine gets completely stiff. The Fleche test may detect an early involvement of cervical spine.

- *Fleche test:* The patient stands with his heel and back against the wall and tries to touch the wall with the back of his head without raising the chin. The inability to touch the head to the wall suggests cervical spine involvement.
- *Thoracolumbar flexion-extension:* The distance between prominent seventh cervical vertebra and the sacro-coccygeal junction is measured in the erect, in full flexion and in full extension.
- *Lumbar flexion and extension:* On the patient's back two points are taken as landmarks: One midway between the spinous processes of fourth and fifth lumbar vertebra and another 10 cm above this. The difference between the 2 points measured in full flexion and extension provides the range of flexion-extension.
- *Lateral flexion:* The distance between the finger tip and the floor with the patient in maximum side flexion is measured.
- *Rotation:* The pelvis is rotated with the patient in supine, with the hips and knees flexed. The movement is then recorded.
- *Spinal flexion with hip flexion:* From erect posture patient bends forward without flexing the knees. The distance between the finger tip and the floor provides combined measure of hip and spinal flexion. Major arc of movement is contributed by hip joints. However, this assessment is important from the point of view of functional activities.
- *Examination of the peripheral joints:* Commonly involved peripheral joints like temporo-mandibular, shoulder, hip and knee should be examined for active and passive ROM.
- *Respiratory function:* An early involvement of costrovertebral joints results in gradual restriction of the movements of ribs and reduces the respiratory capacity. The chest expansion is markedly reduced often less than 2.5 cm. Chest expansion should be recorded at two levels: at xiphoid process (seventh rib) and at the nipple (fourth rib). The vital capacity, peak flow and forced expiratory volume should be recorded.
- *Functional status:* Functional status of the patient in relation to the disability and type of daily work is evaluated.

Radiological Examination

In a suspected case, an X-ray of pelvis and dorso-lumbar spine is required. Oblique views of sacro-iliac joints may be required in the early stages to appreciate their involvement.

Changes Observed in X-ray Pelvis

- Haziness of sacroiliac joints.
- Irregular subchondral erosions in SI joints.
- Sclerosis of articulating surfaces of SI joints.
- Widening of sacroiliac joint space
- Bony ankylosis of sacroiliac joints.
- Calcification of sacroiliac ligament and sacrotuberous ligaments.
- Evidence of enthesopathy—calcification at the attachment of the muscles, tendons and ligaments, particularly around pelvis and around the heel.

Changes Observed in X-ray Lumbar Spine

- *Squaring of vertebrae:* The normal anterior concavity of vertebral body is lost because of calcification of anterior longitudinal ligament.
- Loss of lumbar lordosis.
- Bridging osteophytes (syndesmophytes).
- Bamboo spine appearance.

Changes Observed in X-ray Peripheral Joints

- Formation of large osteophytes.
- Periarticular calcification.
- Bony ankylosis.

Blood Investigations

- Elevated ESR.
- HLA B 27-positive.

Treatment

No specific therapy is available. The aim is to control the pain and maintain maximum degree of joint mobility. These aims are readily achieved by the lifelong pursuit of a structured exercise programme. In some cases surgical intervention is required.

Conservative Methods:

- *Drugs:* NSAIDs are given for pain relief. Indomethacin is effective in most cases; long acting preparations are preferred.
- Physiotherapy.
- Yoga therapy.
- *Radiotherapy:* In some resistant cases.

Surgical Methods:

The role of surgery is in the correction of deformities. As for example:

- Correction of kyphotic deformities of spine by spinal osteotomy.
- Joint replacement for cases with hip or knee joint ankylosis.

Physiotherapy Management

Regular physiotherapy is essential in the management of patient with ankylosing spondylitis. Fibrous tissue is being continuously laid down as a result of mild inflammation and regular physiotherapy with monitored exercise programme moulds these fibrous tissue lines of stress which do not restrict the patient's movements.

Aims of Treatment

- To relieve pain.
- To mobilize the affected joints.
- To minimize deformity.
- To improve respiration.
- To improve body ergonomics.
- Improvement of muscle power and endurance.

Intervention

Pain and muscle spasm:

- The pain and muscular spasm in the acute stage are controlled by superficial modalities such as hydrocollateral packs or cryotherapy which can be applied locally to the specific joints and muscles affected.
- Muscle spasm that persists after the acute inflammation is treated best by hold-relax technique. Deep heating is effective in the chronic stage.
- Steam bath preceding the exercise controls pain and induces relaxation.

Mobility:

The objective is to maintain mobility of spinal intervertebral joints and peripheral joints by various procedures. The most important technique is repeated small range mobilization incorporated in activities of daily routine. The patient should be educated on the correct procedure. Suitable exercises to improve mobility can be enumerated as:

- *Lying:*
  - Physiological relaxation.
  - Practice feeling a position of straight extended spine.
  - Push arms and legs into the floor (Static contractions for quadriceps, glutei and back extensors).

- *Lying with knees bent (crook lying):*
  - Knees rolling from side to side.
  - Raise right arm upwards and outwards, turn head to watch hand. Repeat to left.
  - Deep breathing exercises with hands over upper abdomen—feel air fill under the hands and then sigh out feeling the hands sink down to encourage full use of diaphragm.
  - Pelvic tilting forwards and backwards.
- *Prone lying:*
  - Alternate straight leg raising (SLR) and lowering.
  - Both legs raising and lowering.
  - Hands clasped behind the back, thrust hands towards feet with head and shoulders raising and relaxing.
  - Place hands on the floor, raise head and shoulders:
    - o Walk hands to right and then to left (side flexion in extension).
    - o Arms stretch above head.
    - o Raise arms and ball plus head, shoulders and legs and then lowering.
- *Sitting:*
  - Stretch head and neck upwards (postural correction).
  - Hands on shoulders: trunk turning from side to side.
  - Hands clasp: bend and twist to touch right foot, stretch upwards and backwards to the left and repeat to opposite side.
  - Head and neck turning from side to side.
- *Standing:*
  - Hands on shoulders: trunk turning from side to side.
  - Deep breathing.
  - Trunk bending from side to side.

Deformity:
The body attitudes promoting the deformities should be discouraged. Maximum emphasis needs to be given to the static as well as dynamic postural attitudes.

Respiration:
Free active exercises with deep breathing maintain the mobility and improves respiratory capacity. Localized thoracic breathing without back support improves breathing capacity.

Body ergonomics:
The usual tendency to stoop should be strictly discouraged. Instead, the chest should be held up and forward with the shoulders retracted.
Repetitions of isometric shoulder bracing are valuable and should be made a part of daily routine.
Postural attitudes should be emphasized upon:
- Keep the chin tucked in.
- Repeated prone lying with hyperextension at dorsal spine on forearm supports.
- Hip hyperextension in prone.
- Trunk lateral bending with deep breathing.

Muscle power and endurance:
Muscles which are strong and capable of maintaining contractions will provide the necessary force to sustain correct posture. To induce relaxation and to improve mobility, active free movements play an important role. Muscles will be strengthened by the increase in exercise taken by the patient. Muscle power is retained by working against maximal resistance for a short time. Endurance is improved by working muscles against submaximal resistance for progressively longer times.

Importance of Hydrotherapy in Treatment of Ankylosing Spondylitis

Relief of pain and muscle spasm together with restoration of mobility is readily obtained by hydrotherapy. The warmth of the water effectively reduces protective muscle guarding thereby enabling the patient to make full use of available joint ranges by formal exercises or free swimming. Bad Ragaz patterns for arms, legs and trunk are effective in restoring mobility.

Procedures

- *Float lying:* Relaxation practice.
- *Float lying:* Arms and legs pushing down into water and resting.
- *Lying on half stretches:* Deep breathing exercises
- *Lying on half stretches:* Legs pushing down and out.
- Float lying: Arms stretching sideways and upwards.
- *Sitting:* Trunk turning side to side. Progress by holding arms forwards and grasping a bat.
- *Prone lying grasping rail:* Breast stroke action of legs.
- *Swimming:* Progress to underwater swimming.

CHAPTER 12

RHEUMATOID ARTHRITIS

DEFINITION

This is a non-suppurative, systemic inflammatory disease of unknown cause characterized by a symmetrical polyarthritis affecting peripheral joints and extra-articular structures. The course of the disease is variable but tends to be chronic and characterized by exacerbations and remissions.

Aetiology

The exact aetiology is not known. The following factors have been thought to play important role.

- A genetic predisposition is strongly suspected because of certain histocompatibility markers associated with it (HLA-drw 4/HLA-DRI).
- Agents such as mycoplasma, clostridium and some viruses (EB virus) have been implicated in its aetiology.

Age

The age of onset may be as young as 16 years but is generally in the 20-55 years of age group.

Gender

Women are affected more than men in the proportion of 3:1.

Causes

There are a number of hypotheses related to its causes. These are:

- *Initiating factor therapy:* An initiating factor causes joint inflammation and does not switch off after the acute episode.
- *Infectious theory:* Infections from diptheroids and mycoplasms or from viruses of rubella, herpes zoster or Epstein-Barr may be implicated.
- *Genetic predisposition:* Relatives of people with RA are more prone to develop the disease than the rest of population.
- *Autoimmune disease.*

Pathology

Rheumatoid arthritis is a generalized disorder of connective tissues affecting articular and extra-articular structures.

Articular Changes (Fig. 12.1)

- Initially the synovium becomes oedematous filled with fibrin exudates and cellular infiltrates. The vascular changes include focal areas of necrosis, the living synovial cells multiply and become

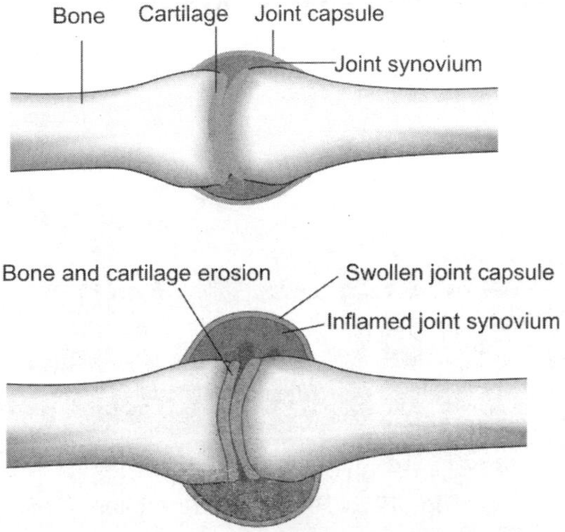

Fig. 12.1: Articular changes in rheumatoid arthritis

several layers thick. As the inflammation persists, the synovium gets hypertrophied and surrounds the periphery of the articular cartilage to form a pannus.

- Articular cartilage loses its smooth shiny appearance. The pannus extends over the cartilage from the periphery and burrows into subchondral bone. With further progress of the disease, the cartilage becomes worn off and the bone surfaces become raw.
- The erosion of subchondral bone leads to joint subluxation and deformity.
- Tendon sheaths behave in the same fashion as synovium and proliferative granulation tissue here may cause tendon rupture or attenuation.

Non-Articular Changes

- Nodules (Fig. 12.2) consist of a central neurotic core surrounded by mononuclear cells, plasma cells and lymphocytes. They develop in areas of pressure and may be subcutaneous or intracutaneous. They may also present in organs such as heart and lungs.
- Vascular changes constitute inflammation of the tunica intima of the arteries of all sizes. The lumen of small vessels can become obliterated.
- Persistent overstimulation of the reticulo-endothelium system occasionally leads to enlargement of spleen.

Stages of Rheumatoid Arthritis

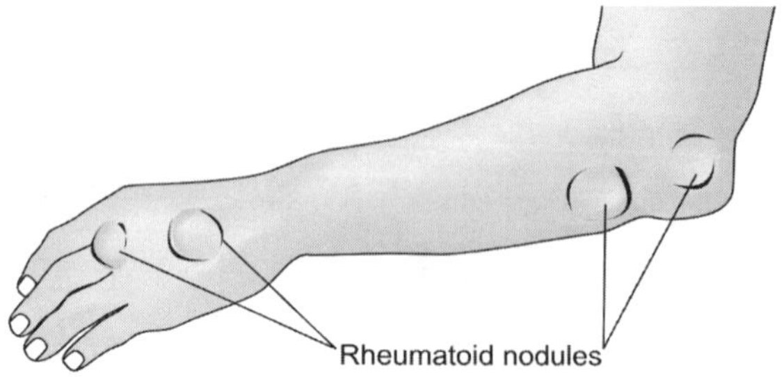

Fig. 12.2: Rheumatoid nodules

From the clinical viewpoint rheumatoid arthritis can be divided into three stages:

- *Potentially reversible soft tissue proliferations:* In this stage, the disease is limited to synovium. There occurs synovial hypertrophy and effusion. No destructive changes are evident on radiographs.
- *Controllable but irreversible soft tissue destruction and early cartilage erosions:* Radiograph shows a reduction in the joint space, but the outline of articular surface is maintained.
- *Irreversible soft tissue and bony changes:* The pannus ultimately destroys the articular cartilage and erodes the subchondral bone. The joint becomes ankylosed usually in a deformed position. It may be subluxated on dislocated.

Clinical Presentations

- *An acute symmetrical polyarthritis:* Pain and stiffness in multiple joints (atleast four) particularly in the morning mark the beginning of the disease. This may be followed by frank symptoms of articular inflammation.
- *Others:* The onset may be with fever, the cause of which cannot be established (PUO), especially in children. Sometimes, the visceral manifestations of the disease such as pneumonitis, rheumatoid nodules etc. may antedate the joint complaints.

Clinical Features

- *Symmetrical:* Peripheral polyarthritis starting distally and progressing proximally with acute episodes and remissions.
- *Palindromic:* Irregular attacks of pain and swelling in one or two joints. The pain may last few days and disappear. Nodules also may be present and then disappear. 50% of these patients progress to RA changes.
- *Polymyalgic:* There is diffuse joint pain and stiffness, but no synovitis. Joint disease and positive rheumatoid factor may follow.

- *Mono and oligoarticular:* There is pain and swelling in both knees. This occurs in young women and usually dies out after a couple of years with no long-term consequences.

Articular Features

There is generally a symmetrical polyarthritis with early involvement of small joints.

Joints affected in rheumatoid arthritis (Fig. 12.3)

Common	• Metacarpophalangeal joints of hand • Proximal interphalangeal joints of fingers • Wrists, knees, elbows, ankles
Less common	• Hip joint • Temporomandibular joint
Uncommon	• Atlantoaxial joint • Facet joints of cervical spine
Joints spared	• Distal interphalangeal joints • Sacroiliac joints

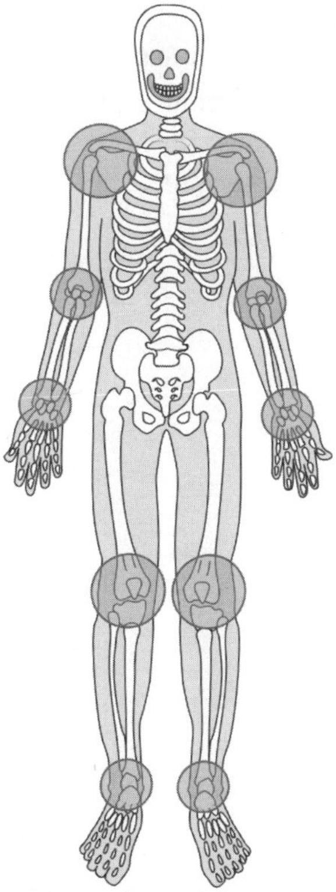

Fig. 12.3: Joints affected in rheumatoid arthritis

- *Pain:* This is present at rest and readily exaggerated by movement. It can be dull ache with sharp overtones.
- *Tenderness:* This is present over affected joints and can be aggravated by pressure of clothes or bed clothes.
- *Swelling:* There is both effusion (intra-articular) swelling and periarticular swelling in the soft tissues. During an acute phase, the swelling is fluid but as the disease progresses the synovial membrane and other soft tissues become thickened so that the joints appear enlarged.
- *Warmth over joints:* The skin over the affected joints is warm during an exacerbation in association with the inflammation of synovial membrane.
- *Loss of movement:* This is initially due to pain but can become permanent as the swelling becomes fibrosed and erosion of the joint surface leads to ankylosis.
- *Muscle atrophy:* Occurs rapidly around the inflammed joints both as part of the disease process and because of disuse.
- *Deformity*: During an acute exacerbation, the joints tend to be held in a position of comfort. As the disease progresses and irreversible joint changes occur, the deformity becomes permanent.

Deformities in RA

Hand	• Ulnar drift of hand • Boutonniere deformity • Swarm neck deformity
Elbow	• Flexion deformity
Ankle	• Equinus deformity
Knee	• Early—Flexion deformity • Late—Triple subluxation
Foot	• Hallux valgus, hammer toe

Non-Articular Features

- *Systemic:* Fatigue, weight loss, malaise, lassitude and sometimes low grade pyrexia.

- *Skin:* Thin, papery and shiny skin.
- *Nodules:* These are common over the elbows but can occur anywhere. They are round and firm but are not generally functionally disabling unless they interfere with tendon movement.
- *Vasculitis:* Inflammation of blood vessels which can be fatal if large arteries become occluded.
- *Cardiac involvement:* Pericarditis is a feature in some patients.
- *Respiratory features:* Pleurisy, pleural effusion and pulmonary fibrosis can all occur.
- *Sjögren's syndrome*: Dry eyes and mouth can occur in some patients.
- *Ocular features:* Inflammation and atrophy of lacrimal ducts leads to scleritis and conjunctivitis.
- *Felty's syndrome:* Enlarged spleen and leucopenia.

Individual Joint Involvement

- *Cervical spine:* Subluxation is common at atlantoaxial joint. It may produce root symptoms, upper motor neuron symptoms, visual disturbances, transient hemiparesis and vertigo.
- *Temporomandibular joint:* Pain and limitation of movement.
- *Cricoarytenoid joint:* It may progress from hoarseness of voice to stridor and thus needs regular and careful watch.
- *Shoulder joint:* Glenohumeral joint and rotator cuff involvement are common.
- *Elbow:* Limitation of extension is common. It may affect forearm movements also. Occasionally compression of the ulnar nerve may be present.
- *Wrist:* Subluxation of distal end of ulna may result in stiffness, deformity and pain. This may also cause rupture of extensor tendons of third, fourth and fifth fingers, ulnar deviation deformity and occasionally carpal tunnel syndrome.
- *Hands:* Palmar subluxation and ulnar deviation are common deformities due to involvement of metacarpophalangeal and proximal interphalangeal joints. A typical swan-neck deformity and boutonniere deformity may occur (Fig. 12.4).
- *Hip:* Erosion of head of femur occurs with its protrusion into acetabulum (protrusio acetabuli). Trochanteric bursitis may also occur. Eventually the hip may become stiff.

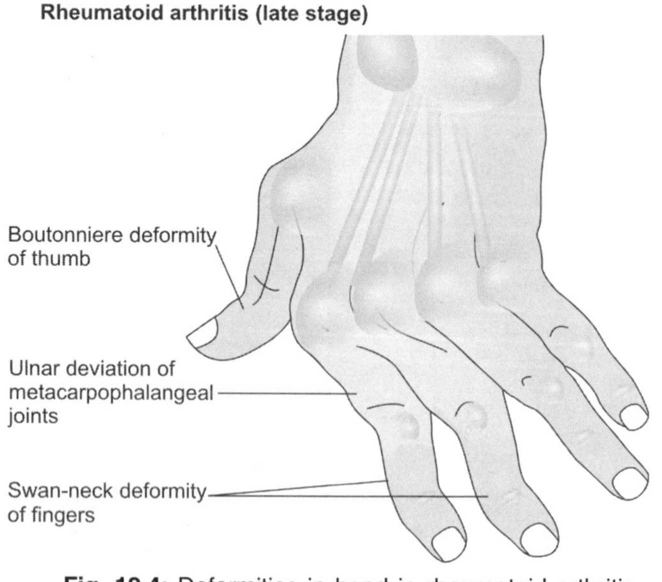

Fig. 12.4: Deformities in hand in rheumatoid arthritis

- *Knee:* Beginning with synovial lining swelling it may lead to severe destructive changes resulting in deformity like fusion or wind-swept deformity. Marked instability and secondary degenerative changes occur in the late stage.
- *Ankle and foot:* Ankle joint may be spared but the distal joint may usually be involved leading to valgus foot.
- *Metatarsophalangeal joint:* Subluxation may occur at these joints with hallux-valgus and toe fanning.

Diagnosis

Criteria for diagnosis of rheumatoid arthritis (American Rheumatism Association):

- Morning stiffness.
- Pain on motion or tenderness in atleast one joint.
- Swelling of one joint either due to soft tissue or effusion or both.
- Swelling of atleast one other joint with an interval free of symptoms no longer than three months.
- Symmetrical joint swelling.
- Positive test for rheumatoid factor in serum.
- Synovial fluid showing poor mucin clot formation when added to dilute acetic acid.
- Histopathology of synovium consistent with rheumatoid arthritis.
- Characteristic histopathology of rheumatoid nodules.
- Radiographic changes—erosion or unequivocal periarticular osteopenia.

If four or more of these are present, it is rheumatoid arthritis.

Investigations

Following are some useful investigations:

- *Radiological examination (Fig. 12.5):* This consists of X-rays of both hands and of affected joints. The following features may be present:
  - Reduced joint space.
  - Erosion of articular margins.
  - Subchondral cysts.
  - Juxta articular rarefaction.

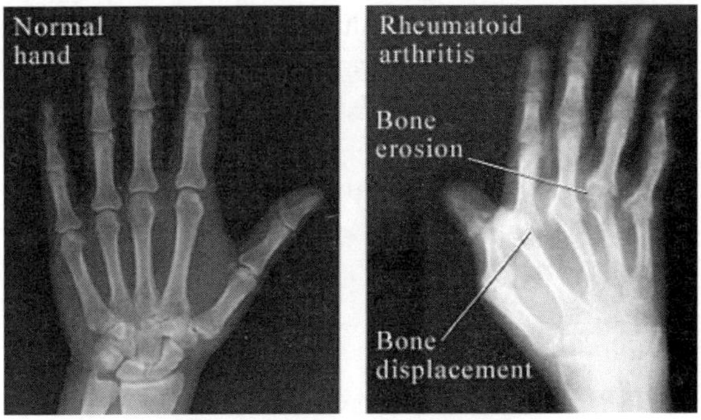

Fig. 12.5: Radiological changes in RA

  - Soft tissue shadow at level of joint because of joint effusion or synovial hypertrophy.
  - Deformities of hands or fingers.
- *Blood investigation:*
  - Elevated ESR.
  - Low haemoglobin value.
  - Positive rheumatoid factor.

Differential Diagnosis

- *Systemic lupus erythematosus (SLE):* In SLE, the joint involvement is not symmetrical, nor is ankylosis and erosions common. The absence of antinuclear antibody factor (ANF) is in favour of RA, although its presence does not confirm SLE. It is present in 25% cases of RA, though in low titres.
- *Osteoarthritis (OA):* This occurs in older patients. There is complete lack of systemic features of RA. The distal interphalangeal joints are often involved. The duration of morning stiffness, joint swelling, ESR are less compared to RA.
- *Psoriatic arthropathy:* Characteristic skin and nail lesions may be present. The distal interphalangeal joints are usually involved. The rheumatoid factor is negative.

Complications

- *Septic arthritis:* It is potentially fatal. It may be suspected when one or two joints are disproportionately inflamed, red, hot and painful especially if patient is generally unwell.

- *Amyloidosis:* Extracellular deposition of fibrillar material in the kidney, spleen, liver, adrenal glands and bowel.
- *Osteoporosis.*
- Atlanto-occipital subluxation.

Treatment

Principles of Treatment

- The induction of remission and its maintenance.
- The preservation of joint functions and prevention of deformities during active phase of the disease and thereafter.
- Repair of joint damage which already exists.

Medical Treatment

Medical treatment essentially consists of anti-rheumatic drugs.

- Non-steroidal anti-inflammatory drugs (NSAIDs).
- Disease modifying antirheumatic drugs (DMARDs).
- Steroids.

Orthopaedic Treatment

Orthopaedic treatment aims at:

- Prevention of deformity.
- Preservation of joint functions.
- Rehabilitation.

It falls essentially into conservative and surgical methods of treatment.

Conservative Methods

- Physiotherapy.
- Occupational therapy.
- Rehabilitation.

Surgical Methods

- *Preventive surgery:* This is done to prevent damage to joint and nearby tendons by the inflamed, hypertrophied synovium. It consists of synovectomy of wrists, knees and metacarpophalangeal joints.
- *Palliative surgery:* This is done in situations where general condition of patient does not permit corrective surgery, but where some relief can be provided by limited surgical procedures such as bone block operations, tendon lengthening etc.
- *Reconstructive surgery:* This has revolutionized the rehabilitation of patients with deformed and painful joints. It includes tendon transfers, interposition arthroplasties and joint replacements.

Physiotherapy Management

Assessment

- *Pain:* Self assessment by patient is valuable indicator to gauge the effect of pain on patient's performance. The pain felt is localized on a body image chart and quantified by the patient at each site identified. Pain is graded at sites identified between the extremes of 'no pain' and 'extreme pain' using some form of scale.
- *Swelling:* An attempt should be made by palpation to determine the source of swelling.
  - Excess synovial fluid is soft to the touch and compressible.
  - Thickened synovium presents with a firm though soggy feel.
  - Calcification produces hard nodules or ridges.
- *Skin condition:* Following should be noted:
  - General texture and condition of skin.
  - Skin lesions.
  - Subcutaneous nodules.
  - Alteration in texture of nails and hair.
  - Local erythema.
- *Deformity:* When recording deformity it is important to note whether it is fixed or correctable by passive means.
- *Joint range:* Both active and passive range of motion is noted.
- *Muscle strength.*
- *Respiratory function:* Following should be noted:
  - Thoracic excursion.
  - Vital capacity.

- Forced expiratory volume.
- Rate and depth of breathing.
- *Posture:* Standing and sitting posture should be noted.
- *Gait analysis:*
  - Use of aids.
  - Presence of abnormalities on weight bearing.
  - Step length.
  - Width of base.
  - Posture of trunk and limbs while walking.
- *Hand function:* Assessment of hand function along with daily activities should be noted, how able the patient is to support weight through upper limb. This is important for influence on choice of walking aids.

Principles of Physiotherapy Treatment

- Relief of pain and inflammation.
- Prevention of deformity.
- Correction of deformity.
- Restoration and maintenance of joint mobility.
- Improvement of muscular strength and endurance.
- Functional training.

Physiotherapeutic Intervention

- *Pain Relief:*
  - Application of heat in form of:
    - o Infra red radiation.
    - o Paraffin wax bath.
    - o Hot packs.
    - o Short wave diathermy.
  - Cryotherapy can be used provided that cooling is sufficiently prolonged to reduce conduction velocities of nerves supplying the muscles in protective spasm.
    - o Ice towelling.
    - o Ice cube massage over the affected joints.
  - Interferential therapy.
  - Isometric contractions of muscles surrounding the painful joint.
- *Prevention of Deformity:*
  - Postural awareness.
  - General exercises on land or in water will improve the strength of antigravity muscles and should be encouraged.
  - Passive stretching of tight structures must be specifically directed towards stretching the structures at risk.
  - Splintage is valuable particularly when joints are acutely affected.
  - Antideformity positioning.
    - o *Hands:* The wrist should be held in neutral position or in few degrees of extension; metacarpophalangeal joints should be just off full flexion; ulnar drift to be corrected; interphalangeal joints in 5° of flexion; thumb abducted and in opposition.
    - o *Knees:* Knees should be held in 5° of flexion.
    - o *Ankle:* The ankle should be held in plantigrade position without any varus or valgus deviation.
- *Correction of Deformity:*
  - Serial plasters.
  - Serial splinting.
  - Orthoses.
  - Dynamic splints.
- *Maintenance of Joint Range:*
  - Active assisted exercises.
  - Active exercises.
  - Proprioceptive neuromuscular facilitation.
    - o Slow reversal.
    - o Hold relax.
    - o Contract relax.
    - o Repeated contractions.
  - Hydrotherapy.
- *Maintenance and Improvement of Muscle Power:*
  - Resisted exercises.
  - Proprioceptive neuromuscular facilitation:
    - o Rhythmic stabilization.
    - o Slow reversal.
    - o Hold relax.
  - Postural reducation.
  - Strengthening of trunk muscles.
  - Resisted walking.
  - Hydrotherapy.

Management of Rheumatoid Arthritic Patient in Acute Phase

- Properly supported positioning of the involved joint and correct bed posture are important.
- Splints and sand bags may provide additional support.
- Deep breathing exercises are important to improve vital capacity.
- The joints and muscles free from immobilization are needed to put through full range of motion and progressive resistive exercises.
- Functional mobility should be encouraged and maintained.
- Postural guidance and methods of performing activities without putting extra strain on affected joints are taught.
- In cases with involvement of weight bearing joints the upper extremities should be prepared for full crutch walking.
- Isometric exercises do not involve the movements of joints and are therefore relatively painless and would be initiated early in the course of the disease.
- Speedy isometrics to affected limb in elevation reduces swelling and effusion.
- TENS, pulsed ultrasound, ice massage, ice packs or IFT reduces muscle spasm and pain.

UNIT FIVE

SHOULDERS COMPLEX CONDITIONS

CHAPTER 13

SHOULDER COMPLEX

FROZEN SHOULDER

Frozen shoulder is a common term used for any painful condition of the glenohumeral joint. The condition is characterized by pain and limitation of all the movements of the affected joint.

Other Names

The condition is also known as periarthritis shoulder, capsulitis.

Age of Onset

The condition usually affects the middle aged patient around 40 years of age.

Causes

- Insidious onset.
- Post traumatic.
- Post surgical.

Predisposing Factors

- Diabetes.
- Shoulder immobilization.
- Hypertension.

Pathology

The pathological changes in the condition are not fully understood. There is loss of resilience of joint capsule with adhesions (Fig.13.1) between the synovial folds causing restriction of movement and pain while attempting any movement. All the changes occurring are reversible.

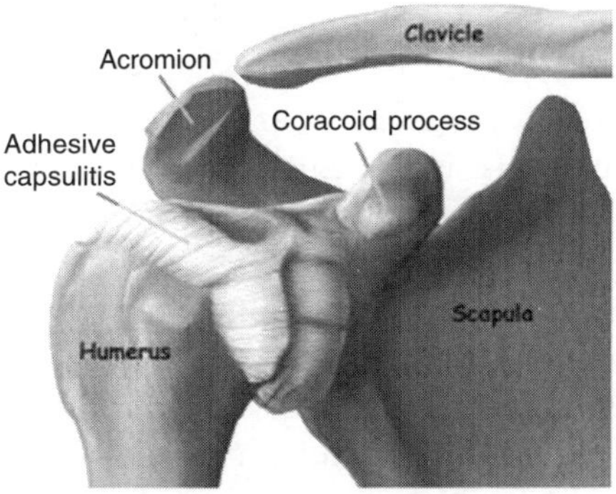

Fig. 13.1: Adhesions in between shoulder joint capsule

Clinical Features

- *Pain:* Patient complains of severe aching pain in the shoulder and upper arm, more common during night and usually disturbs the sleep.
- *Restricted Movements:* The range of motion of all the movements occurring at glenohumeral joint are restricted than the normal. The restriction of the movement usually follows the capsular pattern of the shoulder joint, i.e., lateral rotation, abduction and medial rotation.

Movement	*Normal ROM*	*ROM in frozen shoulder*
Flexion	0-180°	Limited
Extension	0-60°	Limited
Abduction	0-180°	Limited
Adduction	180°-0	Limited
Internal rotation	0-60°	Limited
External rotation	0-80°	Limited

The first movement to be restricted is the lateral rotation followed by abduction and medial rotation. Later, at chronic stage all the movements attempted at the joint are limited and painful.

Diagnosis

The clinical diagnosis of the condition known as frozen shoulder can be done by keeping the following points in mind.

- *Observation:* Bone and soft tissue outlines are normal.
- *Active Range of Motion:* The active range of motion is limited at the affected shoulder joint following the capsular pattern of restriction. Shoulder hiking is practiced by the patient during any of the movements to compensate for resticted range of motion.
- *Passive Range of Motion:* All the movements attempted passively are also limited in a proper capsular pattern. Pain and stretch is felt at the end range of motion as a result of capsular stretch.
- *Resisted Isometric Movement*: It is normal when the arm is by the side of the patient.
- *Resisted Active Movement*: In initial ranges it is pain free but the pain starts shooting up with increasing motion and increasing resistance.
- *Sensory Function and Reflex*: Any of the sensory function or the reflexes is not disturbed.
- *Palpation:* Palpation of the affected joint is not painful but any stretch to the joint capsule leads to immediate pain reaction.
- *Muscular Strength*: All the muscles around the shoulder joint are normal in their strength.
- *Special Test:* Apley's scratch test is positive.
- *Radiographic Diagnosis:* There are no radiographic changes visible in case of frozen shoulder.
- *Arthrography:* Decreased capsular size is identified.

Course of the Diseased Condition

There is tendency towards spontaneous recovery within six to twelve months but it does not hold true for every condition. The pain subsides first, leaving glenohumeral joint stiffness, which thereafter gradually resolves with the active use of limb. In some of the patient restriction of movements remain and spontaneous recovery does not occur and thus needs intensive treatment.

Differential Diagnosis

This condition of frozen shoulder or adhesive capsulitis should be well differentiated from the other conditions resulting in painful shoulder along with restriction of the shoulder joint movements. But in all the differentiating conditions there is no inflammation, adhesions or any changes or damage in the joint capsule. Some of the conditions are as follows:

- Tendinitis of rotator cuff.
- Sprain and tear of rotator cuff.
- Bicipital tenosynovitis.
- Synovitis of shoulder.

Management

The management of the frozen shoulder is basically by physiotherapeutic techniques along with aid of medical treatment which include:

- Analgesics.
- Non-steroidal anti-inflammatory drugs.
- Intra-articular steroid injection as for example: Hydrocortisone.
- Manipulation under general anaesthesia.

Physiotherapy Management

Physiotherapy plays an important role in the management of frozen shoulder. This serves two functions:

- Prevention of the condition.
- Resolution of the condition.

Preventive Programme

The preventive programme is helpful in both primary and secondary capsulitis.

- *Prevention of Primary Capsulitis:* Primary capsulitis is idiopathic in nature and its diagnosis is difficult as the pain and stiffness are not acute in the nature in early stage of the disease. The condition can be diagnosed by observing certain early symptoms like limited end range abduction both actively and passively along with pain in shoulder on lying at the affected side.

- *Prevention of Secondary Capsulitis:* Secondary capsulitis of the shoulder develops mainly due to immobilized shoulder joint usually after:
  - Fractures in upper limb.
  - Paralysed arm following stroke.
  - Unconscious patient.
  - Post surgical, e.g., mastectomy.

Prevention is done in form of early mobilization and movement in available range of motion.

Restorative Programme

Once the patient has established frozen shoulder, early and careful physiotherapy treatment is undertaken so that the patient can gain full functional mobility.

Aims of Restorative Programme

- To induce relaxation.
- To reduce pain.
- To increase range of motion.
- To improve muscular strength.
- To increase extensibility of soft tissues.

Intervention

To Induce Relaxation

Relaxation of the glenohumeral joint and all the structures surrounding the joint is a must before starting with any of the shoulder exercises as to make the exercises easier and pain free. Following measures should be taken in order to relax the glenohumeral joint:

- Shoulder girdle retraction and depression with hold and release should be practiced regularly throughout the day.
- General physiological relaxation before going to sleep.
- Prior heating of the affected joint induces relaxation and makes the exercises much easier. Any heating modality may be used as a suitable measure like short wave diathermy, infra-red therapy or hot packs.
- Axial traction of the glenohumeral joint.
- Relaxed passive mobilization in the form of rhythmic pendular movements in the available range of abduction-adduction makes the joints and muscles relaxed.

To Reduce Pain

Various pain relieving measures are taken before and after exercises in order to make the patient comfortable. Some of them can be enlisted as:

- *Heating modalities:* Short wave diathermy, hot packs, infrared therapy.
- *Interferential therapy*
  - Acute onset high intensity pain: 100-140 Hz.
  - Chronic low intensity aching pain: 50-100 Hz.
- Pulsed electromagnetic energy (PEME).
- Ice therapy is advantageous in relieving pain in patients of acute onset. Ice toweling is usually undertaken.

To Increase Extensibility of Soft Tissues

- Ultrasound therapy provides deep heating and added advantage of increasing extensibility of contracted soft tissues. It is usually applied over the tender spots of the shoulder joint.
- *Stretching of the tightened structures:* Passive stretching of tightened structures like pectoralis minor and/or major along with latissmus dorsi is undertaken. Stretching of the capsule at the end range of motion is done so as to increase the extensibility of the capsule of the shoulder joint.

Postural Correction

The postural correction is advantageous and needful in case of frozen shoulder and can be described as shoulder girdle retraction and depression along with the retraction of the head. It requires regular practice.

Increasing Range of Motion

The enhancement of the range of motion of the affected shoulder is the main requirement of the patient in case of frozen shoulder. Because of the limited motion patient is sometimes unable to perform his/her daily activities and thus faces a whole range of problems. Various measures can be undertaken to increase range like:

- Free active exercises.
- Passive mobilization.
- Proprioceptive neuromuscular facilitation.
- Sling suspension.

Free Active Exercises

- Codman's pendular exercises (Fig. 13.2) are the first set of exercises that are actively performed by the patient. The patient stands in walk standing and lean forwards from hips, bending the front knee and keeping the back knee straight. The affected arm should be hanged down freely from the shoulder. A weight cuff of 0.5 to 1 kg is tied around the wrist of freely hanging limb. This weight provides the traction to the humerus and increases the momentum of the movement. The movement of flexion-extension, abduction-adduction and circumduction are practiced to obtain the good arc of movement.

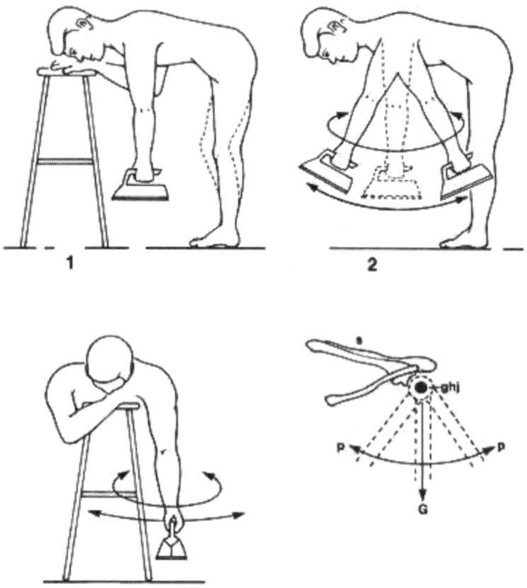

Fig. 13.2: Codman's pendular exercises

- *Ladder wall exercises (Fig. 13.3):* The exercise comprises the movement of the fingers on the wall as 'walking the fingers up the wall'. The exercise is used to gain elevation and monitor the progression of the range of motion. The movement up the wall is made in abduction as well as flexion.

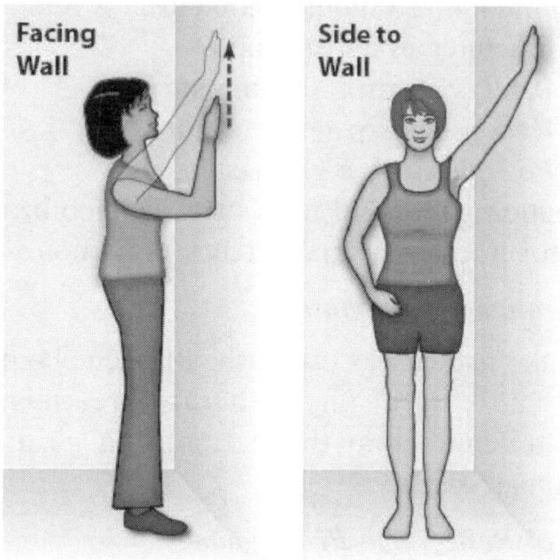

Fig. 13.3: Ladder wall exercises

- *Reciprocal pulley (Fig. 13.4):* It is used for auto-assisted elevation. The patient is in sitting position while performing flexion and back; abduction-adduction. The patient must be carefully instructed not to bend sideways or backwards and also not to over force the shoulder.

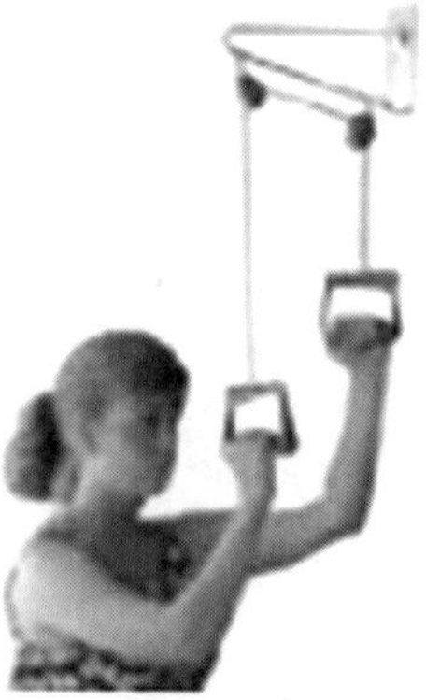

Fig. 13.4: Reciprocal pulley

Passive Mobilization

Accessory movements to the glenohumeral joints are essential for restoring the gliding between the joint surfaces necessary for every movement. Every precaution must be undertaken so as to carefully mobilize the joint without causing any injury or harm. The position of the patient and the therapist is very important along with the mechanism of mobilization (Table 13.1).

Proprioceptive Neuromuscular Facilitations (PNF):

- Stabilizations are appropriate at stage of acute pain. The patient should be taught:
  - Interlink hands together, push together, count 5.
  - Interlink hands together, pull apart without separating hands, count 5.
  - Place one fist on top of other, push together, count 5, Place other fist on top, push together, count 5.
- Hold relax technique is nearly always appropriate to gain lengthening of pectoralis major and latissimus dorsi.
- Repeated contractions are also useful to gain elevation, lateral and medial rotation and to strengthen the muscles producing these movements.
- Graduated relaxed sustained stretching based on PNF patterns designed for various movement combinations is advocated.

Sling Suspension

Abduction or flexion can be practiced in pain free range with gravity counter-balanced and this gives the patient confidence.

To Increase Muscular Strength

In order to increase the muscular strength of the muscles surrounding the shoulder girdle following can be practiced:

- Resisted exercises.
- Isometric strengthening exercises.
- Use of weight cuffs or dumbells.

Home Exercise Programme

There are certain do's and don'ts that the patient must follow so as to aid in effective recovery.

Do's:

- Hot water fomentation.
- Full range available movements of shoulder.

Table 13.1: Glenohumeral joint mobilization

Glide	*Indication*	*Position of patient*
Caudal glide	To increase abduction	Supine with arm in resting position
Caudal glide progression	To increase abduction when range approaches 90°	Supine with arm abducted to end of its available range. External rotation of humerus should be added to end-range position as arm approaches and goes beyond 90°
Elevation progression	To increase elevation beyond 90° of abduction	Supine with arm abducted and elevated to end of its available range. The humerus is then externally rotated to its limit
Posterior glide	To increase flexion and internal rotation	Supine with arm in resting position
Posterior glide progression	To increase horizontal adduction and flexion when reaches 90°	Supine with arm flexed to 90°, internally rotated with elbow flexed. The arm may also be placed in horizontal adduction
Anterior glide	To increase extension and external rotation	Prone with arm in resting position over edge of treatment table
Anterior glide progression	To increase external rotation	Shoulder in resting position

- Pendular exercises.
- Toweling action.

Don'ts:

- Don't sleep on the affected side.
- Don't lift heavy weight from affected arm.
- Don't try out any passive movement at home.
- Don't massage the affected part.

SUPRASPINATUS TENDINITIS

The tendon of the supraspinatus passing underneath the acromion process of the scapula gets inflamed (Fig. 13.5) causing pain and movement restriction at the shoulder joint.

Causes

- Fall on the shoulder tip.
- Over exercises as for example aerobics.
- Series of minor steps as writing.

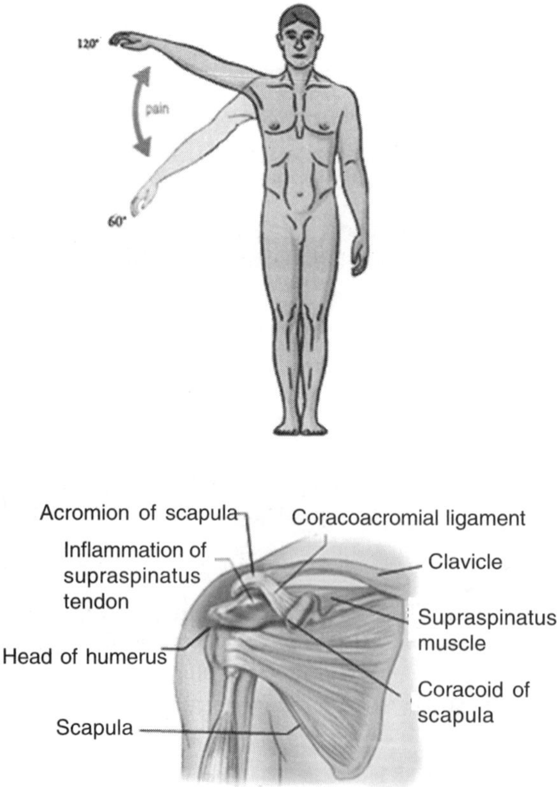

Fig. 13.5: Painful arc in supraspinatus tendinitis

Clinical Features

Pain

- The pain is tooth ache like.
- It radiates from acromion process to the insertion of deltoid.
- The pain is characteristically present in the abduction arc of 60-120° (Fig. 13.5).

Shoulder Movements

- The active range of motion at the affected shoulder joint is full but painful.
- Abduction and flexion shows a characteristic painful arc between 60–120°.
- Resisted abduction is painful.

Tenderness

Tenderness can be elicited while the patient is sitting or standing with shoulder medially rotated i.e. arm at the back. Tenderness is present at anterior aspect of acromion process.

Diagnostic Tests

- While the patient is making an attempt to lower the arm from the elevated position it is very painful but if this attempted as a resisted movement, it becomes pain free.
- While attempting any movement at the glenohumeral joint, the glenohumeral rhythm is reversed.
- *Empty Can or Jobe Test:* The patient's arm is abducted to 90° with neutral rotation and resistance to abduction is provided by the examiner. The shoulder is then medially rotated and angled 30° forwards (empty can position) so that the thumb of the patient points towards the floor (Fig. 13.6). Pain reflects the positive test indicating supraspinatus tendinitis.

Management

- Non-steroidal anti-inflammatory drugs (NSAIDs).
- Hydrocortisone.

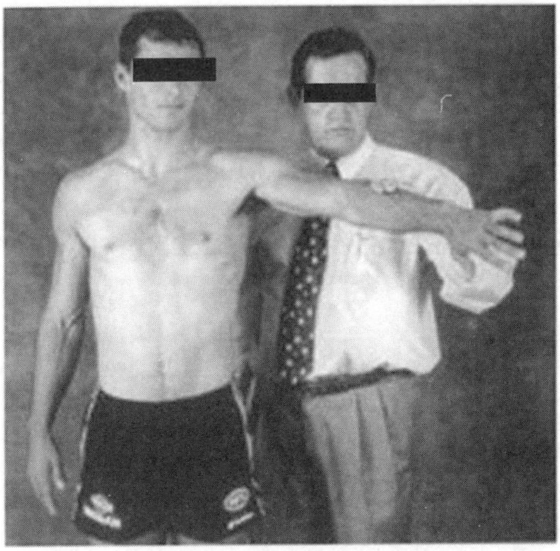

Fig. 13.6: Empty can test

Physiotherapy Management

Physiotherapy management plays an important role in preventing and treating the supraspinatus tendinitis.

Aims of Physiotherapy Management

- To reduce inflammation.
- To reduce adhesions.
- To improve shoulder movements.
- To improve glenohumeral rhythm.
- To prevent the occurrence of frozen shoulder.

To Reduce Inflammation i.e. Pain and Swelling

- Rest in arm sling.
- Ultrasonic therapy to the tendon with arm in extension and medial rotation.
- Cryotherapy in the form of ice toweling applied to superior aspect of shoulder for 10-20 minutes.

To Reduce Adhesions

- Ultrasonic therapy over the tendon of the supraspinatus.
- Transverse friction applied to the supraspinatus tendon in the sub-acute or chronic stage of tendinitis positioning the arm in extension, medial rotation and adduction. With the aid of transverse friction the tendon is mobilized, adhesion are softened and stretched.

To Improve Shoulder Movements

- Auto-assisted elevation through flexion and abduction.
- Active shoulder movements to be practiced in full range.

To Improve Glenohumeral Rhythm

- Slow reversal technique of PNF
- Stabilization techniques of the scapula.
- Teaching the correct pattern of movement.

To Prevent the Occurrence of Frozen Shoulder

Shoulder mobilization exercises are practiced at regular intervals so as to prevent the occurrence of frozen shoulder.

Prevention of Supraspinatus Tendinitis

- Poor posture predisposes to stress on tendon leading to its tendinitis, thus protraction and depression of shoulder girdle is practiced to improve the posture.
- Stretching of the pectoralis major, as its tightness may prevent lateral rotation of humerus during elevation.

INFRASPINATUS TENDINITIS

The infraspinatus tendon if subjected to trauma results in inflammation. It is usually chronic in presentation rather than acute.

Clinical Features

- No pain is usually present at rest.
- Weakness is noticed during the functional use of the shoulder.
- Lateral rotation is usually restricted.
- All other movements at the glenohumeral joint are free.
- Painful arc may be present in initial 30° of lateral rotation.

- *On palpation:* The tendon is thickened and muscle fibers are taught.
- Resisted lateral rotation is usually painful.

Diagnostic Test

- *Spring Back Test:* The patient is seated or in standing position with the arm by the side and the elbow flexed to 90°. The examiner passively abducts the arm to 90° in the scapular plane, laterally rotates the shoulder to end range and asks the patient to hold it. For a positive test, the patient cannot hold the position and hand springs back anteriorly towards the midline.
- *Drop Sign:* The test is performed with arm in 20° abduction of by the side in scapular plane with elbow at 90° and the shoulder laterally rotated, the examiner then takes the arm into maximum lateral rotation and asks the patient to hold the position. The arm drops back to 0° lateral rotation.

Management

Injection of hydrocortisone is given at the site of lesion in the tendon of infraspinatus.

Physiotherapy Management

- Ultrasonic therapy to the affected tendon proves to be very beneficial in reducing pain and inflammation.
- Deep transverse friction massage is very effective.
- Hold-relax technique of PNF is utilized to gain the range of lateral rotation.
- Elevation at the shoulder girdle should be practiced both in flexion and abduction.
- Strengthening of lateral rotators is the important aspect of management of infraspinatus tendinitis. It may be done with aid of resistive exercises or a chest expander (spring resistance for both the arms).

SUBSCAPULARIS TENDINITIS

Causes

- Overstrain or continuous overuse causes stress injury to the tendon resulting in tendinitis.

Clinical Features

- Pain at the terminal range of active internal rotation.
- All the passive movements at the shoulder joint are full and painless.
- Resisted shoulder medial rotation is extremely painful.

Diagnostic Test

- *Lift off sign (Fig. 13.7)*: The patient stands and places the dorsum of the hand on the back pocket or against the mid lumbar spine. The patient then lifts the hand away from the back. An inability to do so indicates the lesion.

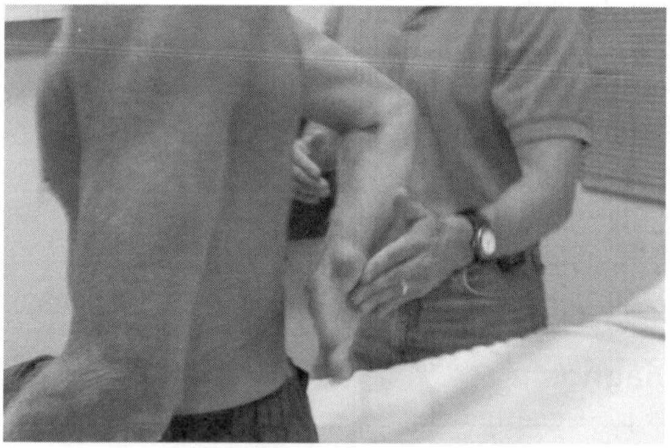

Fig. 13.7: Lift off sign

Management

Hydrocortisone may be injected at the site of the lesion.

Physiotherapy Management

- Rest to the part is important in the acute stage.
- Cryotherapy.

- Ultrasonic therapy.
- Strengthening of internal rotators.
- Relaxed pain free full range passive movements to avoid secondary stiff shoulder.

BICEPS BRACHII TENDINITIS

The tendinitis of biceps brachii is often a rare injury.

Causes

- Overuse or severe strain.
- Frictional irritation to the tendon within its groove.
- Degeneration of the tendon.

Clinical Features

- Pain in front of the shoulder joint becoming worse on the active use of the arm.
- Local tenderness can be elicited in the course of long tendon of biceps in the bicipital groove of the humerus.
- Resisted flexion of the elbow with forearm in supination elicits pain.
- Strength of the muscles during movement of flexion as well as supination is quite normal.
- In chronic case, a bulge is noticed in the arm in the vicinity of muscle bulk of biceps.
- Patient experiences a feeling of giving way during lifting or pulling.

Diagnostic Test

- *Speed's Test or Straight Arm Test (Fig. 13.8):* The examiner resists the shoulder forward flexion by the patient while the patient's forearm is first supinated then pronated and the elbow is completely extended. The test may also be performed by forward flexing the patient's arm to 90° and then asking the patient to resist an eccentric movement into extension first with forearm supinated then pronated. A positive test elicits increased tenderness in the bicipital groove especially with forearm supinated indicating bicipital tendinitis.

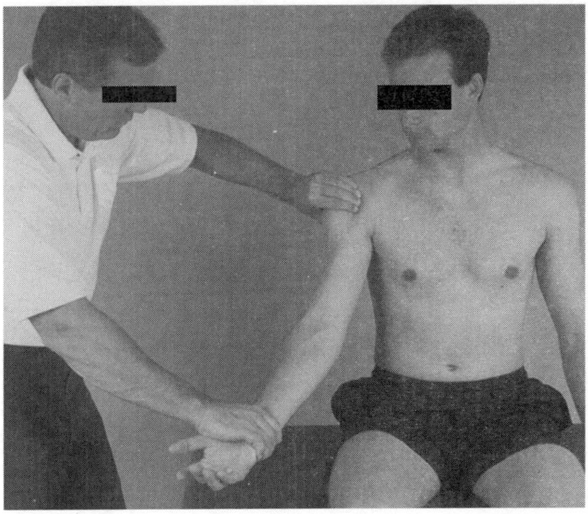

Fig. 13.8: Speed's test

- *Yegarson's test (Fig. 13.9):* The patient's elbow is flexed to 90° and stabilized against the thorax and with forearm pronated, the examiner resist supination while the patient rotates the arm laterally against resistance. The tendon of the biceps will be felt 'Pop out' of the groove along with increased tenderness on palpation indicative of bicipital tendinitis.

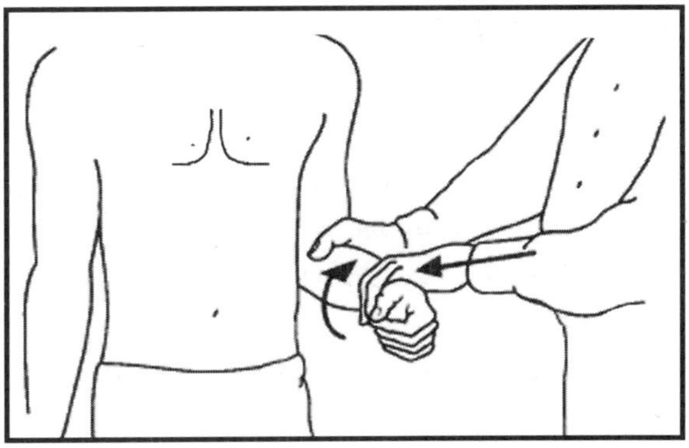

Fig. 13.9: Yegarson's test

Management

- Analgesics.
- Rest in the sling.
- Injection of hydrocortisone in the tendon.

Physiotherapy Management

- Cryotherapy adjuncts are used initially to reduce pain and inflammation.
- Ultrasonic therapy.
- Transverse friction massage is advocated to break adhesions and make the tendon mobile.
- Reciprocal relaxation is tried for the biceps brachii by inducing isometrics to triceps and pronators.
- Graduated strengthening regime for the movements of flexion at elbow and supination at forearm initiating with relaxed passive movements progressing to assisted. As active painless range is achieved, resistive movements should begin.

ROTATOR CUFF INJURIES

Rotator cuff injuries occur because of mechanical abrasion within a decreased glenohumeral joint space. The most frequent cause in an active young adult is excessive anterior translation of the humeral head within the joint space.

Following factors are taken into account while considering the mode of treatment:

- The degree of instability.
- Whether the condition is acute or chronic.
- The strength and endurance of the shoulder girdle musculature particularly the rotator cuff.
- The patient's performance or activity requirements.
- The flexibility of the soft tissues around the shoulder.

The most important caveat to any rotator cuff rehabilitation program is avoiding excessive anterior translation of the humeral head so that dynamic joint stability is restored. In addition, all strengthening exercises should be modified to allow pain free motion.

Conservative Management

Phase I

To reduce inflammation, the patient needs to modify or refrain from activities that aggravate the condition. The therapist will apply modalities as needed and perform or direct range of motion exercises.

Active strengthening exercises for internal and external rotation are performed with the arm at the side and the elbow flexed to 90° using surgical tubing or other elastic bands for resistance. If necessary, modify the external rotation exercise by limiting the degree of rotation; this will avoid excessive translation of the humeral head out of the fossa and reduce discomfort. If pain continues, switch to isometric exercise, keeping the arm in the same position, i.e., at the side with the elbow flexed to 90°. If this still causes discomfort, adjust the shoulder position to allow a bit of abduction and flexion, ie., loose packed position.

As pain decreases and strength increases, progress to free weights. Internal rotation is best done lying on the involved side with a bolster under the lateral chest wall (Fig. 13.10) to decrease the joint compression on the involved shoulder.

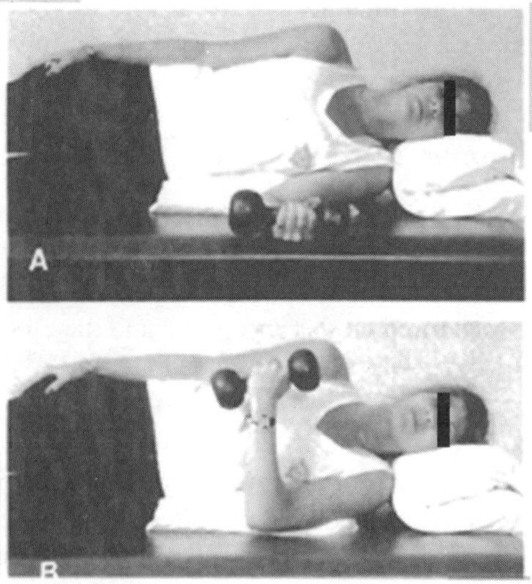

Fig. 13.10: Internal rotation exercise with dumbbell

Limit excursion into external rotation on the eccentric portion of the exercise to minimize stress on the anterior capsule. External rotation is performed while lying on the uninvolved side (Fig. 13.11).

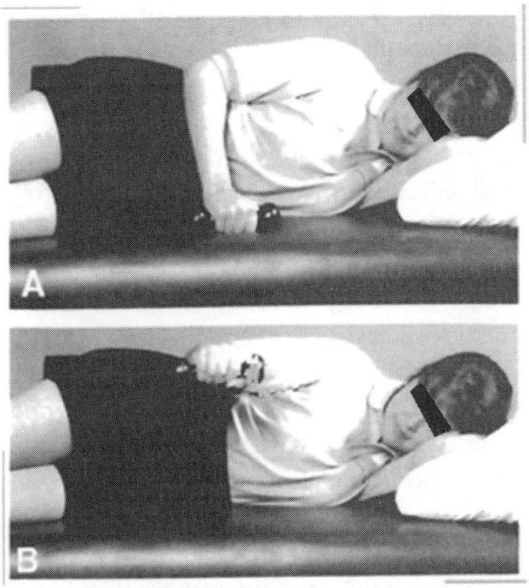

Fig. 13.11: External rotation exercise with dumbbell

If 90° of elevation is available in the scapular plane (20-30° forward of the coronal plane), add supraspinatus exercise (Fig. 13.12).

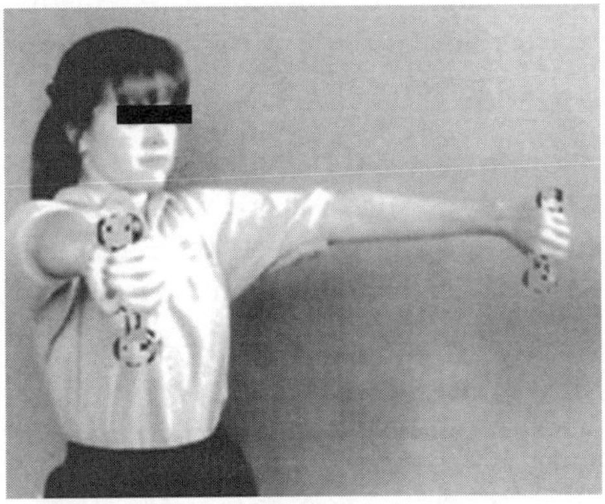

Fig. 13.12: Supraspinatus exercise

Alternate these exercises with active shoulder flexion through the pain-free range of motion and shoulder abduction performed in the scapular plane. Attention should be paid to develop strength and endurance in the anterior and middle deltoid in the overhead (i.e., above 90° of elevation) position. These exercises need to be performed without irritating cuff structures or the long head of the biceps.

Shoulder extension exercise can be done either prone or standing (bending forward from the waist). The involved shoulder should not be moved behind the plane of the body. The shoulder extensors also function as depressors of the humeral head and, thus, resist the upward migration of the humeral head and decrease the likelihood of further impingement. Even early in the rehabilitation program, shoulder endurance exercises should be included. As soon as adequate pain-free range of motion is present, add arm ergometer exercise. Begin with short duration, low intensity, and frequent rest periods; increase duration and intensity and decrease rests as recovery and tolerance proceed.

Phase II

Continue posterior cuff and capsule stretching and shoulder range of motion exercises. As healing progresses, more aggressive stretching may be warranted if adequate range has not yet been obtained.

If there is no pain and no significant edema, begin isokinetic programs for both strength and endurance. Use speeds in excess of 200°/sec for shoulder internal and external rotation. The best and safest patient position is standing with the dynamometer head tilted and the shoulder in the scapular plane (Fig. 13.13), arm at the side.

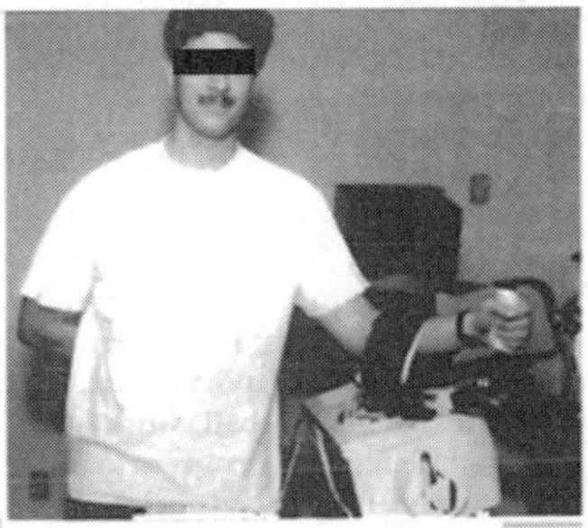

Fig. 13.13: Isokinetic exercises with dynamometer

In the free weight portion of the exercise program at this stage, eccentric contraction of the rotator cuff and the posterior shoulder girdle musculature is emphasized. To this end, add active horizontal adduction exercise, with the starting position in the scapular plane. Both military presses and push-ups are added now.

Initiate wall push-ups concentrating on protraction of the scapula to emphasize serratus anterior function. Pay special attention to getting full extension of the elbows and an extra "push" into full scapular protraction at the end of the exercise. Do not lower the trunk below elbow level. This caution is necessary during the descent phase to avoid excessive anterior translation of the humeral head.

Begin low intensity level for the specific sport or activity, e.g., volleyball, basketball, and progress logically and carefully. Lunges, squats, trunk strengthening and flexibility, and general cardiovascular conditioning should be added now.

Phase III

The culmination of the rehabilitation program involves continuation of the total body conditioning program and progressive throwing program, emphasis on the eccentric phase of rotator cuff strengthening, and progressively more difficult isotonic exercises. Isokinetic flexion/extension and abduction/adduction exercise may be added, along with longer bouts on the arm ergometer. Skill refinement includes work at an increased intensity, sustained for an extended time.

Postoperative Rehabilitation

Surgical procedures will address the underlying pathology of inadequate glenohumeral joint space, or excessive joint laxity or frank muscle tears.

Phase I

If the patient has had an open rotator cuff repair, no active shoulder flexion or abduction is allowed for the first month. Shoulder is immobilized using a sling except for gentle passive range of motion in flexion, abduction, and external rotation. With the arm at the side and the elbows extended, active shoulder internal and external rotation is permitted. Modalities and mobilizations are used for pain control. Active exercises include shoulder shrugs, pendulum exercises, and ball squeezes.

If the patient has had an anterior capsulolabral reconstruction, he or she may be in a pillow abduction splint or an "airplane" type splint for a period of a few days to 2 weeks. While in the splint, the patient should be instructed for active and active- assisted elevation exercises, lifting the arm up and out of the restraint. Elbow flexion and extension, wrist motion, and ball squeezes are also required. After the appropriate time interval for each patient, active assistive exercises, e.g., wall climb, wand, etc., and active range of motion exercises begin, using joint mobilization to improve motion if necessary. Begin isometric internal and external rotation, abduction, flexion, and extension in a number of positions throughout the pain-free range (multiple-angle isometrics). Active resistive exercises begin with shoulder internal and external rotation, arm at the side, using elastic bands or tubing. Add active shoulder extension either prone or standing while bending at the waist and extend the arm to the plane of the trunk. As tolerated, add horizontal adduction in supine. As in the non-operative rehabilitation program, this exercise should be started with the arm in the scapular plane.

Phase II

Continue range of motion exercises and more vigorous stretching of capsular tissues. Hanging from an overhead bar is a more aggressive stretch for shoulder motion. Begin by taking as much weight as tolerated and progress to a full body hang. As strength improves, add elastic band resistance to shoulder internal and external rotation exercises. Keep the arm at the side. Progress to free weights in side lying and remember to position the arm with a bolster under the lateral chest wall for internal rotation. Add active strengthening exercises for elevation: flexion, abduction, and supraspinatus. For flexion, pay special attention to the anterior portion of the deltoid and add work in the 110-125° range. Limit abduction to 90° since deltoid activity peaks at this angle. Supraspinatus exercise and flexion exercise should be performed in a pain-free range of motion only. Begin active horizontal abduction exercise, either prone or leaning over from the waist. Limit motion to the plane of the trunk at the end of the exercise, still allowing the scapular adductors to perform. Make certain that the initial motion is occurring at the glenohumeral joint; scapular adduction and trunk rotation can disguise horizontal abduction, making it appear that more motion is occurring than is actually the case.

Phase III

By this time, the patient should have full passive and active range of motion. Continue isotonic rotator cuff exercises, with emphasis on eccentric strengthening as well as strengthening elbow and wrist musculature as necessary. Begin military press exercise. This should be done with the arm in front of, rather than behind, the chest to decrease the load on the cuff. Begin push-ups with emphasis on protraction at the end of the exercise. Start with wall push-ups, move on to modified hands-and knees push-ups, and, finally, use the full hands and toes variety. When the patient has the ability to lift 5-10 lbs in external rotation and 15-20 lbs in internal rotation, is pain free, and has no significant edema, begin isokinetic strength and endurance training at 200+°/sec. Add arm ergometer work and include conditioning for the rest of the body as well. Include significant workouts for lower extremity and trunk musculature.

Phase IV

It is important for isokinetic testing to demonstrate that the involved shoulder has at least 90% of the strength and endurance of the uninjured shoulder before progressing to sports- or activity-specific exercise. Throwing athletes may then proceed to a throwing program, and others may proceed to their appropriate programs. Meanwhile, total body conditioning continues, and abduction/adduction, horizontal abduction/adduction may be added.

IMPINGEMENT SYNDROME

The space between the undersurface of the acromion and the superior aspect of humeral head is called the impingement interval. This space is anatomically narrow and is maximally narrowed when the arm is abducted. Any condition that further narrows this space can cause impingement. Impingement can result from extrinsic compression or from loss of competency of the rotator cuff.

Risk Factors

Impingement is common in both young athletes and middle-aged people. Young athletes who use their arms overhead for swimming, baseball and tennis are particularly vulnerable. Those who do repetitive lifting or overhead activities using arm, such as paper hanging, construction or painting are also susceptible. Pain may also develop as a result of minor trauma or spontaneously with no apparent cause.

Causes

Primary Impingement

- Increased subacromial loading.
- Acromial morphology (Type 2 and Type 3 acromions).
- Acromioclavicular arthrosis (inferior osteophytes).
- Coracoacromial ligament hypertrophy.
- Coracoid impingement.
- Subacromial bursal thickening and fibrosis.
- Prominent humeral greater tuberosity.
- Trauma (direct macrotrauma or repetitive microtrauma).
- Overhead activity (athletic or non-athletic).

Secondary Impingement

- Rotator cuff overload/soft tissue imbalance.
- Eccentric muscle overload.
- Glenohumeral laxity/instability.
- Long head of biceps tendon laxity/weakness.

- Glenoid labral lesions.
- Muscle imbalance.
- Scapular dyskinesia.
- Posterior capsular tightness.
- Trapezius paralysis.

Stages of Rotator Cuff Impingement

Neer described the following three stages in the spectrum of rotator cuff impingement:

- *Stage I:*
  It commonly affects patients younger than 25 years of age. The stage is depicted by acute inflammation, edema and haemorrhage in the rotator cuff. This stage is usually reversible with conservative treatment.
- *Stage II:*
  It usually affects patients aged 25-40 years, resulting as a continuum of Stage I. The rotator cuff tendon progresses to fibrosis and tendonitis, which commonly does not respond to conservative treatment and requires surgical intervention.
- *Stage III:*
  It commonly affects patients older than 40 years of age. As this condition progresses, it may lead to mechanical disruption of the rotator cuff tendon and the changes in the coracoacromial arch with osteophytosis along with anterior acromion. Surgical intervention in the form of anterior acromioplasty and rotator cuff repair is commonly required.

Outlet Impingement

The supraspinatus outlet is a space formed on the upper rim, humeral head and glenoid by the acromion, coracoacromial arch and acromioclavicular joint. This outlet accommodates the passage and excursion of the supraspinatus tendon. Abnormalities of the supraspinatus outlet have been attributed to a cause of impingement syndrome and rotator cuff disease. Impingement implies extrinsic compression of the rotator cuff in the supraspinatus outlet space. Variations in acromial size and shape can also contribute to impingement. Other sites of impingement in the supraspinatus outlet space include the coracoacromial ligament (thickening) and the undersurface of acromioclavicular joints (osteophyte formation). These impingement sites in the supraspinatus outlet are compressed further when the humerus is placed in the forward flexed and internally rotated position, forcing the greater tuberosity of the humerus into the undersurface of the acromion and acromioclavicular arch.

Nonoutlet Impingement

Causes of nonoutlet impingement includes loss of humeral head depression either from a large rotator cuff tear or from weakness in the rotator cuff muscles due to C5/C6 neural segmental lesion or a suprascapular mononeuropathy. This condition may also occur because of thickening or hypertrophy of the subacromial bursa and rotator cuff tendons.

Symptoms

- Mild pain present both at rest and on activity.
- Radiating pain from front of the shoulder to side of the arm.
- Sudden pain with lifting and reaching movements.
- Athletes in overhead sports may have pain when throwing or serving a tennis ball.
- Local swelling and tenderness in front of the shoulder.
- Pain and stiffness in lifting the arm.
- Pain can be present at night which can even disturb the sleep.
- Reduced range of motion with difficulty in the activities like placing the hand behind the back.
- In advanced cases loss of motion may progress to a frozen shoulder.

Rehabilitation Following Conservative Treatment of Shoulder Impingement

Acute Phase

Aims:

- To reduce inflammation (pain, swelling).

- To maintain flexibility.
- To retard muscle atrophy.

Intervention:

- Cryotherapy can be used to reduce inflammation.
- Use of transcutaneuos electrical nerve stimulation and high voltage galvanic stimulation is also advised.
- Pendulum exercises in limited symptom free range are advocated to improve and maintain range of motion.
- Active assisted exercises with rope and pulley and L-bar can be initiated.
- Inferior and posterior grade 1 and 2 glides in scapular plane improves joint play.
- Sub maximal isometric strengthening exercises are prescribed for external and internal rotators, biceps and deltoid.
- Educate patient about the pathology and elimination of any activity that causes increase in symptoms (over head activities, reaching, lifting, throwing).

Subacute Phase

The patient is considered to be in sub-acute phase if the symptom improves importantly range of motion and muscle function.

Aims:

- To improve range of motion.
- To retard muscle atrophy.

Intervention:

- Initiate abduction range of motion exercise upto 90° with aid of L-bar and rope and pulley.
- Initiate range of motion exercise for external and internal rotation, initially with arm in 45° abduction progressing to 90° abduction.
- Anterior and posterior capsular stretching to improve flexibility and to gain range of motion.
- Progress joint mobilization (inferior, anterior and posterior glides) to grade 2, 3 and 4.
- Modalities like ultrasound and cryotherapy can be used if inflammation still persists.
- Continue with isometric exercises.
- Scapulothoracic strengthening exercises are advised to improve the dynamics and control.
- Proprioceptive neuromuscular facilitation can be used.

Chronic Phase

Chronic phase of rehabilitation deals with strengthening exercises, which has to be progressive in nature. The phase is further divided into two phases:

Phase 1

Patient is considered in this phase of rehabilitation, as there occurs reduction in pain and symptoms, achievement of normal active-assisted range of motion with improvement in muscular strength.

Aims:

- To normalize range of motion.
- To improve muscular performance.

Intervention:

- Continue with self-anterior and posterior capsular stretching to improve flexibility and range of motion.
- Aggressive L-bar exercises in all planes.
- Initiate isotonic dumbbell exercises for strengthening serratus anterior.
- Initiate endurance exercise using arm ergometer.

Phase 2

Patient is progressed to phase 2 will full non-painful range of motion, no pain or tenderness.

Aims:

- To improve strength and endurance
- To improve neuro-muscular control.

Intervention:

- Initiate isokinetic strengthening exercises
- Initiate plyometric exercises

Return to Activity Phase

Patient can return to normal activity with satisfactory clinical examination having no pain or tenderness, non-painful full range of motion and normal isokinetic testing. Patient can perform all unrestricted symptom free activities and is advised to follow the maintenance program.

Return to Play:

Return to play is restricted until full pain free range of motion is restored, both rest and activity related pain are eliminated, and provocative management signs are negative. Isokinetic strength testing must be 90% compared to the contralateral side. When the patient is symptom free, resuming activities is gradual, first during practice to build up endurance while working on modified techniques/mechanics, and then in simulated game situations. The athlete should continue flexibility and strengthening exercises after returning to sports to prevent recurrence.

Prognosis

Prognosis after correct diagnosis and treatment of shoulder impingement syndrome is good and 60–90% of patients improves and are symptom free with conservative treatment. Surgical outcomes are promising in patients who fail to respond to conservative treatment.

Complications

- Rotator cuff degeneration and eventual tear.
- Adhesive capsulitis.
- Rotator cuff tear arthropathy.
- Reflex sympathetic dystrophy.

SLAP LESIONS

SLAP lesion indicates an injury located within the superior labrum extending anterior to posterior (Fig. 13.14).

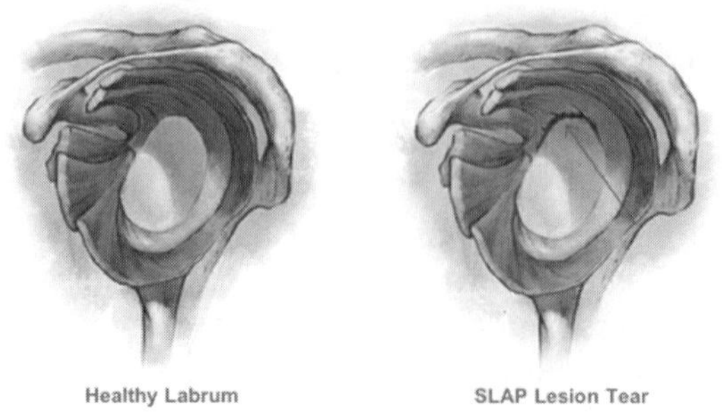

Fig. 13.14: SLAP lesion

Anatomy and Biomechanics of the Glenoid Labrum

Glenohumeral stability is the result of the interplay between multiple anatomical structures that include the capsule, ligaments, muscles, tendons, osseous configuration, and glenoid labrum. The glenoid labrum plays an important role in this process.

The labrum is a fibrous structure strongly attached around the edge of the glenoid that serves to increase the contact surface area between the glenoid and the humeral head. The glenoid labrum enhances shoulder stability in 4 distinct ways:

- It produces a ''chock-block'' effect between the glenoid and the humeral head that serves to limit humeral head translation.
- It increases the ''concavity-compression'' effect between the humeral head and the glenoid.
- It contributes to the stabilizing effect of the long head of the biceps anchor.
- It increases the overall depth of the glenoid fossa.

Pathomechanics of SLAP Lesions

There are several injury mechanisms that are speculated to be responsible for creating SLAP lesions. These mechanisms range from single traumatic events to repetitive microtraumatic injuries. Traumatic events, such as falling on an outstretched arm or bracing oneself during a motor vehicle accident, may result in SLAP lesions due to compression of the superior joint surfaces superimposed with subluxation of the humeral head. Snyder *et al.* referred to this as a pinching mechanism of injury. Other traumatic injury mechanisms include direct blows, falling onto the point of the shoulder, and forceful traction injuries of the upper extremity. Repetitive overhead activity, such as throwing a baseball, is another common mechanism of injury frequently responsible for producing SLAP injuries.

In theory, SLAP lesions most likely occur in overhead athletes from a combination of these two previously described forces. The eccentric biceps activity during deceleration may serve to weaken the biceps-labrum complex, while the torsional peel-back force may result in the posterosuperior detachment of the labral anchor.

Classification of SLAP Lesions

- Type I SLAP lesions (Fig. 13.15) were described as being indicative of isolated fraying of the superior labrum, with a firm attachment of the labrum to the glenoid. These lesions are typically degenerative in nature.

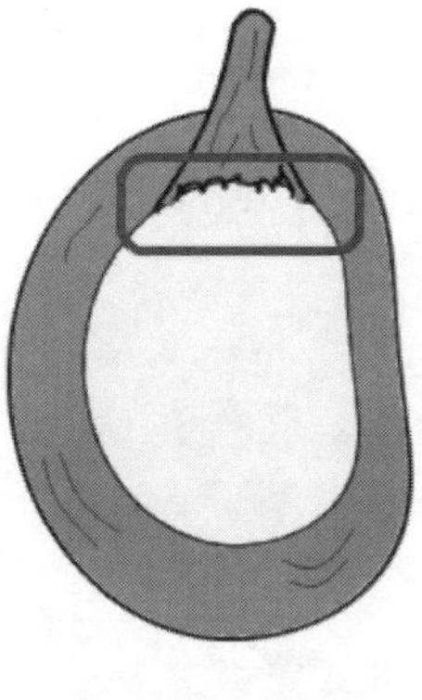

Fig. 13.15: SLAP lesion type I

- Type II SLAP lesions (Fig. 13.16) are characterized by a detachment of the superior labrum and the origin of the tendon of the long head of the biceps brachii from the glenoid resulting in instability of the biceps-labral anchor.

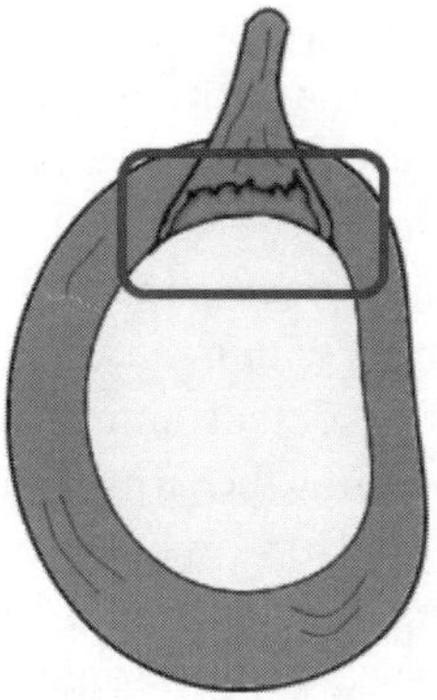

Fig. 13.16: SLAP lesion type II

- A bucket-handle tear of the labrum with an intact biceps insertion is the characteristic presentation of a type III SLAP lesion (Fig. 13.17).

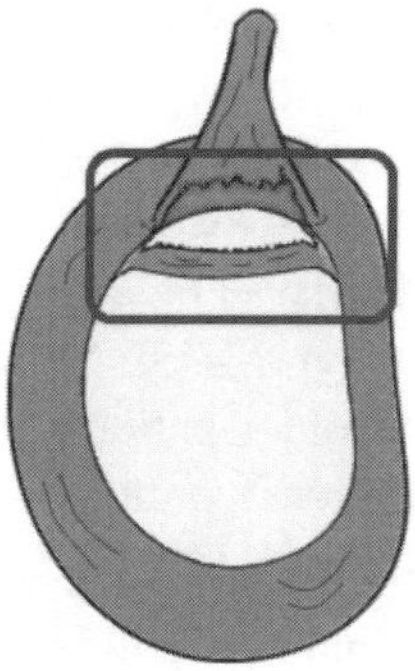

Fig. 13.17: SLAP lesion type III

- Type IV SLAP lesions (Fig. 13.18) have a bucket-handle tear of the labrum that extends into the biceps tendon. In this lesion, instability of the biceps-labrum anchor is also present, similar to that seen in the type II SLAP lesion.

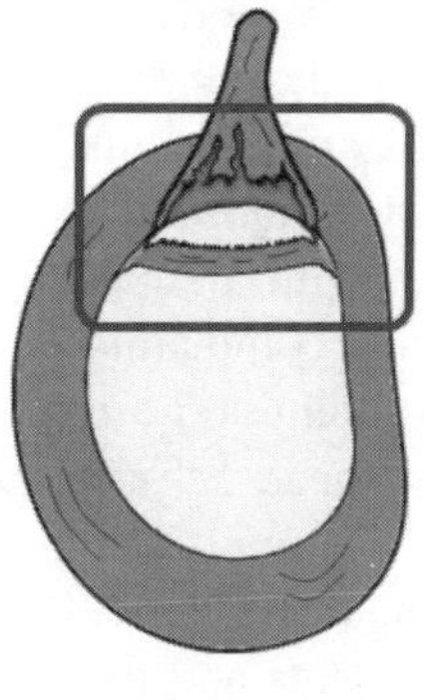

Fig. 13.18: SLAP lesion type IV

- Type V SLAP lesions are characterized by the presence of a Bankart lesion of the anterior capsule that extends into the anterior superior labrum.
- Disruption of the biceps tendon anchor with an anterior or posterior superior labral flap tear is indicative of a type VI SLAP lesion.
- Type VII SLAP lesions are described as the extension of a SLAP lesion anteriorly to involve the area inferior to the middle glenohumeral ligament.

Clinical Evaluation

Clinical examination to detect SLAP lesions is often difficult because of the common presence of concomitant pathology in patients presenting with this type of condition. Type I SLAP lesions are typically associated with rotator cuff pathology, while types III and IV are associated with traumatic instability. The injuries presenting concomitant with type II SLAP lesions vary by patient's age, with older patients presenting more often with rotator cuff pathology and younger patients with instability.

The clinical examination should include subjective history, physical examination, specific special tests, and an enhanced MRI. A comprehensive history, including the exact mechanism of injury, must be obtained and should clearly define all overhead activities and sports participation. The clinician should keep in mind that while labral pathologies frequently present as repetitive overuse conditions, such as those commonly seen in overhead athletes, the patient may also describe a single traumatic event such as a fall onto the outstretched arm or an episode of sudden traction, or a blow to the shoulder. A patient with a superior labral injury may have non-specific complaints. Pain complaints are typically intermittent and are most frequently associated with overhead activity. Often patients exhibit mechanical symptoms of painful clicking or catching of the shoulder. Pain is typically elicited with specific movements and the condition is not painful at rest.

The physical examination should include a complete evaluation of bilateral passive and active range of glenohumeral motion with particular emphasis on determining the presence, persistence, and behaviour of any painful arc of motion. Patients with a SLAP lesion will often exhibit pain with passive external rotation at 90° of shoulder abduction, especially with overpressure. Special test maneuvers include:

- *Active-Compression Test:* The active compression test, as described by O'Brien *et al.*, is used to evaluate labral lesions and acromioclavicular joint injuries. The shoulder is placed into approximately 90° of elevation and 30° of horizontal adduction across the midline of the body. Resistance is applied, using an isometric hold in this position, with both full shoulder internal rotation and external rotation (altering humeral rotation against the glenoid in the process). A positive test for labral involvement (Fig. 13.19) is when pain is elicited during testing, with the shoulder in internal rotation and forearm in pronation (thumb pointing toward the floor). Symptoms are typically decreased when tested in the externally rotated position or the pain is localized at the acromioclavicular (AC) joint.

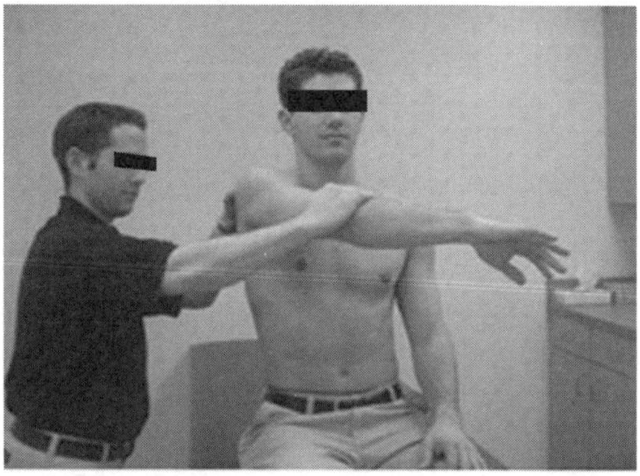

Fig. 13.19: Active compression test

- *Compression-Rotation or Grind Test:* The compression-rotation test is performed with the patient in the supine position. The glenohumeral joint is manually compressed through the long axis of the humerus while the humerus is passively rotated back and forth in an attempt to trap the labrum within the joint. The examiner may attempt to detect anterosuperior labral lesions by placing the arm in a horizontally abducted position while providing an anterosuperior-directed force. In contrast, the examiner may also horizontally adduct the humerus and provide a posterosuperior directed force when performing this test.

- *Speed's Test:* The Speed's biceps tension test has been found to accurately reproduce pain in instances of SLAP lesions. It is performed by resisting downwardly applied pressure to the arm when the shoulder is positioned in 90° of forward elevation with the elbow extended and forearm supinated (Fig. 13.20). Clinically, a new test for SLAP lesions is also performed which is a variation of the original Speed's test, refer to as the ''dynamic Speed's test'' (Fig. 13.21). During this manoeuvre, the examiner provides resistance against both shoulder elevation and elbow flexion simultaneously as the patient elevates the arm overhead. Deep pain within the shoulder is typically produced with shoulder elevation above 90° if this test is positive for labral pathology.

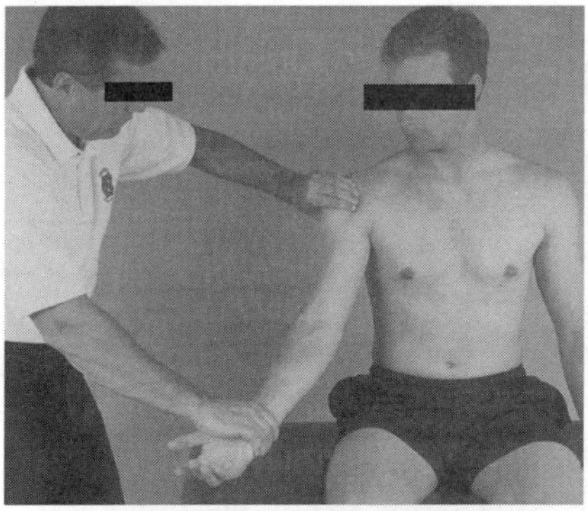

Fig. 13.20: Speed's test

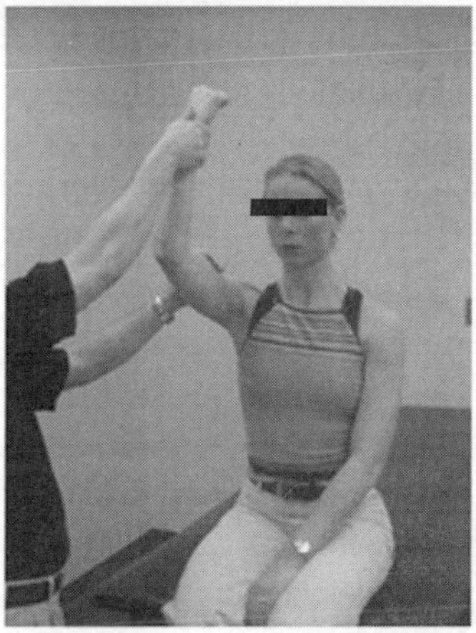

Fig. 13.21: Dynamic Speed's test

- *Clunk test:* The clunk test is performed with the patient supine. The examiner places one hand on the posterior aspect of the glenohumeral joint while the other grasps the bicondylar aspect of the humerus at the elbow. The examiner's proximal hand provides an anterior translation of the humeral head while simultaneously rotating the humerus externally with the hand holding the elbow. A positive test is produced by the presence of a clunk or grinding sound and is indicative of a labral tear.
- *Crank Test:* The crank test can be performed with the patient either sitting or supine. The shoulder is elevated to 160° in the plane of the scapula. An axial load is then applied by the examiner while the humerus is internally and externally rotated in this position (Fig. 13.22). A positive test typically elicits pain with external rotation. Symptomatic clicking or grinding may also be present during this maneuver.

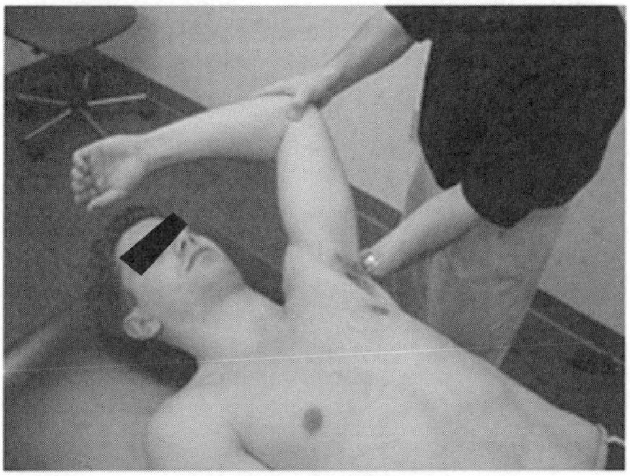

Fig. 13.22: Crank test

- *Anterior-Slide Test (Fig. 13.23):* To perform this test the arm to be examined is positioned with the hand on the ipsilateral hip with the thumb forward. The examiner then stabilizes the scapula with one hand and provides an anterosuperiorly directed axial load to the humerus with the other hand. The test is considered positive if there is a click or deep pain in the shoulder during this manoeuvre.

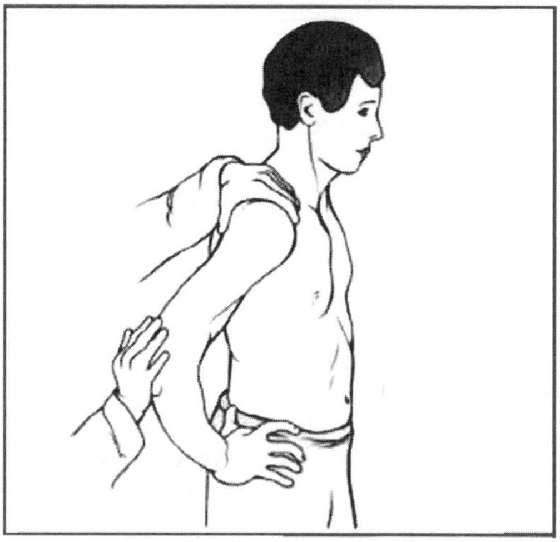

Fig. 13.23: Anterior Slide test

- *Biceps Load Test (Fig. 13.24):* The shoulder is placed in 90° of abduction and maximally externally rotated. At maximal external rotation and with the forearm in a supinated position, the patient is instructed to perform a biceps contraction against resistance. Deep pain within the shoulder during this contraction is indicative of a SLAP lesion.

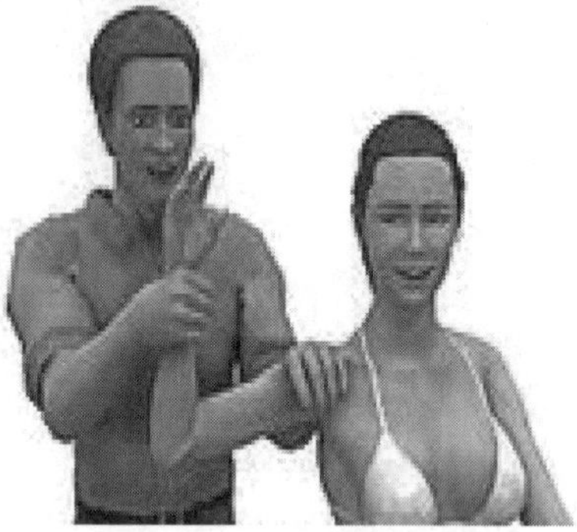

Fig. 13.24: Biceps load test

- *Pain Provocation Test:* During this manoeuvre, the shoulder is passively abducted 90° to 100° and passively externally rotated with the forearm in full pronation and then full supination. The authors determined that a SLAP lesion was present if pain was produced with shoulder externally rotated with the forearm in the pronated position or if the severity of the symptoms was greater in the pronated position. It has been noted that positive symptoms with this test are due to the additional stretch placed on the biceps tendon when the shoulder is externally rotated with the forearm pronated.
- *Pronated Load Test (Fig. 13.25):* It is performed in the seated/supine position with the shoulder abducted to 90° and externally rotated. However, the forearm is in a fully pronated position to increase tension on the biceps and subsequently the labral attachment. When maximal external rotation is achieved, the patient is instructed to perform a resisted isometric contraction of the biceps to simulate the peel-back mechanism.

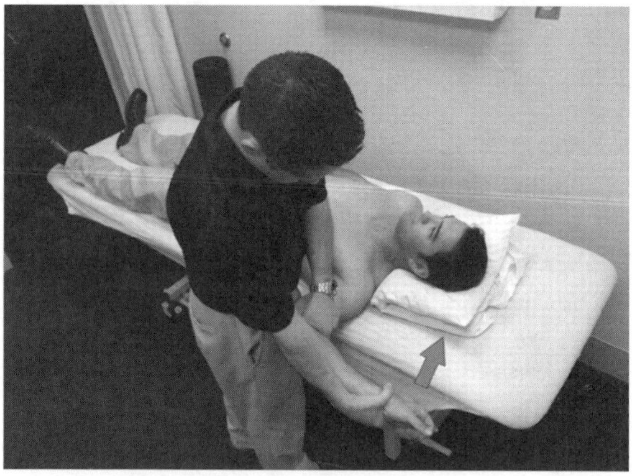

Fig. 13.25: Pronated load test

- *Resisted Supination External Rotation Test (Fig. 13.26):* During this test, the patient is positioned in 90° of shoulder abduction, and 65° to 70° of elbow flexion, and the forearm in neutral position. The examiner resists against a maximal supination effort while passively externally rotating the shoulder. Myers *et al.* noted that this test simulates the peel-back mechanism of SLAP injuries by placing maximal tension on the long head of the biceps.

Table 13.2: Selection of SLAP tests based on mechanism of injury

Mechanism	*Test*
Compressive Injury	• Active Compression Test • Compression-Rotation Test • Clunk Test • Anterior Slide Test
Traction Injury	• Speed's Test • Dynamic Speed's Test • Active Compression test
Peel-back Injury	• Pronated Load test • Resisted Supination – External Rotation Test • Biceps Load I and II Test • Pain Provocation Test • Crank Test

Surgical Management

Conservative management of SLAP lesions is often unsuccessful, particularly of type II and IV lesions with labral instability and underlying shoulder instability. Therefore, surgical intervention is most often warranted to repair the labral lesion while addressing any concomitant pathology. The goal of surgical repair of a SLAP lesion is to obtain a strong repair that allows the patient to aggressively rehabilitate the shoulder and return to full activities or sports participation.

In the presence of a type II SLAP lesion, the superior labrum should be reattached to the glenoid and the biceps anchor stabilized. Treatment of type IV SLAP lesions is generally based on the extent to which the biceps anchor is involved. When biceps involvement is less than approximately 30% of the entire anchor, the torn tissue is typically resected and the superior labrum reattached. If the biceps tear is more substantial, a side-to-side repair of the biceps tendon, in addition to reattachment of the superior labrum, is generally performed. However, if the biceps tear is extensive enough to substantially alter the biceps origin, a biceps tenodesis is more practical than a direct repair.

Rehabilitation Protocol Following Arthroscopic Debridement of Type I and III SLAP Lesions

Phase 1: Motion Phase (Days 1-10)

Goals:

- Re-establish non-painful range of motion.
- Retard muscular atrophy.
- Decrease pain/inflammation.

Range of Motion (Passive ROM/Active-assisted ROM):

- Pendulums exercise.
- Rope and pulley.
- L-bar exercises:
  - Flexion/extension
  - Abduction/adduction
  - External Rotation/Internal Rotation (begin at 0° Abduction, progress to 45°, then 90°)
- Self-stretches (capsular stretches).

Exercises:

- Isometrics to the shoulder girdle musclature except biceps.
- No biceps isometrics for 5 to 7 days postoperative.
- Initiate tubing for External Rotation/Internal Rotation at 0° Abduction (usually 7 to 10 days postoperative)

Decrease pain/inflammation:

- Ice, NSAIDs, modalities

Phase 2: Intermediate Phase (Weeks 2-4)

Goals:

- Regain and improve muscular strength.
- Normalize arthrokinematics.
- Improve neuromuscular control of shoulder complex.

Criteria to Progress to Phase 2

- Full passive ROM.
- Minimal pain and tenderness.
- Good muscle strength of flexors, internal and external rotators.

Week 2

Exercises:

- Initiate isotonic program with dumbbells for following:
  - Shoulder musculature.
  - Scapulothoracic muscles
- Tubing External Rotation/Internal Rotation at 0° abduction.
- Side lying External Rotation.
- Prone rowing External Rotation.
- PNF manual resistance with dynamic stabilization.
- Normalize arthrokinematics of shoulder complex:
  - Joint mobilization
  - Continue stretching of shoulder (External Rotation/Internal Rotation at 90° of abduction).
- Initiate neuromuscular control exercises.
- Initiate proprioception training.
- Initiate trunk exercises.
- Initiate upper extremity endurance exercises.

Decrease pain/inflammation:

- Continue use of modalities, ice, as needed.

Week 3

Exercises:

- Thrower's ten program.
- Emphasize rotator cuff and scapular strengthening.
- Dynamic stabilization drills.

Phase 3: Dynamic-Strengthening Phase, Advanced-Strengthening Phase (Weeks 4-6)

Goals:

- Improve strength, power and endurance.
- Improve neuromuscular control.
- Prepare athlete to begin to throw, etc.

Criteria to enter Phase 3:

- Full non-painful active ROM and passive ROM.
- No pain or tenderness.
- Strength 70% compared to contralateral side.

Exercises:

- Continue thrower's ten program.
- Continue dumbbell strengthening (supraspinatus, deltoid).
- Initiate tubing exercises in the 90°/90° position for External Rotation/Internal Rotation (slow/fast sets).
- Exercises for scapulothoracic musculature.
- Tubing exercises for biceps.
- Initiate plyometrics (2 hand drills progress to 1 hand drills).
- Diagonal patterns (PNF).
- Initiate isokinetic strengthening.
- Continue endurance exercises: neuromuscular control exercises.
- Continue proprioception exercises.

Phase 4: Return-to-Activity Phase (Week 7 and Beyond)

Goals:

- Progressively increase activities to prepare patient for full functional return.

Criteria to progress to Phase 4:

- Full passive ROM.
- No pain or tenderness.
- Isokinetic test that fulfills criteria to throw.
- Satisfactory clinical examination.

Exercises:

- Initiate interval sport program (i.e., throwing, tennis, etc).
- Continue all exercises as in Phase 3 (throw and train on same day, lower extremity and ROM on opposite days).
- Progress interval program.

Follow-up visits:

- Isokinetic tests.
- Clinical examination.

Rehabilitation Protocol Following Arthroscopic Type II SLAP Repair

Phase 1: Immediate Postoperative Phase "Protected Motion" (Day 1-Week 6)

Goals:

- Protect the anatomic repair.
- Prevent negative effects of immobilization.
- Promote dynamic stability.
- Diminish pain and inflammation.

Week 0-2

- Sling for 4 weeks.
- Sleep in immobilizer for 4 weeks.
- Elbow/hand passive ROM.
- Hand-gripping exercises.
- Passive and gentle shoulder active assistive ROM exercise.
  - Flexion to 60° (week 2, flexion to 75°).
  - Elevation in scapular plane to 60°.
  - External rotation/Internal rotation with arm in scapular plane.
  - External rotation to 10°-15°.
  - Internal rotation to 45°.
  - No active external rotation, extension or abduction.
- Submaximal isometrics for shoulder musculature.
- No isolated biceps contractions.
- Cryotherapy, modalities as indicated.

Week 3-4

- Discontinue use of sling at 4 weeks.
- Sleep in immobilizer until week 4.
- Continue gentle ROM exercises (Passive ROM and Active-assistive ROM).
  - Flexion to 90°.
  - Abduction to 75°–85°.
  - External Rotation in scapular plane to 25°–30°.
  - Internal rotation in scapular plane to 55°–60°.
- No active external rotation, extension, or elevation.
- Initiate rhythmic stabilization drills.
- Initiate proprioception training.
- Tubing external rotation/internal rotation at 0° abduction.
- Continue isometrics.
- Continue use of cryotherapy.

Week 5-6:

- Gradually improve ROM:
  - Flexion to 145°.
  - External rotation at 45° abduction: 45°-50°.
  - Internal rotation at 45° abduction: 55°-60°.
- May initiate stretching exercises.
- May initiate light (easy) ROM at 90° abduction.
- Continue tubing external rotation/internal rotation (arm at side).
- PNF manual resistance.
- Initiate active shoulder abduction (without resistance).

- Initiate "full can" exercise (weight of arm).
- Initiate prone rowing, prone horizontal abduction.
- No biceps strengthening.

Phase 2: Intermediate Phase: Moderate-Protection Phase (Weeks 7-12)

Goals:

- Gradually restore full ROM (week 10)
- Preserve the integrity of the surgical repair
- Restore muscular strength and balance

Week 7-9:

- Gradually progress ROM:
  - Flexion to 180°.
  - External Rotation at 90° abduction: 90°-95°.
  - Internal Rotation at 90° abduction: 70°-75°.
- Continue to progress isotonic strengthening program.
- Continue PNF strengthening.
- Initiate thrower's ten program.
- May begin active ROM biceps.

Week 10-12:

- May initiate slightly more aggressive strengthening.
- Progress external rotation to thrower's motion:
  - External rotation at 90° abduction: 110°-115° in thrower's (weeks 10-12).
- Progress isotonic strengthening exercises.
- Continue all stretching exercises:
  - Progress ROM to functional demands (i.e., overhead athlete).
- Continue all strengthening exercises.

Phase 3: Minimal Protection Phase (Weeks 12-20)

Goals:

- Establish and maintain full passive ROM and active ROM.
- Improve muscular strength, power and endurance.
- Gradually initiate functional activities.

Criteria to Enter Phase III:

- Full non-painful Active ROM.
- Satisfactory stability.
- Muscular strength (good grade or better).
- No pain or tenderness.

Weeks 12-16:

- Continue all stretching exercises (capsular stretches).
- Maintain throwers motion (especially External Rotation).
- May begin resisted biceps and forearm supination exercises.
- Continue strengthening exercises:
  - Thrower's ten program or fundamental exercises.
  - PNF manual resistance.
  - Endurance training.
  - Initiate light plyometric program.
  - Restricted sport activities (light swimming, half golf swings).

Weeks 16-20:

- Continue all exercise listed above.
- Continue all stretching.
- Continue thrower's ten program.
- Continue plyometric program.
- Initiate interval sport program (throwing, etc).

Phase 4: Advanced Strengthening Phase (Weeks 20-26)

Goals:

- Enhance muscular strength, power and endurance.
- Progress functional activities.

- Maintain shoulder mobility.

Criteria to enter Phase IV:

- Full non-painful active ROM.
- Satisfactory static stability.
- Muscular strength 75%-80% of contralateral side.
- No pain or tenderness.

Weeks 20-26:

- Continue flexibility exercises.
- Continue isotonic strengthening program.
- PNF manual-resistance patterns.
- Plyometric strengthening.
- Progress interval sport programs.

Phase 5: Return-to-Activity Phase (Months 6 to 9)

Goals:

- Gradual return to sport activities.
- Maintain strength, mobility and stability.

Criteria to enter Phase V:

- Full functional ROM.
- Muscular performance isokinetic (fulfills criteria).
- Satisfactory shoulder stability.
- No pain or tenderness.

Exercises:

- Gradually progress sport activities to unrestrictive participation.
- Continue stretching and strengthening program.

Repair of Type IV SLAP Lesion

The surgical repair of a type IV SLAP lesion with either a biceps repair, biceps resection of frayed area, or tenodesis follows much the same postoperative rehabilitation course as that outlined for a type II lesion, in that the range of motion and exercise activities are progressed similarly. However, there are substantial differences related to controlling both active and resistive biceps activity, based on the extent of bicipital involvement. In cases where the biceps is resected, biceps muscular contractions may begin between 6 and 8 weeks post-surgery. Conversely, in the cases of repaired biceps tears or biceps tenodesis, noresisted or active biceps is recommended for 3 months following surgery, when the soft tissue is most likely healed. Light isotonic strengthening for elbow flexion is initiated between weeks 12 and 16 postoperatively and progresses gradually, as tolerated from that point. Full resisted biceps activity is not incorporated until weeks 16 to 20. Progression to sport-specific activities, such as plyometrics and interval sport programs, follows similar guidelines to those outlined for type II SLAP repairs.

SUBDELTOID BURSITIS

Subdeltoid bursa is situated between the deltoid and the capsule of shoulder joint and it may get inflammed due to various reasons.

Causes

- Direct trauma.
- Infection.
- Rheumatism.
- Local deposition of calcium salts.

Clinical Features

- Severe pain.
- Tenderness.
- Painful shoulder movements.
- Warmth over the surface of bursa.

Onset: It may be gradual or sudden.

Treatment

- Rest in a triangular sling.
- Local infiltration with hydrocortisone.

Physiotherapy Management

- Pain relieving heat modality is used.
- Ultrasonic therapy.
- Relaxed passive movements in available pain free range should be encouraged to avoid stiff shoulder.
- Deep friction massage is also effective.

UNIT SIX

ELBOW AND WRIST COMPLEX CONDITIONS

CHAPTER 14

ELBOW AND WRIST COMPLEX

TENNIS ELBOW

Definition

It is a common clinical entity characterized by pain and tenderness at lateral epicondyle of the humerus. It is due to non-specific inflammation at origin of extensor muscles of the forearm.

Aetiology

Age of onset: 30 to 60 years.
Gender: It is equally distributed amongst both genders.

Causes

- Strain.
- Incomplete rupture of forearm extensor muscles.
- Incomplete rupture of aponeurotic fibres.
- Carrying heavy case.
- Wrong technique at sports (e.g., tennis, golf, badminton, fencing).
- Unaccustomed gardening or carpentry.

Pathology

A tear occurs at tendo-muscular or tendo-periosteal junction (Fig. 14.1), resulting in inflammation that produces exudate in which fibrin forms to heal the torn tissue. Excessive fibrin formation results in adhesion between the tendon and the neighboring tissues. Repeated use and minor injury to the tendon prevent healing and formation of excessive scar tissue.

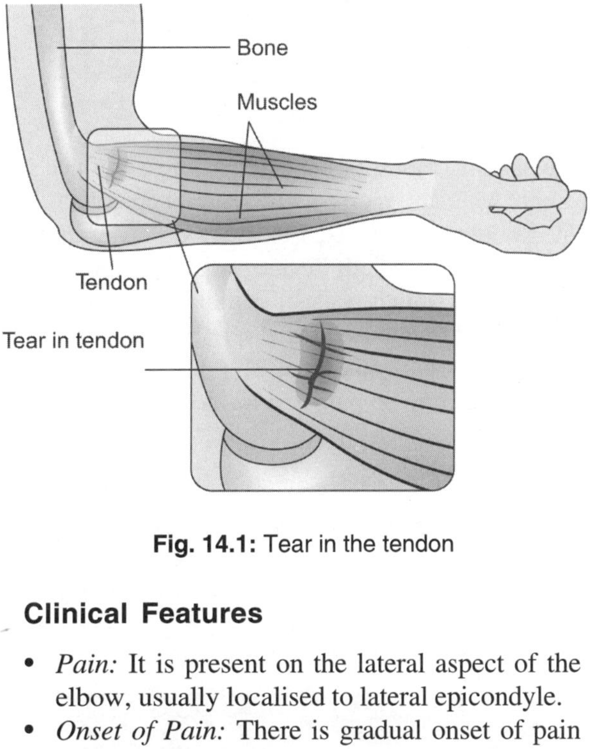

Fig. 14.1: Tear in the tendon

Clinical Features

- *Pain:* It is present on the lateral aspect of the elbow, usually localised to lateral epicondyle.
- *Onset of Pain:* There is gradual onset of pain present after activity and disappears with rest.
- *Referred Pain:* The pain refers from elbow to wrist on the extensor aspect. The pain is of aching and sharp character.
- *Tenderness:* It is localized to the front of lateral epicondyle of the humerus.
- *Range of Motion:*
  - In acute cases: Range of motion is normal.
  - In chronic cases: Accessory movements of elbow and superior radioulnar joints may be reduced.

Clinical Diagnosis

Cozen's Test (Fig. 14.2)

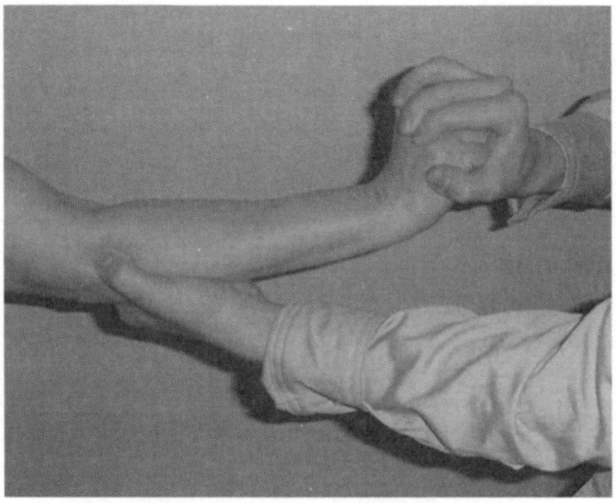

Fig. 14.2: Cozen's test

The patient's elbow is stabilized by the examiner's thumb, which rests on patient's lateral epicondyle. The patient is then asked to make a fist, pronate the forearm and radially deviate and extend the wrist while the examiner resists the motion. A positive sign is indicated by sudden severe pain in the area of lateral epicondyle of the humerus. The epicondyle may be palpated to indicate origin of pain.

Mill's Test (Fig. 14.3)

While palpating the lateral epicondyle, the examiner passively pronates the patient's forearm, flexes the wrist fully, and extends the elbow. A positive test is indicated by pain over the lateral epicondyle of humerus.

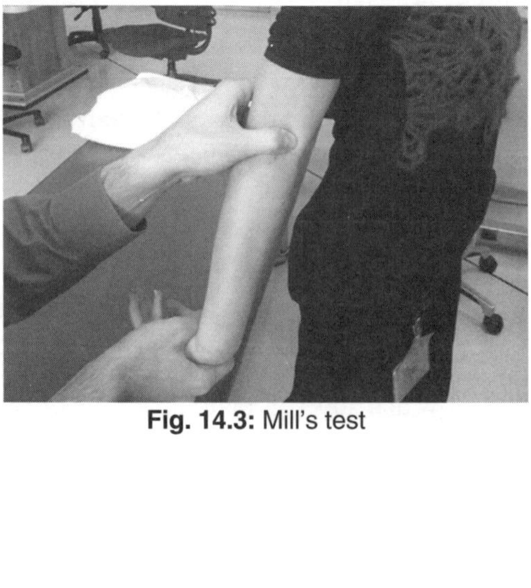

Fig. 14.3: Mill's test

Resisted Extension Test (Fig. 14.4)

The examiner resists extension of third digit of hand distal to proximal inter-phalangeal joint, stressing extensor digitorum muscle and tendon. A positive test is indicated by pain over lateral epicondyle of humerus.

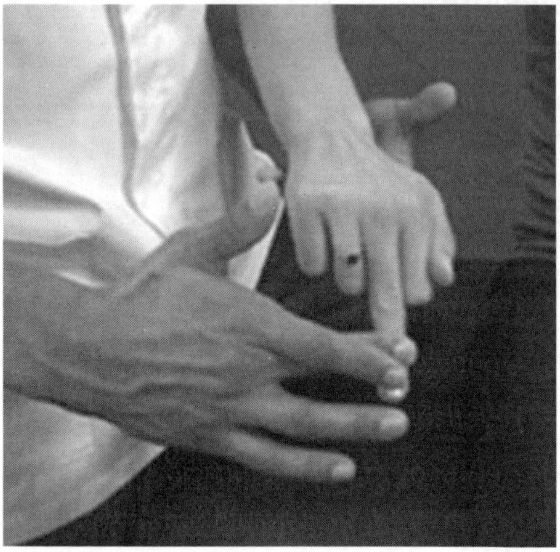

Fig. 14.4: Resisted extension test

Radiological Examination

The radiological diagnosis of the affected elbow does not show any alterations from normal.

Course

If left untreated, the symptoms may subside spontaneously but can even persist for two years or more.

Treatment

Conservative Treatment

- Non steroidal anti-inflammatory drugs (NSAIDs).
- Injection of hydrocortisone with local anaesthetic solution is given at the point of maximum tenderness.

Surgical Treatment

It is rarely indicated but if conservative treatment fails and disability is severe surgery has to be done.

Surgical procedure includes stripping of the extensor origin from its attachment to lateral epicondyle and is allowed to fall back into place. This completes the detachment of pain-sensitive fibers from the bone and allows healing to occur.

Physiotherapy Management

The physiotherapy management plays an important role in preventing the occurrence of tennis elbow and also in restoring the functions, once the inflammation has already set in.

Preventive Physiotherapy Regime

The preventive programme for the tennis elbow helps to those mechanical professionals or sports persons who have to perform repeated forceful jerky movements to the common extensor origin which is the main cause of the inflammatory changes.

Various preventive measures include:

- Proper conditioning.
- Specific warm up before starting with the sports activity.
- Specific strengthening exercises for the following muscle groups:
  - Extensor carpi radialis longus.
  - Extensor carpi radialis brevis.
  - Supinator.
- Education about the proper technique of the sport so as to avoid any strain on the extensor origin.
- Use of proper sports equipment with proper calibrations.

Restorative Physiotherapy Regime

The restorative physiotherapy regime in case of tennis elbow or lateral epicondylitis depends upon the condition of the patient, i.e., acute or chronic.

Acute Condition

- *Rest to the Part:* Rest to the affected area is the primary and the most important need to the patient in the acute stage. The rest will help in subsiding the inflammatory process and will proceed towards early healing. Following immobilization techniques can be used:
  - Posterior slab for 2-3 weeks.
  - Splint which holds the wrist in mild degree of extension, forearm in supination and elbow in flexion can be used for 2-3 weeks.
  - Tennis elbow brace (Fig. 14.5).

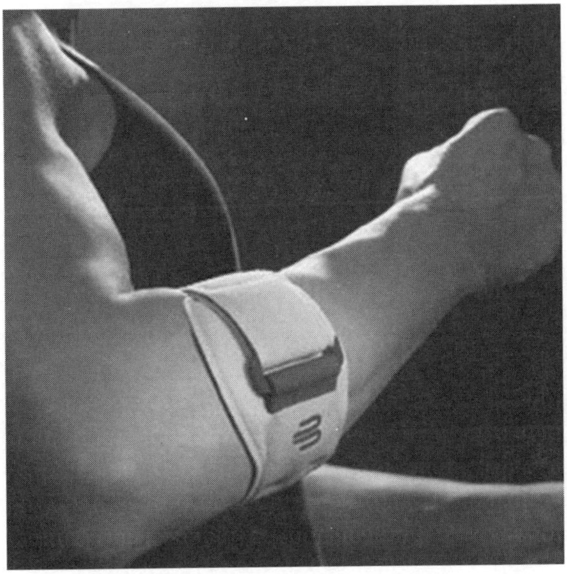

Fig. 14.5: Tennis elbow brace

- *Cryotherapy:* Ice in the initial stages proves to be a good adjunctive to reduce pain and inflammation.
  Ice could be applied over the painful area or the entire muscle belly in any of the following forms:
  - Ice towelling for 15-20 minutes.
  - Ice pack for 10-15 minutes.
  - Ice massage for 7 minutes.
- *Elevation:* The limb should be kept in an elevated position.
- *Electrical Stimulation:* The painful area is stimulated with the use of sinusoidal waves for 20 minutes. During stimulation the arm should be kept in elevation. The electrical stimulation serves the following purposes:
  - Relieves muscle spasm.

- Prevents adhesion formation.
- Reduces oedema.
- Iontophoresis could also be used to reduce pain and inflammation.

Chronic Condition

- Ultrasonic therapy is advocated over the tender spot for 8 minutes at the dosage of 1wb/cm^2 on pulsed mode. The use of hydrocortisone cream of 0.05% concentration is also advised during ultrasonic therapy.
- *Soft tissue manipulation:* Lysian advocates gentle effleurage and kneading for first two weeks, succeeded by deep friction massage (transverse) for 5-10 minutes.
- Pulsed electromagnetic energy (PEME) can be used after transverse frictions to ease off the tenderness.
- Transcutaneous electrical nerve stimulator (TENS) is used over the extensor aspect of the forearm relieves pain and muscle spasm.
- Gentle active movements at the elbow to be initiated with emphasis over the extension.
- Isometerics are carried out at the terminal ranges. Precaution should be taken that it should never be painful.
- Self resistive exercises are initiated once the movements are pain free.
- *Manipulation:* Manipulation by Mills maneuver is effective in cases where pain is provoked with active use of extensor muscles but it is contraindicated in the following cases:
  - Pain at rest.
  - Stiffness after rest.
  - Fibrositis.
- Taping of the elbow

The function of taping for tennis elbow is to limit wrist flexion, radial and ulnar deviation along with limiting the tendon stretch.

Technique

The patient is in sitting position with wirst in neutral position and forearm pronated on the table. Three anchors are used, one on proximal forearm, second around the wrist and third around the hand, leaving the thumb over the metacarpophalangeal joints. Four strips are applied over the dorsal aspect of forearm extending from the proximal anchor to hand anchor limiting the finger flexion with wirst in slight extension. The distal end of the strips are from second the fifth metacarpal. The strips are supported by the anchors placed over the original ones. A long strip is taken whose centre is over the palmar aspect of metacarpal heads. The radial aspect of the strip passes over the dorsum and is applied to the lateral epicondyle at proximal anchor while the ulnar strip is also attached to proximal anchor crossing over the radial strip. This longer strip is locked by proximal and wirst anchors. A strip is applied over the mid-dorsal aspect of wrist anchor wind around ulnar to palmar aspect and pulled up to the epicondyle with moderate tension. At last the fill in strips are applied from proximal to wirst anchors.

Post-Surgical Physiotherapy Management

During Immobilization:

- The limb should be kept in elevation.
- Full range active movements to the free joints.

During Mobilization:

- To reduce pain.
  - Ultrasonic therapy.
  - Diapulse.
  - TENS.
- Shoulder and shoulder girdle should be mobilized to full range of motion to avoid adhesive capsulitis.
- Relaxed passive range of motion to elbow, forearm and wrist.
- Functional mobilization of the joints is advocated.
- Following repeated and jerky movements to be avoided:
  - Supination.
  - Wrist extension.
  - Strong gripping movements.

The patient has fully functional and painless elbow, forearm and wrist within 5-6 weeks.

Differential Diagnosis

- Strain of lateral ligament.
- Synovial fringe entrapment between head of radius and capitulum.
- Arthritis of radiohumeral or superior radioulnar joint.
- Strain of tenoperiosteal attachment of extensor carpi radialis longus.
- Radial nerve entrapment possibly within brachioradialis or supinator muscles.
- Nerve root pressure C5-C6.

DEQUERVAIN'S DISEASE

The disease is characterized by the inflammation of the first dorsal extensor compartment of wrist (Fig.14.6). The compartment encloses the tendon of extensor pollicis brevis and abductor pollicis longus in a single sheath. The inflammation usually occurs at the point where the tendons cross the styloid process of radius.

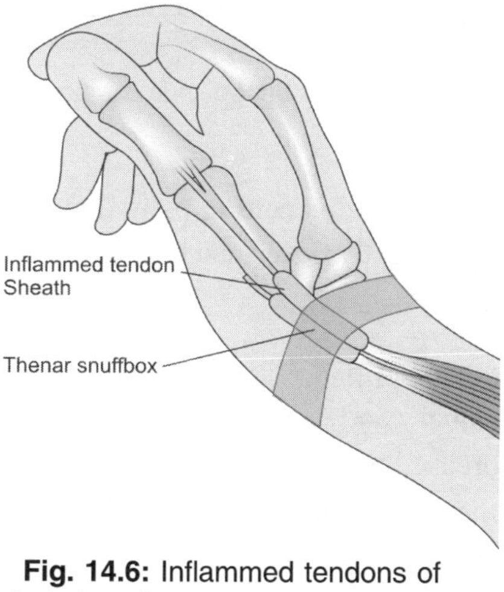

Fig. 14.6: Inflammed tendons of first dorsal extensor compartment

Other Name

The disease is also known as stenosing tenosynovitis.

Cause

The common cause of occurrence of the disease is overuse of wrist and hand particularly in movements requiring radial deviation while thumb is stabilized in a grip.

Precipitating Factor

Summation of micro-trauma due to friction.

Aetiology

The problem is particularly evident in middle aged women. There occurs repeated microtrauma due to household work like wringing clothes. Women are affected 3-10 times more than men.

Clinical Features

- The main complaint of patient is the pain on radial aspect on the wrist in the region of radial styloid.
- *On palpation:*
  - Tenderness is noticed over the tendons of first dorsal extensor compartment (Fig. 14.7), usually localised to thenar anatomical snuffbox.
  - Sometimes nodule can be palpated in the course of tendons of extensor pollicis brevis and abductor pollicis longus.
  - Crepitus may be evident on palpation due to thickening of tendon sheaths.

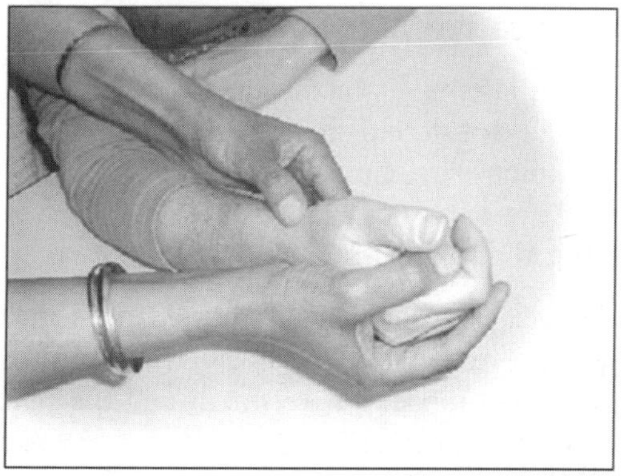

Fig. 14.7: Site of tenderness

- *Movements:*
  - Flexing the thumb across the palm is quite painful.

- Resisted abduction and extension may be painful.
- Radial and ulnar deviation may produce clicking or pain.
- Pinch and grip are weak and painful.

Clinical Diagnosis Test

Finkelstein's Test (Fig. 14.8): The patient makes the fist with thumb inside the fingers. The examiner stabilizes the forearm and deviates the wrist towards ulnar side. A positive test is indicated by pain over the region of tendons of abductor pollicis longus and extensor pollicis brevis at the wrist.

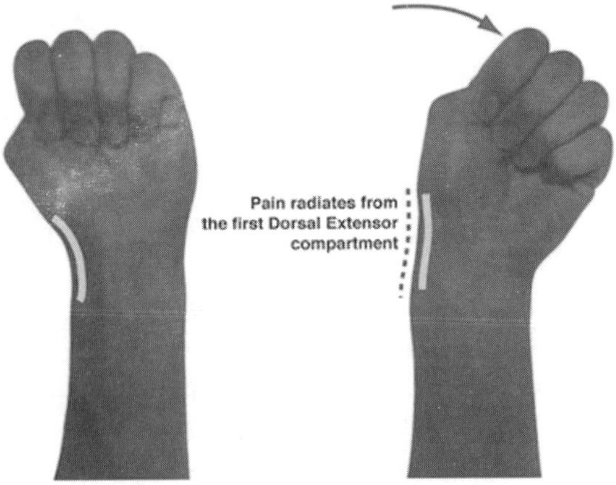

Fig. 14.8: Finkelstein's test

Conservative Management

- Antiinflammatory medication.
- Injection of steroid or analgesic medication over the point of maximum tenderness.

Surgical Management

The surgical management is indicated in the chronic cases where the patient is not responding to conservative modes of treatment and the pain is disabling the patient. Following surgical procedures could be undertaken:

- Splitting of the lateral wall of the tendon sheath.
- Surgical removal of tendons of the first extensor compartment of wrist.

Physiotherapy Management

- Immobilization techniques to support the inflammed tendons and make them to rest comfortably so as to provide time for the reduction of inflammation.
- Immobilization using forearm based thumb spica splint (Fig. 14.9) to prevent further overuse of tendons during initiation of rehabilitation programme. It should be worn during asymptomatic times or periods of high activity.
- Thumb spica taping is used to provide support and rest to inflammed tendons.

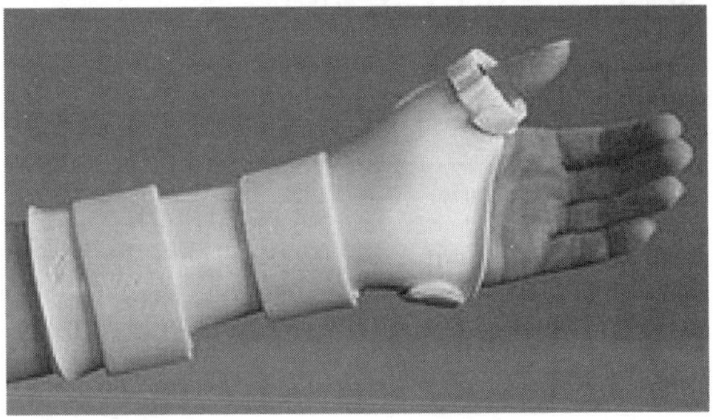

Fig. 14.9: Forearm based thumb spica splint

Taping Procedure

Position: The hand is held in palm down position with thumb slightly flexed and phalanges adducted.

Application

Apply anchor strip of adhesive tape down the wrist. Start at ulnar condyle. Cross the dorsal aspect of distal forearm and encircle the wrist.

Apply the first of three support strip for the first metacarpophalangeal joint.

Starting at ulnar condyle, cross the dorsum of the hand, cover the lateral joint line and encircle the thumb. Proceed across palmar aspect of hand and finish at ulnar condyle. This is commonly referred to as thumb spica.

Repeat this step twice. Overlap the tape by one half its width, moving distally each time.

Apply a final anchor strip around the wrist to help hold the procedure in place.

- Interventions to reduce pain and inflammation:
  - Cryotherapy.
  - Iontophoresis.
  - Ultrasound therapy.
- Cross friction massage over the first dorsal compartments breaks down adhesion and helps in the provision of free range of motion.
- Stretching exercises should be incorporated in the treatment regime to gain mobility and flexibility of following muscles:
  - Extensor pollicis brevis.
  - Abductor pollicis longus.
  - Extrinsic wrist flexor.
  - Extensor muscles.
- Strengthening should be initiated after full pain free range of motion has been achieved.
- Gripping exercises should be incorporated.

Education to Patient

- Avoiding or limiting the situation contributing to symptoms is essential for the prevention of recurrence.
- Work, hobby or sport modifications are necessary to decrease the frequency and forces involved with wrist and thumb motion.

TRIGGER FINGER

Definition

The condition is characterized by momentary locking of flexor tendon on attempting extension of the digit following flexion. It gets released with sudden snap by passively moving the finger into extension.

It is a common condition resulting in thickening and constriction of mouth of fibrous digital sheath (Fig. 14.10) which interfere with free gliding of contained flexor tendons.

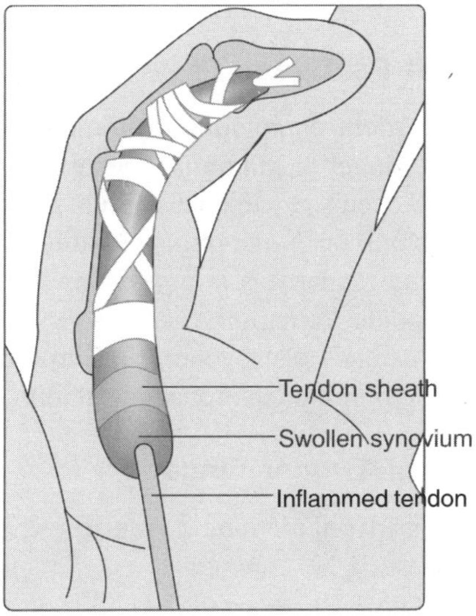

Fig. 14.10: Inflammed tendon in trigger finger

Causes

The thickening of the fibrous sheath may result from repetitive trauma or by direct pressure over metacarpophalangeal joint in palm as while performing grasping movements.

Pathology

There occurs thickening of proximal part of fibrous sheath at the base of finger or thumb resulting in the constricted mouth of the sheath. The flexor tendons get wasted associated with marked swelling. These swollen segments enter the mouth of the sheath only with difficulty when an attempt is made to straighten the finger from flexed position.

Other Names

The condition is also termed as:

- Digital tenovaginitis stenosans.
- Snapping finger.

Common Site of Affection

Flexor pollicis longus.

Associated Disease

Rheumatoid arthritis.

Clinical Features

- The patient complains of momentary locking of the finger or thumb into flexion.
- There occurs a palpable nodule at the base of the thumb or in line of distal palmar crease.
- Marked tenderness is present over the site of the nodule formation.
- Pain extends from volar metacarpophalangeal joint to proximal interphalangeal joint.

Types of Trigger Finger

The condition may be categorized into two categories:
- Adult type.
- Infantile type.

Characteristic Features of Adult Type–Trigger Finger

- Tenderness at the base of the affected finger.
- Palpable nodule at base of the affected finger.
- There occurs locking of the affected finger into full flexion.
- Locking can be overcome by strong effort (actively) or by extending the finger with other hand (passively). In either of the above-mentioned procedures flexion is released with distinct snap.

Characteristic Features of Infantile Type—Trigger Finger

- Thumb is usually affected in the infants.
- Infant is unable to straighten the thumb which is locked into flexion.
- Palpable nodule is present at the base of thumb in position of mouth of fibrous sheath that is at the level of head of metacarpal bone.
- It is possible to extend the thumb passively with snap.
- In many cases the flexed position cannot be corrected even by moderate force.

Differential Diagnosis

- Dislocated thumb.
- Congenital deformity.

Management

The management of the trigger finger could either follow a conservative or surgical path.

Conservative Management:

- Injection of hydrocortisone at the site of tenderness (Fig. 14.11).

Physiotherapy Management:

- Cryotherapy in the form of icing could be used in acute cases.

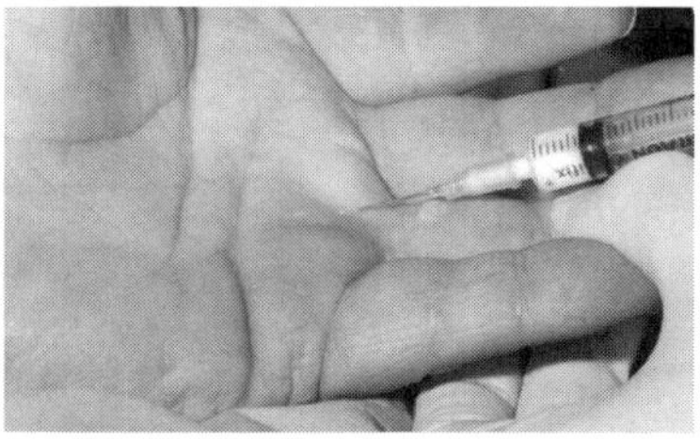

Fig. 14.11: Hydrocortisone injection

- In chronic cases paraffin wax bath may form suitable adjunct in order to release the spasm developed at the site of the flexor tendon.
- Ultrasonic therapy over the nodule formed at metacarpophalangeal joint or proximal interphalangeal joint.
- Friction massage is advocated in order to make the adhesions loose and decrease the swelling.
- Exercise regime to be followed:
  - *Active exercise program:* Interphalangeal flexion and extension.
  - Tendon gliding exercises.

Surgical Management:

The surgical procedure for treating the condition is incising the mouth of fibrous flexor sheath longitudinally.

Post-operative Physiotherapy Regime

- Potential splinting
  - Hand based splint/Digital splint can be used. It holds the metacarpophalangeal joint in full

extension (Fig. 14.12) leaving all the other joints free. It should be worn for a period of three weeks post-operatively. Thereafter it should be used for the periods of high activity.

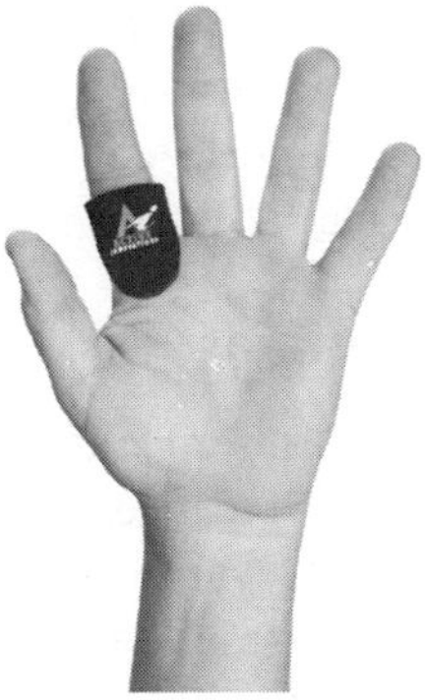

Fig. 14.12: Hand based splint

- Active exercise program.
- Progressive grip strengthening exercises.
- Work modification is necessary to avoid or limit the repetitive grasping and releasing activities of the hand.

CARPAL TUNNEL SYNDROME

Carpal tunnel syndrome (CTS) results from compression of the median nerve within the carpal tunnel at the wrist. CTS is a common upper extremity entrapment neuropathy and is estimated in one study to occur in 1% to 3% of the general population.

Signs and Symptoms of CTS

- Paresthesia, tingling, numbness, and/or pain within the cutaneous distribution of the median nerve to the thumb, index, middle, and radial half of the ring digits (Fig. 14.13).
- Nocturnal paresthesia is a frequent complaint; this tingling in the hand that interrupts sleep may be partially relieved by shaking the hand back and forth.
- Pain may radiate into the palm and up the forearm and arm.

With compression of the median nerve in the carpal tunnel, the skin overlying the thenar eminence is

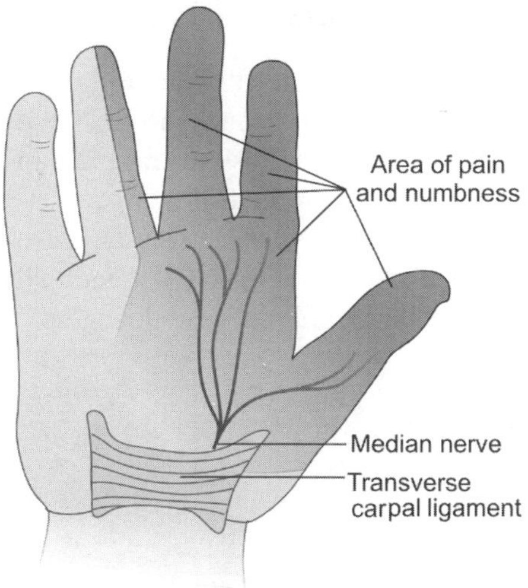

Fig. 14.13: Area of pain and numbness in CTS

usually spared because this area is innervated by the median nerve's palmar cutaneous branch. The branch originates from the median nerve before it enters the carpal tunnel and lies volar to the tunnel. While many cases of CTS are idiopathic in nature, a recent report suggests that there may be a genetic predisposition for developing the disorder. There are certain other hand disorders which occur concomitantly and/or are associated with CTS.

Some Conditions Associated with Carpal Tunnel Syndrome

Localized to upper quadrant:

- Basal (thumb carpometacarpal) joint arthritis.
- Distal radius fracture.
- Dupuytren's contracture.
- Proximal compression on median nerve.
- Scaphotrapeziotrapezoid (STT) arthritis.
- Trigger finger/thumb.

Systemic conditions:

- Diabetes mellitus.
- End-stage renal disease on renal dialysis.
- Long-term haemodialysis.
- Pregnancy.
- Rheumatoid arthritis.
- Thyroid disease (hypothyroidism).

Diagnostic Criteria

Harrington *et al.* suggested that surveillance criteria for carpal tunnel syndrome should be pain or paraesthesia or sensory loss in the median nerve distribution and one of the following:

- *Tinel's test positive (Fig. 14.14):* Percussion of the median nerve at the wrist creating tingling in the median nerve innervated fingers.

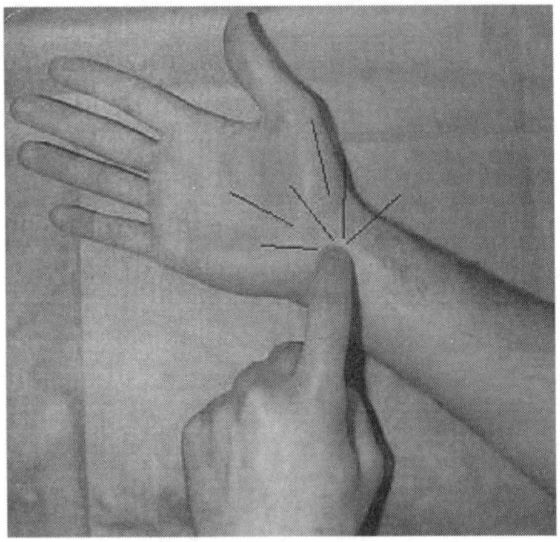

Fig. 14.14: Tinel's test

- *Phalen's test positive (Fig. 14.15):* Wrist flexion provoking tingling in median nerve innervated fingers within 60 seconds.

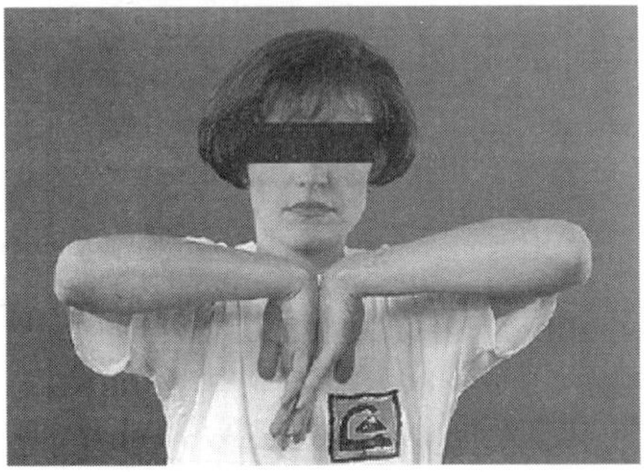

Fig. 14.15: Phalen's test

- Nocturnal exacerbation of symptoms.
- Motor loss with wasting of the abductor pollicis brevis.
- Abnormal nerve conduction studies.

Associated Features

Obesity, rheumatoid arthritis, pregnancy, diabetes, thyroid dysfunction, renal dialysis (amyloid), and radial malunion can be associated with carpal tunnel syndrome. The double crush phenomenon may play a part with minor compression at neck and wrist summating to create significant clinical complaints. Oral contraceptives, or other medications, which tend to cause fluid retention may also provoke carpal tunnel syndrome.

Severity of Symptoms

Patients commonly present with numbness and tingling in the median nerve innervated fingers which wakes them at night. Symptoms are mild and infrequent at the onset and may resolve spontaneously for months or years. Untreated carpal tunnel syndrome gradually deteriorates with increasing frequency of numbness and tingling and sleep disturbance. The tingling becomes unremitting and then progresses to numbness. Weakness and finally wasting of the abductor pollicis brevis is usually a late feature of severe compression.

- Mild cases are those with a short history of intermittent episodes of paraesthesia.
- Moderate cases may be considered those with frequent episodes of paraesthesia or numbness.
- Severe cases have persistent paraesthesia or numbness or wasting of the abductor pollicis brevis.

Outcome Measures

Following outcome measures can be used to evaluate the patient's condition following carpal tunnel syndrome:

- Boston Carpal Tunnel Scales questionnaires.
- Grip and pinch strength.
- Manual muscle testing (particularly of the thenar muscles).
- Light touch with monofilaments.

Conservative Nonsurgical Intervention Options for CTS (Table 14.1)

With entrapment neuropathy, the microcirculation of the nerve is compromised, venous congestion occurs, and axoplasmic transport is reduced. The

Table 14.1: Suggested conservative non-surgical interventions for a patient with carpal tunnel syndrome

Intervention	*Rationale for Intervention*	*Clinical suggestion*
Wrist splint	• Lowers carpal tunnel pressure	• Splint with wrist in neutral rotation • Wear at night
Heat modality	• Enhance circulation, reduce pain and paresthesia	• Continuous low-level heat wrap during the day
Nerve- and tendon-gliding exercises	• Intermittent exercises reduce carpal tunnel pressure	• Suggested every hour if doing repetitive activity
Activity modification	• Reduce compression in carpal tunnel • Minimize external pressure on palm • Assess activities of the individual and modify	• Minimize lumbrical incursion
Yoga program	• Improve posture and reduce compression on median nerve	• For patients able to participate in a regular exercise program
Corticosteroid injection into carpal canal	• Reduce pain and inflammation • May be used in conjunction with other techniques • May be used as screening to determine candidates for surgery	• May be used in conjunction with other techniques

neutral (0°) wrist position minimizes pressure within the carpal tunnel, while wrist flexion and extension increase pressure. Other factors that increase pressure within the carpal tunnel include:

- External pressure on the palm.
- Incursion of the lumbricals into the carpal tunnel
- Forearm position of full supination.
- Sustained grip.
- Isolated finger flexion against resistance.

The focus of intervention techniques is to lower the pressure within the carpal tunnel and enhance neural circulation and nutrition. Conservative treatment has focused on splint wear, modality application (e.g, heat, laser, ultrasound), exercise, activity modification and corticosteroid injection.

Splinting

Wrist splinting is a commonly employed intervention to relieve symptoms of digital paresthesia due to carpal tunnel syndrome. A properly fitted splint can assist in controlling symptoms of carpal tunnel syndrome and should be offered to most patients as a first line of care. Splints should also be considered for recurrence of symptoms. Splinting the wrist in a neutral (0°) flexion/extension rotation (Fig.14.16) position is generally agreed upon as the favoured technique. Wearing instructions for splints have varied. Splints have been recommended to be worn during the day for activity and at night.

Cortisone Injection

Steroid injection into the radial or ulnar side of the median nerve proximal to the wrist (Fig. 14.17) appears to be effective in the short term for those people who have mild symptoms of Carpal tunnel syndrome. For carpal tunnel syndrome occurring during the last trimester of pregnancy, this may be a viable alternative to control symptoms until after delivery, when many of the symptoms typically resolve.

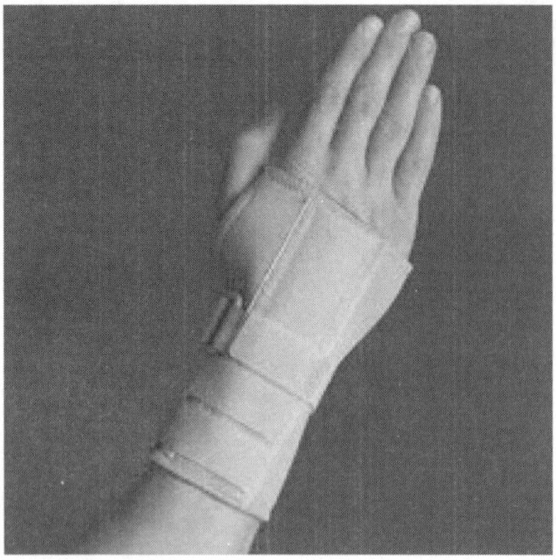

Fig. 14.16: Carpal tunnel splint

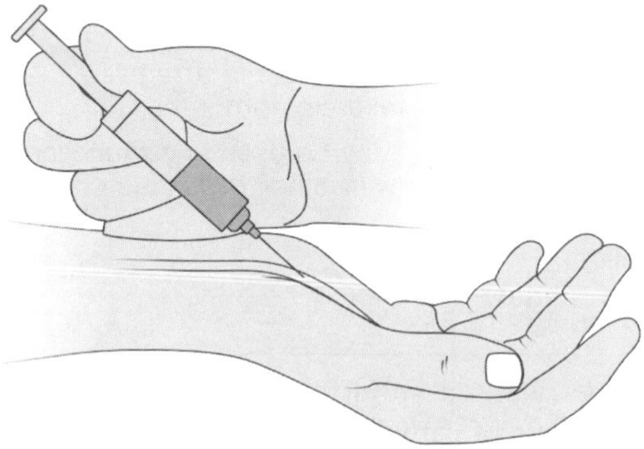

Fig. 14.17: Cortisone injection

Exercises

One of the first instincts of a physical therapist when presented with a patient who has pain and reported loss of function due to carpal tunnel syndrome is to reduce the pain and to give the patient exercises for mobility and strength. Tendon gliding of the finger flexor tendons and nerve gliding of the median nerve exercises are recommended for conservative management of symptoms related to Carpal tunnel syndrome.

Nerve and Tendon Gliding Exercises (Fig. 14.18)

Wilgis and Murphy have popularised the concept of some cases of nerve compression arising from an adhesive neuritis, with tethering of the nerve with limited excursion of the nerve through wrist and finger flexion extension range. The normal excursion of the median nerve at the wrist is approximately 14 mm. Tethering of the nerve reduces the perfusion within the nerve and compromises function. Digital flexor tendon mobilizing techniques are particularly valuable in the management of postoperative carpal tunnel patients. Care should be taken that the frequency and force of the exercises is not so great that exacerbation of symptoms is provoked. The beneficial effect of gliding exercises may be the mobilization of the nerve directly or facilitation of venous return or oedema dispersal.

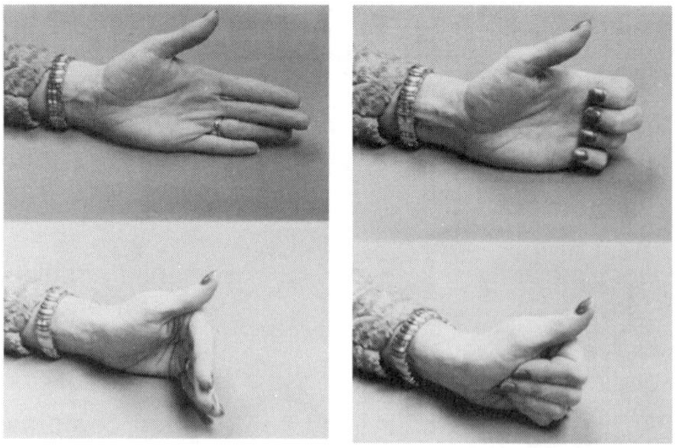

Fig. 14.18: The sequence of tendon- and nerve-gliding exercises recommended for carpal tunnel syndrome. Flexion and extension of the digits will glide the median nerve through the carpal tunnel

These exercises may have a positive effect on carpal tunnel syndrome, in part, by facilitating venous return or edema dispersion in the median nerve. Grip-strengthening exercises with therapy putties or hand grippers are not appropriate in the conservative management of Carpal tunnel syndrome. This form of exercise increases pressure within the carpal tunnel.

Modalities

Reduced circulation to the nerve can adversely affect nerve function. Heat, therapeutic ultrasound, and laser to the wrist have been used to reduce the symptoms of Carpal tunnel syndrome. Perhaps an effect of these modalities is to increase circulation or to provide an environment to decrease expression of tumor necrosis factor beta.

Work Place Task Modification

Task modification that reduces metacarpophalangeal joint flexion range will reduce lumbrical incursion and may control symptoms. The ergonomics of the workplace can be assessed to avoid protracted hand use at extremes of joint range. The position of the wrist during work is crucial in controlling symptoms of carpal tunnel syndrome. Adjustment of work height or tools can optimise the wrist position and avoid extremes of range. The diameter of tool handles may also be adjusted to minimise grip forces. Tasks may be varied or rotated to spread the most forceful or repetitive activities evenly throughout the shift. Rest breaks should be applied in a similar manner. Often simple and obvious alterations to working practice can be beneficial in controlling milder symptoms of carpal tunnel syndrome.

Activity Modification and Patient Education

Activities can be modified to maintain the wrist in neutral for as many activities as practical and to reduce repetitive and forceful gripping and pinching. Increases in carpal tunnel pressure have been measured during fingertip loading (example, active flexor tendon loading during depression of keyboard keys). As the wrist is moved from neutral during fingertip loading, pressure within the carpal tunnel increases. There is ongoing controversy of whether keyboard use causes carpal tunnel syndrome; but if carpal tunnel syndrome is present in keyboard users, it would be prudent to advise activity modification to control symptoms. These modifications can include avoiding resting the wrist on a hard surface, such as a desk edge, regular breaks to perform nerve- and tendon-gliding exercises, and using a split keyboard to avoid full pronation while typing. Sustained-grip activities should be discouraged as it increases carpal tunnel pressure. Lumbrical incursion into the carpal tunnel can also occur during gripping activities.

Surgical Intervention

Surgical decompression, an option offered to the patient if conservative care fails involves transaction of the transverse carpal ligament (TCL) to relieve pressure on the median nerve. Surgery is performed via an open carpal tunnel release (OCTR) or endoscopically assisted carpal tunnel release (ECTR). Ideal outcomes of carpal tunnel release include resolution of preoperative symptoms and restoration of hand function to a pre-morbid level.

Post-Surgical Care

A bulky dressing is usually applied following surgery. Some patients, though, may have a wrist splint applied. The rationale is to splint the wrist in about 20° extension. Scar desensitization and hand strengthening should be emphasized upon.

Postoperative exercises usually include flexor-tendon-gliding and nerve-gliding exercises. The finger flexion and extension exercises will also produce proximal and distal gliding, respectively, of the median nerve through the carpal tunnel and minimize risk of adherence to the nerve to surrounding tissues. The median nerve has a mean excursion of 1 cm after CTR with full finger flexion and extension. Grip and pinch-strengthening exercises begin 3 to 4 weeks after surgery.

GOLFER'S ELBOW

Golfer's elbow is a pathological condition causing inflammation of pronator teres and flexor carpi radialis at the medial epicondyle. The condition is also known as medial epicondylitis. The condition is less frequent than lateral epicondylitis.

Causative Factors

- Repetitive trauma resulting in microtears.
- Overuse syndrome (repetitive flexor forearm pull).
- Repetitive wrist flexion.
- Repetitive valgus stress on elbow especially in throwing athletes.
- Sports activities: Tennis, racquetball, squash, throwing.

Clinical Features

- Pain and tenderness localised to the medial epicondyle.
- Reduced grip strength.
- Pain can be clicited by:
  - Flexion of the wrist followed by forearm pronation actively by the patient elicits pain at medial epicondyle.
  - Making a tight fist.
  - Passive extension of elbow, forearm supination and valgus strain.

Clinical Diagnostic Test

While palpating the patient's medial epicondyle, the patient's forearm is passively supinated and the elbow and wrist are extended. A positive sign is indicated by pain over the medial epicondyle of humerus.

Differential Diagnosis

- Ulnar neuropathy.
- Rupture of ulnar collateral ligament in throwers.

Rehabilitation

General concepts of rehabilitation for medial epicondylitis:

- Controlled activity with appropriate rest.
- Stretching of flexor and pronator muscles (stretching should not reproduce the symptoms).
- Strengthening program should begin as the symptoms resolve.

Physiotherapy Treatment

Phase 1 : Acute Phase

Aims

- To decrease pain and inflammation.
- To promote tissue healing.
- To retard muscle atrophy.

Therapeutic Intervention

- Cryotherapy.
- Phonophoresis.
- HVGS.
- Iontophoresis.
- Friction massage.
- Avoid painful movements such as gripping.
- Stretching to increase flexibility.
  - Elbow extension-flexion.
  - Wrist extension-flexion.
  - Forearm pronation-supination.

Phase 2 : Subacute Phase

Aims

- To improve flexibility.
- To improve muscular strength and endurance.
- To increase functional activities and return to function.

Therapeutic Intervention

- Continue flexibility exercises.

- Emphasise on concentric-eccentric strengthening.
- The patient is advised to use counterforce brace.
- The patient is educated to gradually reinitiate previously painful movements.
- Initiate the gradual return to stressful activities.
- The patient must continue the use of cryotherapy after exercise or any function.

Phase 3 : Chronic Phase

Aims

- To improve muscular strength and endurance.
- To enhance and maintain the available flexibility.
- Gradual return to sports.

Therapeutic Intervention

- Continue flexibility exercises.
- Continue strengthening exercises.
- Emphasize on maintenance program.
- Gradually reduce the use of counterforce brace.
- Equipment modifications (grip size, string tension, playing surface).
- Initiate gradual return to sports.

MALLET FINGER

Mallet finger is the name given to the condition where the extensor tendon is avulsed from its insertion at the base of the distal phalanx. Sometimes a bone fragment is avulsed along with extensor tendon. The condition is also known as Baseball finger.

Mode of Injury

The injury occurs due to sudden passive flexion of distal interphalangeal joint. As for example if the ball strikes on the dorsal aspect of tip of finger.

Clinical Features

- The distal phalanx remains in flexion.
- The patient is unable to attempt passive flexion at the distal interphalangeal joint.
- There is marked tenderness over the avulsion site.

Management

Conservative Treatment

The affected distal interphalangeal joint is immobilised in a position of hyperextension with aluminium splint or plaster cast for a period of six weeks.

Surgical Treatment

The surgical treatment is recommended if the bone fragment is avulsed along with the tendon. Either of the following techniques can be utilized:

- Percutaneous fixation using k wires.
- Open reduction and internal fixation.

OLECRANON BURSITIS

Olecranon bursa is present on the posterior aspect of the elbow behind the olecranon process.

Other Names: Student's ellow, Minor's ellow.

Causes

- Trauma.
- Infection.
- Gout.

Associated Diseases: Rheumatoid arthritis.

Clinical Features

- *Pain:* Olecranon bursitis is painful only if there is associated infection.
- *Swelling:* Swelling is discrete, being more sharply demarcated as 'goose egg' over olecranon process.
- *Position of ellow:* The elbow is usually held in a position of 70° of flexion.

- The bursa is distended with clear fluid.
- Whitish deposits of sodium biurate (tophi) may be visible through walls of the bursa.

Treatment

- Aspiration of bursa.
- Injection of hydrocortisone into the bursa.
- Incision and drainage of the bursa.
- Excision of bursa.

Physiotherapy Management

- Active physiotherapy is contraindicated initially.
- Gradual mobilization is to be started as infection subsides.

MEDIAN NERVE NEUROPATHIES

Causes of Median Nerve Neuropathies

- Diabetes.
- Human immunodeficiency virus.
- Nutritional deficiencies.
- Entrapment/compression of the nerve.

Median nerve compression proximal to the carpal tunnel may be divided into two major categories:

- Pronator Syndrome (PS).
- Anterior Interosseous Nerve Syndrome (AINS).

PRONATOR SYNDROME

It was first described by Seyfferth in 1951. It has been expanded to encompass compression of the median nerve at:

- Ligament of struthers.
- Laceratus fibrosees.
- Pronator teres.
- Arch of flexor digitorum superficialis.

Pronator syndrome usually presents in the fifth decade and is four times more common in women than men. It has been related to repetitive exertional grasping work performed commonly by:

- Assembly line workers.
- Carpenters.
- Weightlifters.
- Tennis players.

Clinical Presentation

The onset of symptoms is insidious. The patient with pronator syndrome typically complain of:

- Pain in the proximal volar aspect of the forearm. It is aggravated by activities which involves repetitive pronation and supination.
- Parasthesia in the thumb, index and long fingers.
- Numbness in palm consistent with distribution of palmar cutaneous branch of median nerve.

Clinical Diagnostic Tests

These tests are based on creating maximal tension on the anatomical sites that can contribute to compression of the median nerve as it courses from elbow to wrist, so as to determine the site of proximal median nerve entrapment.

Source of Compression	Clinical Test
Pronator teres	Reproduction of symptoms with resisted pronation with forearm in neutral as the elbow is gradually extended.
Laceratus fibrosus	Reproduction of symptoms with resisted elbow flexion at 120° to 130° with forearm in maximal supination.
Flexor digitorum superficialis	Reproduction of symptoms with resisted flexion of proximal interphalangeal joint of the long finger.

Pronator Compression Test

The test is performed by placing pressure over the pronator muscles in both upper extremities. A positive test is indicated by reproduction of parasthesia in the lateral 3-$^{1/2}$ digits in 30 seconds or less while the uninvolved limb remains asymptomatic.

ANTERIOR INTEROSSEOUS NERVE SYNDROME

It was first described by Kiloh and Nevin in 1952. It is a rare entity as it accounts for fewer than 1% of all upper extremity neuropathies. It has been expanded to encompass compression of the median nerve at:

- Deep head of pronator teres, flexor digitorum superficialis.
- Gantzer's muscle (accessory head of flexor pollicis longus).
- Tendinous origin of palmoris profundus.
- Accessory laceratus fibrosus.

Compression of the anterior interosseous nerve can also occur by direct physical compression of the nerve or the nerve's vascular supply by a blood vessel. The blood vessels that can act as sources of compression include:

- Ulnar recurrent vessels.
- Aberrant radial artery.
- Anomalous median artery.
- Anterior interosseous versels.

Clinical Presentation

- Pain in the proximal volar forearm which tends to increase with repetitive forearm motion.
- Difficulty in writing or picking up small objects due to weakness in flexor pollicis longus, flexor digitorum profundus of the index and long finger and the pronator quadratus.
- Lack of parasthesia is the key characteristic.
- The patient presents with 'classic attitude' of weak pinch when attempts to touch the tip of the thumb to tip of index finger. The change in pinch is considered to be an indicator of late stages of AINS.

The diagnosis of AINS is confirmed by electromyographic testing in 80% to 90% of cases.

Intervention

Rest/Immobilization

- Instruct the patient to avoid aggravating activities such as repetitive promotion/supination and aggressive physical activities involving forceful grip (weightlifting, tennis).
- Posterior elbow splint to be worn for two weeks with elbow in 90° flexion and forearm in mid rotation. The splint should be removed for gentle range of motion activities.

Soft Tissue Mobilization

The soft tissue mobilization to the area of suspected entrapment is done to induce muscle relaxation and/or to decrease muscle tension. In patients with pronator syndrome, soft tissue mobilization to the pronator teres is performed. This decreases mechanical force imparted to the nerve at the area of entrapment and therefore decreases the probability of inducing histologic damage to the nerve.

- Superficial heating modalities are used to induce muscle relaxation and/or decrease muscle tension.

Nerve Mobilization

Nerve gliding/mobilization should be proceeded by superficial heating modalities and soft tissue mobilization.

To mobilize the median nerve at the level of pronator teres, the tension on median nerve should be established proximally by side bending and rotating the cervical spine to the contralateral side and established distally by extending the wrist and fingers. The median nerve is gently mobilized by flexing and extending the elbow while supinating the forearm.

During the procedure, any exacerbations of symptoms should be avoided. The physiotherapist should not proceed past the point of pain and symptom reproduction.

- Cortisone injection into the region of pronator teres if conservative therapy is unsuccessful.
- Surgical decompression of median nerve involves compression of all possible sites of nerve compression. Surgery is only indicated if there is no significant change in symptoms after 8 to 12 weeks of conservative treatment.

UNIT SEVEN

HIP JOINT CONDITIONS

15. HIP JOINT CONDITIONS

CHAPTER 15

HIP JOINT CONDITIONS

AVASCULAR NECROSIS OF HIP

Avascular necrosis (AVN) of the femoral head is a pathological process that results from interruption of blood supply to the bone. AVN of the hip is poorly understood, but this process is the final common pathway of traumatic or non-traumatic factors that compromise the already precarious circulation of the femoral head. Femoral head ischemia results in the death of marrow and osteocytes and usually results in the collapse of the necrotic segment.

EPIDEMIOLOGY

AVN of the femoral head is a debilitating disease that usually leads to osteoarthritis of the hip joint in relatively young adults. The disease prevalence is unknown, but estimates indicate that 10,000-20,000 new cases are diagnosed in the United States per year. Furthermore, it is estimated that 5-18% of the more than 500,000 total hip arthroplasties performed annually are for osteonecrosis of the femoral head.

FUNCTIONAL ANATOMY

By the time an individual reaches age of 13-14 years, the partially ossified bone of the ilium, ischium, and pelvis coalesce to form a Y-shaped triradial cartilage, which proceeds to fuse by age of 15-16 years. The acetabulum is chiefly spherical in its superior margin and allows for approximately 170° of coverage of the femoral head. The femoral head is not perfectly spherical, and joint congruity is precise only in the weight-bearing position.

The internal trabecular system (Fig. 15.1) of the femoral head is oriented along lines of stress. Thick trabeculae that arise from the calcar extend into the weight-bearing dome of the femoral head and help to resist compressive loads across the joint.

The arterial supply to the femoral head is principally provided by 3 sources:

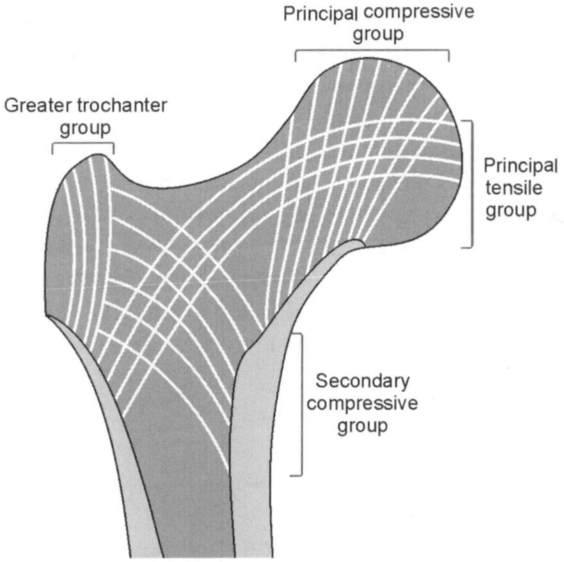

Fig. 15.1: Trabecular system of femoral head

- An extracapsular arterial ring at the base of the femoral neck.
- Ascending branches of the arterial ring on the femoral neck surface.
- Arteries of the round ligament.

This arterial supply is well affixed to the femoral neck and is easily damaged with any femoral neck fracture-displacement. Furthermore, nutrient vessels to the femoral head terminate in small arterioles that are easily occluded with small embolic matter (i.e., lipids).

SPORT-SPECIFIC BIOMECHANICS

Forces that act on the femoral head in vivo are appreciable. Standing on one leg generates a force of approximately 2.5 times the body weight across the loaded hip. Running increases femoral head forces to roughly 5 times the body weight, whereas simply performing a supine straight-leg raise generates 1.5 times the body weight across the hip joint. During gait, the maximum pressure occurs in the anterosuperior femoral surface and superior acetabular dome.

CAUSES

- Traumatic AVN is simply a result of mechanical disruption of blood flow to the femoral head. During sports endeavours, hip dislocation or subluxation is the most frequently reported traumatic means of AVN. A tackle from behind may cause an anterior hip subluxation in a ball carrier. Likewise, extreme abduction or external rotation may result in an anterior dislocation in a fallen water-skier.

  Similarly, a displaced femoral neck fracture can damage the fragile retinacular vessels, which supply the femoral head and result in femoral head necrosis.
- Traumatic causes of femoral head AVN include the following:
  - Femoral neck fractures
  - Hip dislocation
  - Slipped capital femoral epiphysis
- Most cases of AVN are atraumatic and include the following:
  - Excessive corticosteroid usage and alcohol abuse account for as many as 90% of new cases.
  - Intravascular coagulation appears to be the central event associated with non-traumatic AVN. Coagulation may occur secondary to extravascular compression (eg, marrow fat enlargement), vessel wall injury (e.g., chemotherapy, radiation), or a thromboembolic event (e.g., fat emboli).
  - Ischemic insult to the femoral head results in infarcted subchondral bone. In this situation, weakened and unrepaired necrotic bony trabeculae fail under a compressive load, leading to subchondral collapse (ie, crescent sign) and, ultimately, articular collapse.

Atraumatic osteonecrosis causes include the following:

- Alcohol abuse – Patients who consume less than 400 ml of alcohol per week have a 3-fold higher risk for AVN than individuals who do not drink. The risk rises to an 11-fold risk if more than 400 ml per week is consumed.
- Coagulopathies
- Chemotherapy
- Chronic liver disease
- Corticosteroids
- Decompression sickness
- Gaucher disease
- Gout
- Hemoglobinopathy (e.g., sickle cell disease)
- Idiopathic hyperlipidemia
- Idiopathic atraumatic osteonecrosis
- Metabolic bone disease
- Pregnancy
- Radiation
- Smoking
- Systemic lupus erythematosus
- Vasculitis

Clinical Course of The Disease

Patient with AVN usually present with nonspecific signs and symptoms. Early in the disease process, the condition is painless; however, patients ultimately present with pain and limitation of motion. The pain is most commonly localized to the groin area, but it may also manifest in the ipsilateral buttock, knee, or greater trochanteric region.

Painful symptoms are usually exacerbated with weight bearing but are relieved by rest.

Physical Examination

- Passive range of motion of the hip is limited and painful, especially forced internal rotation.
- A distinct limitation of passive abduction is usually noted.
- A straight-leg raise against resistance provokes pain in most symptomatic cases.
- Passive internal and external rotation of the extended leg ("log roll test") may elicit pain that is consistent with an active capsular synovitis.

Differential Diagnosis

- Femoral Neck Fracture
- Femoral Neck Stress Fracture
- Groin Injury
- Hip Dislocation
- Hip Fracture
- Hip Overuse Syndrome

Imaging Studies

Plain radiographs:

- Anteroposterior and frog-leg lateral views of both hips are obtained. The high incidence of bilateral involvement (>60%) and occult disease in cases of femoral head AVN warrant imaging of the unaffected leg.
- Early radiographic findings include:
  - Femoral Head Lucency
  - Subchondral Sclerosis
- With disease progression, following changes become evident:
  - Subchondral Collapse (Crescent Sign)
  - Femoral Head Flattening
  - Joint Space Narrowing (end result of untreated femoral head AVN)
- Radiographic staging of AVN was first proposed by Ficat and Arlet in the 1960s and later amended in the 1970s. This 4-stage system delineates the natural history of AVN:
  - Stage I: Normal Radiographs
  - Stage II: Cystic Changes and Sclerosis
  - Stage III: Subchondral Collapse or Femoral Head Flattening
  - Stage IV: Joint Space Narrowing

  However, this system does not differentiate among certain phases in disease progression (eg, subchondral vs femoral head collapse), nor does it quantify the size and extent of the lesion.
- Steinberg proposed the Steinberg Classification System, which is concise and delineates the progression and extent of AVN involvement more accurately.
  - Stage I – Normal radiographs; abnormal MRI or bone scan
  - Stage II – Abnormal lucency or sclerotic site in femoral head
  - Stage III – Subchondral collapse (ie, crescent sign) without flattening of femoral head
  - Stage IV – Flattening of the femoral head; normal joint space
  - Stage V – Joint space narrowing, acetabular changes, or both
  - Stage VI – Advanced degenerative changes
  - Stages I-IV are further subdivided according to the percentage of femoral head involvement: A (< 15%), B (15-30%), or C (>30%).

Magnetic Resonance Imaging (MRI):

- MRI is the study of choice in patients who demonstrate signs and symptoms that are suggestive of AVN but whose radiographs are normal.
- MRI is the most sensitive and specific means of diagnosing AVN. MRI may detect disease as early as 5 days subsequent to an ischemic insult.
- Characteristic MRI findings for AVN of the hip include a low signal intensity band (seen on T1 and T2 images) that demarcates a necrotic anterosuperior femoral head segment. The extent and location of femoral head necrosis on MRIs have been studied as predictors of femoral

head collapse. Smaller lesions (less than one fourth the diameter of the femoral head) and more medial lesions (away from primary weight-bearing areas) predict a better outcome.

Bone Scanning:

- Abnormalities may show up on a bone scan before they do on plain radiographs. Bone scan findings should be supplemented with MRI findings.
- The presence of a photopenic area that is surrounded by increased tracer uptake is the typical scintigraphic picture for radionuclide imaging.
- Bone scans are considerably less sensitive and less specific than MRI, but the images may be useful if the use of MRI is contraindicated.

Computed Tomography (CT) Scanning:

- CT scans confer significant radiation exposure to the patient and are less sensitive than MRI in diagnosing AVN.
- CT scanning may help delineate early subchondral collapse because the resolution of bony architecture with this modality is unsurpassed.

Angiography:

Angiography is an invasive mean of diagnostic confirmation of AVN; it is most useful as an investigational modality.

Arthroscopy:

The role of arthroscopy to better stage the extent of disease has emerged. Arthroscopic evaluation of the joint can help better define the extent of chondral flaps, joint degeneration and even joint collapse and may help with the temporary relief of synovitis.

Surgical Management

Surgical treatment of AVN can be broadly categorized as either prophylactic measures (to retard progression) or reconstruction procedures (after femoral head collapse).

Prophylactic Measures:

- *Core Decompression:* The most commonly performed prophylactic surgical intervention is core decompression, whereby one or more cores of necrotic femoral head bone is removed in order to stimulate repair.
  - Core decompression is often supplemented with bone grafting (cancellous autograft or structural allograft) to enhance mechanical support and augment healing.
  - Biologic augmentation of core decompression includes the addition of demineralised bone matrix, bone morphogenic proteins, or electric/electromagnetic stimulation. These agents are purported to either enhance bone formation or decrease bone resorption in the hope of maintaining the structural integrity of the femoral head. Biologic augmentation of core decompression alone offers therapeutic benefit—if it is instituted before subchondral collapse (Steinberg stage III).
  - The addition of a vascularized fibular graft to core decompression offers promise in cases with more advanced lesions, but this procedure involves considerable morbidity. One study indicated that vascularized fibular grafts were more effective in preventing femoral head collapse than non-vascularized fibular autografts.
- *Osteotomies:* Osteotomies are performed in attempt to move necrotic bone away from primary weight-bearing areas in the hip joint. Osteotomies can be angular or rotational, with the latter proving to be much more technically difficult. These techniques may delay arthroplasty, but they are best suited for small pre-collapse or early post-collapse of the femoral head in patients who don't have an ongoing cause of AVN. However, osteotomies make subsequent arthroplasty more challenging and, unfortunately, these procedures are associated with an appreciable risk of non-union.

Reconstruction Procedures

Despite aggressive management, most hips that undergo collapse ultimately require reconstruction (i.e., replacement). Prosthetic replacement offers the most predictable means of pain relief in advanced AVN; however, many arthroplasty options are available to meet the challenge of painful arthropathy in younger patients.

- *Femoral Resurfacing Arthroplasty:* Femoral resurfacing arthroplasty is gaining acceptance for younger patients. Both the femoral head and acetablum are "resurfaced" with metal, indicating minimal bone resection. This procedure circumvents the problem of polyethylene wear. However, technical and design problems with surface replacements may explain the relatively high failure rate in some clinical series. Nonetheless, refinements in both technique and design predict improved outcomes.
- *Resurfacing Arthroplasty:* Resurfacing arthroplasty remains a controversial procedure that likely will not last a patient's lifetime. Current recommendations are that resurfacing is contraindicated if the avascular area exceeds one third of the femoral head. Furthermore, there is a 1% incidence of femoral neck fracture with this procedure. Lastly, the issue of metal ion release has spurred much debate, although there are no good data available to suggest injurious effects. Fortunately, resurfacing arthroplasty likely confers no significant compromise for subsequent arthroplasty.
- *Bipolar Arthroplastty:* Bipolar arthroplasty theoretically decreases shear stress and impact load on acetabular cartilage, although this concept has not been born out clinically. Persistent groin pain, high rates of polyethylene wear, and early loosening have mitigated the appeal of this option.
- *Resection Arthroplasty:* Resection arthroplasty should only be considered in very young patients and in debilitated patients who are at high risk for infection (e.g., patients on dialysis).
- *Total Hip Arthroplasty:* Total hip arthroplasty is perhaps the most commonly performed and successful surgery for advanced AVN of the hip. Cementless prostheses with an improved design may afford increased longevity relative to cemented counterparts. Despite recent improvements in prosthetic replacement, replacement arthroplasty precludes further participation in impact activities (e.g., running, jogging) because these activities greatly decrease implant longevity.

Physiotherapy Intervention

The physiotherapeutic intervention for the patients treated with total hip arthroplasty has been explained in detail in the chapter dealing with replacement surgeries.

HIP OSTEOARTHRITIS

PREVALENCE

Osteoarthritis is the most common cause of hip pain in older adults. Prevalence studies have shown the rates for adult hip OA range from 0.4% to 27%.

Pathoanatomical Features (Fig. 15.2)

In osteoarthritis of the hip the entire joint structure and function is affected, with joint capsular changes (shortening and lengthening) creating limitation in hip joint range of motion (ROM) along with subsequent articular cartilage degeneration. Later in the disease process osteophytes or spurs may develop from excessive tensile force on the hip joint capsule or from abnormal pressure on the articular cartilage. Other changes also develop including sclerosis of the subchondral bone from increased focal pressure, and sometimes the formation of cysts. Muscle weakness often develops around a joint with osteoarthritis, specifically the abductor muscles of the hip. Most

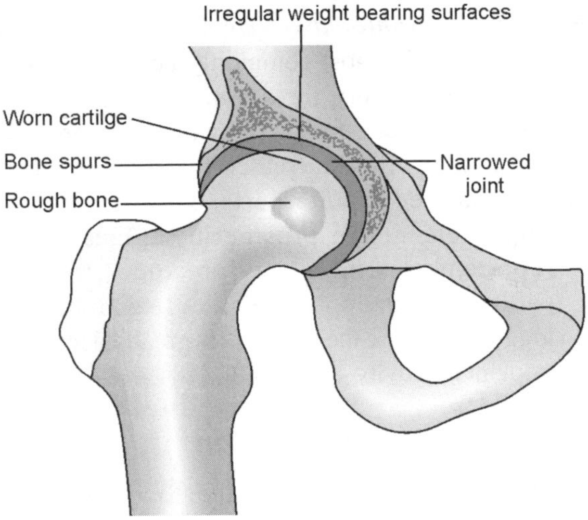

Fig. 15.2: Pathoanatomical changes in OA hip

significantly, the hip abductor muscles progressively weaken in the later stages of hip osteoarthritis, which may create a Trendelenberg gait pattern over time.

Risk Factors

Age: The most common predisposing factor for hip osteoarthritis is age. The condition primarily affects middle-aged and elderly people, most often those over 60 years.

Developmental Disorders: Many studies have demonstrated a link between developmental disorders and pre-mature osteoarthritis of hip. Developmental disorders can be enlisted as:

- Legg-Calve-Perthes disease
- Congenital Hip Dislocation
- Slipped Capital Femoral Epiphysis
- Dysplasia of the Femur and the Acetabulum. Types of dysplasia include:
  - Coxa Vara
  - Coxa Valga
  - Femoral Anteversion
  - Femoral Retroversion
  - Acetabular Anteversion
  - Acetabular Retroversion
  - Coxa Plana
  - Coxa Profundus

Occupation: Lifting very heavy loads over a prolonged period of time. Regular heavy lifting, tractor driving (vibration) and walking on uneven ground are commonly associated with hip osteoarthritis.

Sports Exposure: High intensity, direct impact activities, such as American football and hockey, appear to increase the risk of hip osteoarthritis.

Previous Injury: Proximal hip fracture results in changes to the articular surfaces of the hip joint that creates abnormal joint load bearing and has been shown to be related to the development of hip OA. A history of a previous hip injury is also associated with hip osteoarthritis.

Body Mass index: Obesity is probably associated with the progression of hip osteoarthritis rather than onset and the therapeutic value of weight loss is important.

Natural History of the Disease

The changes that occur around the arthritic hip include a decrease in the joint space between the femur and acetabulum, shortening of the fibrous joint capsule, flattening of the femoral head, the appearance of osteophytic growth around the margins of the femoral head and acetabulum, a superior-lateral or medial migration of the femoral head, and the development of subchondral sclerosis or cysts in the femoral head and acetabulum.

Changes that occur outside of the hip joint include a decreased amount of hip joint ROM (mostly affecting internal rotation and then flexion) and muscle weakness (particularly the abductor muscles), which eventually may result in difficulty with ambulation.

Classification

Hip osteoarthritis is classified as primary in the absence of any obvious underlying joint abnormality, or secondary if degeneration occurs as a result of a pre-existing abnormal joint problem.

Diagnosis

The diagnosis of hip osteoarthritis can be made with a reasonable level of certainty on the basis of the history, physical examination and radiographic evaluation.

Following changes on a plain film radiographs is considered the definitive diagnosis.

- Joint Space Narrowing
- Osteophytes
- Subchondral Sclerosis

The Kellgren/Lawrence scale has been used to classify degenerative findings associated with hip OA. The scale consists of 4 grades:

- Grade 1: No radiographic evidence of OA
- Grade 2: Doubtful narrowing of joint space and possible (minute) osteophytes
- Grade 3: Moderate definite osteophytes, definite moderate narrowing of joint space
- Grade 4: Large osteophytes, severe joint space narrowing, subchondral sclerosis, and definite deformity of bone contour.

The following clinical criteria are typically present in individuals who have radiographic findings consistent with hip osteoarthritis:

- Patient reported moderate pain in the lateral or anterior hip with weight bearing. This pain may progress to the anterior thigh or knee region.
- Adults, greater than 50 years of age.
- Limited passive hip joint ROM in at least 2 of its 6 directions (Flexion, extension, abduction, adduction, internal rotation and external rotation).
- Morning stiffness, which improves in less than 1 hour.

Differential Diagnosis

The following differential diagnoses should be considered in an individual with signs or symptoms suggestive of hip OA:

- Bursitis or tendinitis
- Chondral damage or loose bodies
- Femoral neck or pubic ramus stress fracture
- Labral tear
- Muscle strain
- Neoplasm
- Osteonecrosis of the femoral head
- Paget's disease
- Piriformis syndrome
- Psoriatic arthritis
- Rheumatoid arthritis
- Sacroiliac joint dysfunction
- Septic hip arthritis
- Referred pain as a result of an L2-3 radiculopathy.

Functional Assessment

Clinicians should use validated functional outcome measures before and after interventions intended to alleviate the impairments of body function and structure, activity limitations, and participation restrictions associated with hip osteoarthritis. Following functional outcome measures can be used:

- Western Ontario and McMaster Universities Osteoarthritis Index
- Lower Extremity Functional Scale
- Harris Hip Score

Interventions

A variety of interventions have been described for the treatment of hip osteoarthritis and there is fair evidence from randomized clinical trials and systematic reviews to support the benefits of physical therapy intervention in these patients.

Anti Inflammatory Agents:

Anti inflammatory agents including NSAIDs, Cox-2 inhibitors, and steroid injections are recommended as part of a multidisciplinary treatment approach to hip OA. These can be effective for the temporary relief of symptoms and improvement in function in patients with hip osteoarthritis.

Alternative / Complemetary Medication:

Glucosamine and other similar supplements are commonly suggested for individuals with hip osteoarthritis. These medications results in short-term improvement in pain and in function.

There is some evidence to support the short-term use of injectable viscosupplementation with hyaluronic acid into hip joint of patients with hip osteoarthritis. It works best in mild to moderate hip osteoarthritis, especially when conservative therapy has failed.

Patient Education:

Studies have shown the benefit of patient education in the self-management of patients with arthritis in decreasing pain, improving function, reducing stiffness and fatigue. Clinicians should consider the use of patient education to teach activity modification, exercise, weight reduction when overweight, and methods of unloading the arthritic joints.

An approach, called Hip School that includes primarily patient education as an intervention has been shown to be effective in a preliminary study for patients with signs and symptoms of hip osteoarthritis. The Hip School highlights the need for educating patients with hip osteoarthritis, especially understanding the importance of preserving hip range of motion and muscle function, understanding what therapy is effective and what is not, and when surgery is likely indicated.

Functional, Gait and Balance Training:

Patients with hip osteoarthritis often have gait abnormalities such as asymmetry in weight bearing and step length. Assistive device are often used in patients with hip osteoarthritis to reduce the pain and activity limitations associated with this condition. A cane in the contralateral hand and choosing to carry loads in the ipsilateral hand has been shown to be effective in reducing hip abductor muscles activity and acetabular contact pressures. One study has shown a cane in the opposite hand can reduce hip load, reduce hip pain, and improve function in patients with hip osteoarthritis.

Functional, gait, and balance training is recommended to address impairments of proprioception, balance, and strength, which are all commonly found in individuals with lower extremity arthritis. These deficits can contribute to higher fall risk scores in older individuals.

Manual Therapy:

Some evidence exists for using manual therapy to improve hip joint range of motion, function and reduce pain for short-term in patients with hip osteoarthritis. The manual therapy session consisted of:

- Stretching techniques of shortened muscles surrounding the hip joint.
- Traction of the hip joint.
- Traction manipulation (high velocity thrust technique) in each limited position.

Flexibility, Strengthening and endurance exercises:

The focus of the therapeutic exercise intervention is to improve hip range of motion, muscle length, and strength along with walking endurance.

There are three categories of exercise therapy employed for osteoarthritis:

- ROM/flexibility exercises: Exercise to regain or maintain motion and flexibility is achieved by routines of low-intensity, controlled movements that do not cause increased pain.
- Muscle strengthening exercises: Muscle weakness around an osteoarthritic joint is a common finding. Progressive resistive/ strengthening exercises load muscles in a graduated manner that allow strengthening while limiting tissue injury.
- Aerobic conditioning/endurance exercises: Aerobic exercise has been shown to be helpful in patients with hip osteoarthritis. Aerobic exercises are usually designed to provide a workload to the cardiovascular and pulmonary system at 60% to 80% of maximal capacity and sustained for duration of at least 20 minutes.

Often all 3 types of exercises are utilized jointly for patients with hip OA. Adequate joint motion and elasticity of periarticular tissues are necessary for cartilage nutrition and health, protection of joint structures from damaging impact loads, function, and comfort in daily activities.

Stretching Exercises:

The emphasis of the stretching was on hip muscles, including the iliopsoas, rectus femoris, and hip adductors. Before stretching it is advised to heat the specific muscle and then stretch gently without excessive force for 15 to 30 seconds, performed 5 to 10 times preferably daily, at least 3 times a week.

PERTHE'S DISEASE

It is a painful disorder of childhood, osteochondritis of epiphysis of femoral head characterised by its avascular necrosis.

OTHER NAMES

- Legg Calve Perthes disease.
- Coxa plana.
- Pseudo coxalgia.
- Osteochondritis of femoral capital epiphysis.

Aetiology

Age group: The common age group affected by the disorder is 4-8 years.
Gender: Boys are more commonly more affected than girls in the ratio of 4:1.
Cause: Local disturbance of the blood supply to the femoral head.

Pathogenesis

The cardinal step in pathogenesis is the ischaemia of the femoral head leading to partial or complete avascularization and deformation of femoral head.

In children of age group 4-7 years the blood supply of femoral head is completely dependent on the lateral epiphyseal vessels running in the retinacula. Their anatomical position makes them susceptible to stretching and pressure from effusion. This pressure may cause venous stasis resulting in rise in intraosseous pressure and consequent ischaemia.

The bony nucleus of epiphysis of femoral head undergoes necrosis either in whole or part, presumably from ischaemia. This sets up a sequence of changes which occupies two to three years. In this stage femoral head is susceptible to get deformed if subjected to stresses of weight bearing.

Bony Changes: As the bone is constantly suffering deformation, the femoral head as a whole may become much flattened (Fig. 15.3). At the same time there is often some enlargement of femoral head. As the acetabulum grows, it tends to follow the contours of femoral head, so that it may end up abnormally large and shallow.

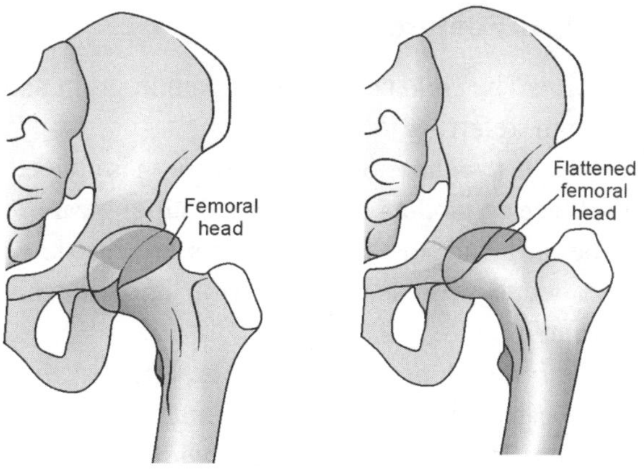

Fig. 15.3: Flattened femoral head

Stages

Stage I: Ischaemia and bone death - The femoral head is either partially or completely dead. The cartilaginous part of femoral head being nourished by synovial fluid remains viable and becomes thicker than normal. There may also be thickening and oedema of synovium and capsule.

Stage II: Revascularisation and repair - Dead marrow is replaced by granulation tissue within weeks of infarction. The bone is revascularised and the new bone is laid down.

Stage III: Distortion and remodeling - This stage depends upon the repair process.

- If repair is rapid and complete: The bony architecture may be restored before the femoral head loses its shape.
- If repair is tardy: Collapse of bony epiphysis, distortion of femoral head and neck occurs.

Clinical Features

- *Pain:* The child complains of pain in groin and thigh, referring to the knee.
- *Hip musculature:* Sometimes wasting is noticed.
- *Range of motion:* The affected hip appears to be stiff and all the movements are restricted especially those of abduction and internal rotation.
- *Limb length discrepancy:* The affected limb appears to be shorter than normal.
- *Limp:* The child usually walks with a limp. The patient demonstrates difficulty in swing through and limp may be accompanied by exaggerated trunk and pelvic movement. Classic manifestations of limp are lateral rotation, flexion and adduction of hip. The patient exaggerates movement of pelvis and trunk to help move the thigh into flexion.

Radiological Examination

- Asymmetry of ossific centres.
- Collapse and sclerosis of epiphysis of femoral head.
- Increase in joint space.
- Flattening and lateral displacement of epiphysis.
- Rarefaction and widening of metaphysis.
- 'Sagging rope' sign may be positive on the anteroposterior radiograph of the affected hip joint. The sign indicates damage to the growth plate with marked metaphyseal reaction. Its presence indicates a severe disease process.

Bone scan reveals decreased uptake by femoral head.

Catterall describes the disease in four groups based on appearances in both anteroposterior and lateral radiographs:

- Group 1: Epiphysis has retained its height and less than half the nucleus is sclerotic.
- Group 2: Upto half the nucleus is sclerotic and there may be some collapse of central portion.
- Group 3: Most of the nucleus is sclerotic. There occurs fragmentation and collapse of femoral head.
- Group 4: Whole head is involved; the ossific nucleus is flat and dense with marked metaphyseal resorbtion.

Prognosis

The prognosis of the disease varies with the amount of involvement of femoral head and also with the age of the patient. The outlook of the disease and the prognosis is excellent if the child is under 6 years of age. After that with increasing age, the prognosis becomes poorer.

There are certain radiographic features which act as adverse prognostic signs:

- Progressive uncovering of epiphysis.
- Calcification in the cartilage later to ossific nucleus.
- Radiolucent area at lateral edge of bony epiphysis.
- Severe metaphyseal resorption.

Management

The management of the Perthe's disease depends upon the stage of the disease:

Acute stage: In the acute stage when all the pathological process has set in, the child is in extreme pain and discomfort. The hip at this stage is regarded as irritable. In this stage the child must be immobilized so as to avoid any weight or pressure on the affected hip. The immobilization is done with the help of skin traction. The hip is maintained in a position of little flexion and external rotation.

Sub-acute stage: Once the irritability has subsided which usually takes around three weeks symptomatic treatment is encouraged.

- Pain control by further spells of traction if necessary.
- Gentle exercises are initiated to maintain movement.

Precautions: Although ambulation is allowed, child is not supposed to play sports or do any strenuous activity.

The subacute stage is of basically group 1 and 2 patients who need supervised neglect.

Chronic Stage: It is group 3 and 4 patients in which the head is not deformed but demands the utmost care. Containment of the femoral head into the acetabular cavity is the main aim of the treatment. It could either follow a conservative or the surgical pathway.

- *Conservative means of containment:* The hips are held in a position of abduction so that the femoral head is totally covered by the acetabulum. This could be attained by either of the following means:
  - Plaster of paris cast.
  - Brace.
  - Splint.
- *Surgical means of containment:*
  - Varus osteotomy of proximal femur.
  - Innominate osteotomy of pelvis.

Physiotherapy Management

The physiotherapeutic intervention plays an important role in Perthe's disease so as to make the patient self-ambulatory and maximizes his abilities.

Aims of Physiotherapy Management:

- Maximizing range of motion.
- Improving muscular strength.
- Ambulation of patient.

Physiotherapy during the application of Skin Traction:

- Application of cryotherapy techniques or moist heat to the affected hip in order to reduce muscular spasm. It is important to reduce this muscular spasm as it leads to pain and deformity.
- Mild isometric contractions are initiated which should be painless to the following muscle groups: glutei, hip abductors and quadriceps.
- If the skin traction is intermittent, then small range passive movements can be performed in the traction free intervals as it improves the nourishment to the joint surface.

Physiotherapy following Skin Traction:

- *Postural correction of the limb:* Proper posture of the affected limb is to be maintained so that the limb does not rests in an unwanted position for a longer period of time causing stretch and stress on the muscles and the joint.
- *Range of motion exercises:* The affected hip is to be moved through full arc of movement so as to maintain the muscle's flexibility and physiological properties. Special attention to be paid on the movements of abduction and internal rotation.
- *Prevention of contractures:* The affected hip joint is at the risk of developing contractures especially at the flexor aspect. This tendency

of the flexor tightness at the hip joint is due to the positioning of the limb. This flexor tightness or the contracture will complicate ambulation and gait pattern whenever the child is allowed to bear weight on the affected limb. Following measures can be taken to prevent the above-mentioned problems:

- Continuous stretching of hip flexors.
- Sessions of prone lying.

• *Increasing muscular strength:* Following measures should be taken to increase the muscular strength depending upon the degree of comfort of the patient:

  - Active-assisted, active or resisted exercises.
  - Eccenteric exercises.
  - Isometerics at the terminal range of movements.

• *Ambulation and gait training:* Initially non-weight bearing standing and walking is taught in the parallel bars when the limb is immobilized into the POP cast or brace. Then progression is made to walker and then to axillary crutches. Transfer activities should be taught.

UNIT EIGHT

KNEE JOINT CONDITIONS

16. KNEE CONDITIONS

CHAPTER 16

KNEE CONDITIONS

CHONDROMALACIA PATELLAE

Chondromalacia patellae is the condition affecting the knee joint leading to softening of the articular cartilage of knee cap, i.e., patella. The condition is also referred as Runner's knee. The softening of the articular cartilage leads to its break down producing irregularities along undersurface of patella (Fig. 16.1).

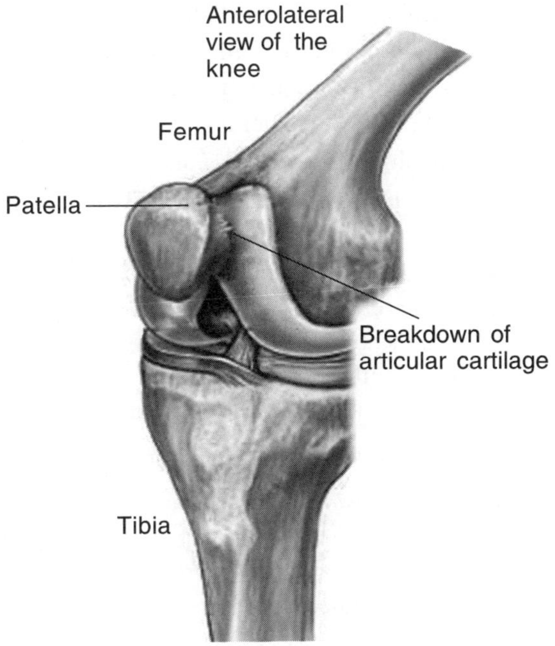

Fig. 16.1: Chondromalacia patellae

Causes

The condition is more prevalent in either the teenagers and the patients of older age group with different causative factors.

In Older Age Group: This group consists of patients more than 40 years of age. The condition is slowly progressive due to natural wear and tear of the bones ultimately leading to osteoarthitis.

In Teenagers: In this age group, the condition commonly affects the teenager girls who are involved in active sports. The softening of the articular cartilage is due to excessive and uneven pressure on the cartilage due to following:

- *Structural changes in legs:* Due to the growth spurt, various structural changes occur in the lower limb bones of young girls commonly accentuating the knee valgus, i.e., knock knees due to which Q-angle increases leading to increase tendency of patella to dislocate laterally with knee flexion.
- *Muscular imbalance around knee:* Vastus lateralis component of the quadriceps femoris muscle is more powerful than vastus medialis thus increasing the tendency of patella to track or dislocate laterally thus inducing undue pressure on lateral facet leading to cartilage softening and breakdown.

Clinical Features

- Pain in front of the knee is the most common complain by the patient. The nature of the pain is deep seated radiating to the back of knee joint.

The pain increases with the repeated knee flexion. Following are the postures that aggravate the pain:
  - Squatting.
  - Kneeling.
  - Negotiating steps especially descending the stairs.
- The patient complains of visible lateral tracking or dislocation of the patella on attempting knee flexion.
- Locking of the knee joint.
- Mild knee effusion may be present.
- Slight atrophy of quadriceps is also evident.
- The range of motion of affected knee joint is normal.

Radiographic Examination

Antero-posterior (AP) and lateral view of the knee joint on a radiograph appears to be normal. The lateral displacement of the patella is noticed on the sunrise or patellar view.

Management

Conservative Management

Usually the patients of chondromalacia patella are treated with the help of physical therapy without any further intervention. But in the patients who complain of very painful knee, immobilization in a POP cylinder cast is needed. The period of immobilization is till the pain subsides.

The non-steroidal anti-inflammatory drugs (NSAIDs) are prescribed in the initial acute stage.

Surgical Management:

- Arthroscopic release of lateral muscles, i.e., vastus lateralis. This release leads to weakness of vastus lateralis. So the strengthening of quadriceps muscle is required.
- *Open surgery:* Extensive open realignment of quadriceps mechanism and bone work is done. The open surgery is done only in the patients with:
  - Severe structural damage or dislocation of patella.
  - Increased Q-angle.
  - Lateral subluxation or dislocation of patella.

Prevention of Chondromalacia Patellae

The prevention of the condition should be initiated in young patients having:
- Anterior knee pain.
- Knock knees.
- Tightness in lateral knee muscles.

Following Measures Should Be Taken

- Warm up and stretching of quadriceps and hamstrings before initiating the game.
- Avoid squatting, kneeling and stairs.
- Consistent and persistent knee exercises should be practised.

Physiotherapy Management

Goal of physiotherapy treatment is to restore the normal patellar alignment with the help of exercises.

Physiotherapy Intervention

- Strengthening of vastus medialis obliqus (VMO).
- Intervention to reduce pain: Pulsed short-wave diathermy ultrasonic therapy.
- Stretching of vastus lateralis.
- Strengthening of quadriceps and hamstrings.
- Patellar taping to prevent lateral redisplacement of patella.
- *Knee brace:*

Patients who are active in sports should use knee brace: Patella stabilizing brace consisting of knee sleeve with patella cutout and horse shoe based laterally to prevent patella from tracking laterally.

Following Exercises Should Be Practised

- *Short arc extension:*

In supine lying, use a rolled up towel to support the thigh while the leg and foot are in air for 5 sec. Lower the foot as knee is flexed slowly. Repeat 10 times each leg.

- Quadriceps isometric exercises.
- Stationary bicycling on low effort.

- *Straight Leg Raises (SLR):* The patient in supine lying - lift the whole lower limb at hip with knee extended. Keep in air for 5 sec. Repeat 10 times. The contralateral hip and knee are flexed with foot supported.

MEDIAL COLLATERAL LIGAMENT (MCL) INJURY

The medial collateral ligament of the knee is attached superiorly to the medial epicondyle of the femur just below the adductor tuburcle (Fig. 16.2). Inferiorly it is divided into anterior and posterior parts. The anterior (Superficial) part is attatched below to the medial border and posterior part of medial surface of tibial shaft. The posterior (deep) part of the ligament blends with medial meniscus. It is attatched to medial condyle of tibia above the groove for semimembranous.

Functions of MCL

- The MCL resists valgus stress occuring at the knee joint being especially effective in extended knee when the ligament is taut.

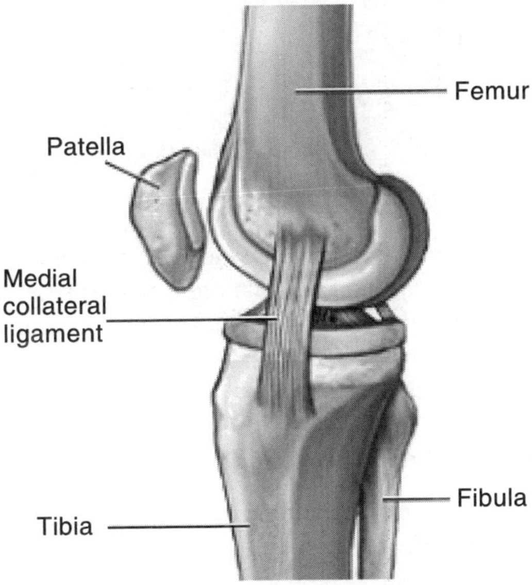

Fig. 16.2: Medial collateral ligament

- MCL plays critical role in resisting valgus stress in slightly flexed knee when other structures make a lesser contribution.
- The alignment of MCL checks the lateral rotation of tibia.
- MCL is a restraint to pure anterior displacement of tibia when primary restraint of anterior cruciate ligament (ACL) is absent.

Causes of MCL Injury

- Direct injury to lateral aspect of knee creating valgus force.
- Forced abduction of tibia.
- Abduction force when the foot and tibia are fixed and the femur is forced medially.
- Rotational force of femur on fixed tibia.

MCL injuries are common in sports activities such as football, high jumping and skiing. It can also occur in swimming due to forceful kick in breast stroke.

Nature of Injury

Most of the MCL injuries occur at the femoral origin or in the mid substance over the joint line (Fig. 16.3), tibial avulsions do occur. The difference over the injury site is due to difference in insertion site structures.

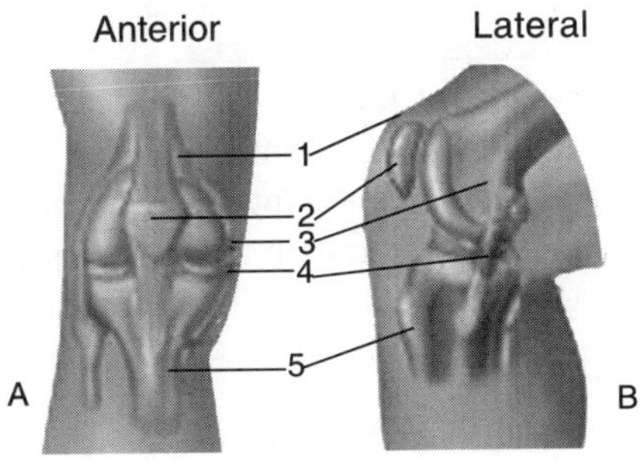

1. Femur
2. Patella
3. Medial collateral ligament
4. Tear
5. Tibia

Fig. 16.3: Medial collateral ligament tear

The MCL injuries could be isolated, being pure MCL injury or could be associated with cruciate ligament injury. The associated injuries occur only if the causative force is rotational in nature.

Classification of MCL Injury

Grade	*Ligament disruption*	*Clinical features*
Grade 1	Micro trauma	Knee is stable Tenderness present No valgus laxity
Grade 2	Elongated but intact ligament	Increased valgus laxity Involuntary guarding present
Grade 3	Complete disruption	↑↑ Valgus laxity

Physical Examination

Examination of the patient begins with detailed history taking which is important in order to determine the mechanism of the injury. The patient complains of pain at the medial aspect of the knee joint.

Pain

There is sharp, sudden pain over the medial side of the knee. The pain might restrict the range of motion of the affected knee in case of severe injury.

On Inspection

- Localized oedema over MCL.
- Prominent medial femoral epicondyle due to injury to the ligament at femoral origin.
- Large effusion indicating intra-articular injury.
- The affected knee is held in a position of slight flexion, as MCL is taut in full extension.

On Palpation

While palpating through full length of ligament from femoral origin to tibial insertion, maximal tenderness is revealed over the injured portion of ligament, which is usually near the upper end at the attachment of medial condyle of femur.

On Movement

If the knee is forcefully attempted to be in full extension it produces medial knee pain.

Clinical Diagnostic Test

Valgus Laxity Test: The patient is positioned in supine. The examiner supports the leg with one hand under the heel and with the other hand applies a gentle valgus force to the fully extended knee (Fig. 16.4). In a normal knee the examiner feels firm resistance with virtually no separation of femur and tibia. In an abnormal knee, the femur and tibia will be felt to separate in response to valgus force and to clink back together when the force is relaxed.

If the valgus stress test is normal with knee in full extension, the examiner flexes the knee about

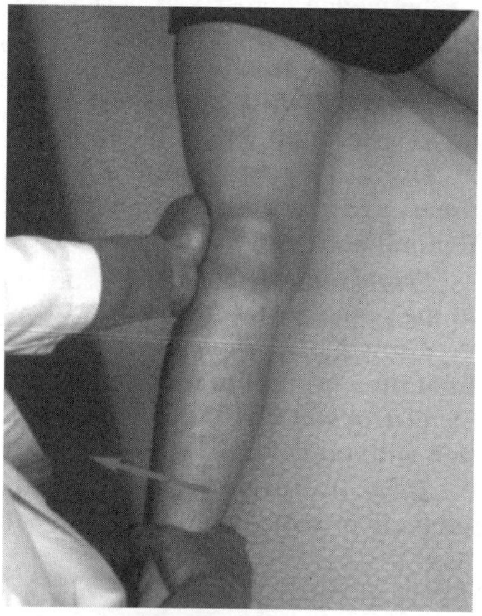

Fig. 16.4: Valgus laxity test

30° and repeats the test. The flexion relaxes the posterior capsule and permits more isolated testing of MCL. With the knee flexed, the examiner again evaluates the firmness of resistance and the amount of joint separation.

Radiographic Examination

The affected knee is examined radiographcially in order to exclude any bony injury.

Differential Diagnosis

- Medial knee contusion.

- Medial meniscal tear.
- Patellar subluxation or dislocation.

Prognosis

MCL has good capacity for repair without any surgical intervention. It heals well without any long-term damage to knee but some valgus laxity does remains.

Management

The treatment of medial collateral ligament depends upon the nature of the injury, whether isolated or combined. In case of isolated injury of MCL only conservative treatment is adequate but in case of combined injury (with meniscus or cruciate ligament) surgical intervention is required.

Conservative Treatment:

It is indicated in case of isolated injury of medial collateral ligament. The affected knee is immobilized either using a long leg plaster, knee immobilizer or full leg braces. But in the present scenario, these methods are discouraged as they tend to inhibit range of motion at the knee joint and prolonged the period of disability.

Now-a-days a light weight hinged brace is used to protect the knee against valgus stresses of function. The brace is worn at all times during initial 3-4 weeks. The brace should not restrict motion or inhibit muscle function.

Surgical Treatment:

The surgical intervention is required in case of combined injury. The structures injured in the medial compartment of the affected knee other than MCL are repaired and then the repair of MCL is done.

Physiotherapy Management

Aims of Physiotherapy Treatment:

- To reduce inflammation
- To decrease pain
- To maintain and gain range of motion.
- To increase muscular strength.
- To aid ambulation and balance.
- To enhance the mobility of the injured ligament.
- Maintenance program.

Physiotherapeutic Intervention

- *To reduce inflammation:*
  This is an important aspect in the acute phase of injury and "PRICE" is the best modality to control inflammation.
  P - Prevention of any further injury.
  R - Rest to the affected area (Affected knee joint).
  I - Ice.
  C - Compression bandage.
  E – Eleveation of the affected leg.
  Ice is introduced either as cold packs, ice toweling or cryotherapy to the medial aspect of the knee joint for 20 min. after every 3-4 hours for initial 48 hours. Cryotherapy provides pain relief and helps in reducing the oedema along with elevation.
- *To decrease pain:*
  In order to decrease pain cryotherapy is the best treatment modality in first 48 hours. After 48 hours interferential therapy (IFT) acts as an adjunct to reduce pain and swelling.
- *To maintain and gain range of motion:*
  For the initial two days the patient should only attempt non-painful motion at the knee joint. As the acute episode ceases, active and active-assisted exercises play an important role in gaining range of motion at knee joint. Following sets of exercises should be practised.
  - The patient is in prone lying attempting knee flexion at the affected joint firstly active and then it could progress to active-assisted where the contralateral leg could assist in the flexion of the affected knee to a greater extent by exerting pressure.
  - The patient must practice knee flexion-extension in high sitting position. The patient is positioned at the end of a table with hip flexed to 90° and knee in the available range

of flexion. This is the best position to gain knee flexion upto 90º as the gravity assists in the motion. For better results, a weight cuff could be tied at the patient's ankle of the affected leg. In this position, knee extension should be practised both in active and active-assisted (the contralateral leg helps in gaining extension) manner.

- When all the signs of inflammation disappears and there is no instability at the affected knee joint, the physiotherapist must begin with passive mobilization of the knee joint to gain maximum range of motion.

- *To increase muscular strength:*

  Exercises and activity that aids in gaining muscular strength especially for the quadriceps femoris must begin at the earliest in order to prevent the atrophy of quadriceps muscle. Strengthening of hamstrings is also important. The strengthening exercises for both the muscles must begin as isometrics progressing to isotonic and to eccentric exercises.

  - Isometeric Exercises

- Towel extension exercises are performed to prevent any atrophy to the quadriceps muscles.
- In prone lying hamstring isometrics could be performed by tightening the buttoks.
- Hamstrings isometric exercises could also be performed in supine lying with towel under the heel.
  - Isotonic and eccentric exercises should be performed for quadriceps, hamstrings and hip abductors.
  - Progressive resistive exercises must be practised to gain further strength.

- *To aid ambulation and balance:*

  The patient is made ambulatory soon after the injury with the help of a walking aid. The choice of the initial walking aid depends upon the severity of the injury. It could either be a walker or crutches. In the initial period weight bearing is allowed on the affected limb as tolerated by the patient. The walking aid is discarded as soon as full extension is gained at the affected knee joint. Walking re-education is important for a proper gait.

  Weight bearing and balance drills are important to gain proper balance and ambulation. Weight bearing exercises are practised after the cessation of inflammatory period and when there is no laxity in the ligament. Following weight bearing exercises and balance drills can be practiced:
  - Single leg standing.
  - Mini squats progressing to complete squats.
  - Star jumps.
  - Stepping on and off a form.
  - Proprioception training.
  - Balance board exercises.

- To enhance the mobility of injured ligament:

  It is important to enhance the mobility and pliability of the injured ligament so that it could not be easily injured in future. Following physiotherapeutic adjuncts helps in gaining mobility and pliability:
  - Transverse friction to the superficial fibers with knee in extended positison and deep fibers with knee in flexed position. The transverse friction is also required to the part of capsule between patella and femur.
  - Ultrasonic therapy to the affected area.

- Maintenance program:

  The maintenance program is required to make the knee as normal as possible and to prevent any further damage. The maintenance program could be made enjoyable and relaxing for the patient while improving and maintaining the flexibility, range of motion, strength and proprioception at the affected joint.

  Following could be practised:
  - Whirlpool bath.
  - Stationary bike.
  - Self stretching exercises.
  - Isokinetic strengthening.
  - Leg press (machine or self).
  - Lunges (forward and lateral).
  - Swimming.

LATERAL COLLATERAL LIGAMENT INJURY

The lateral collateral ligament of the knee also known as fibular collateral ligament, is strong and cord like. Superiorly it is attached to lateral epicondyle of femur just above the popliteal groove (Fig. 16.5). Inferiorly it is attached to head of fibula embraced by tendon of biceps femoris. The tendon of popliteus separates the lateral collateral ligament from meniscus.

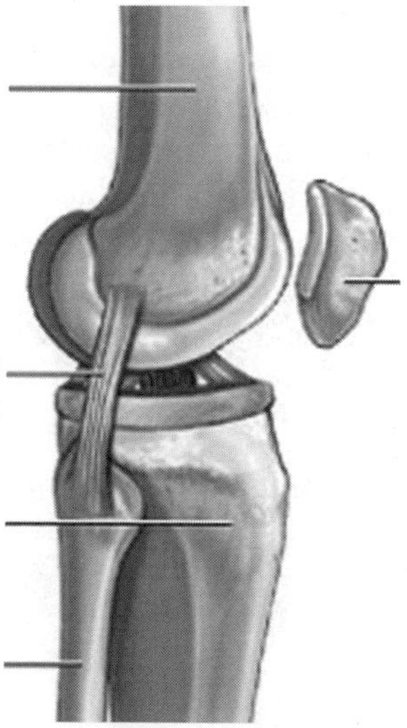

Fig. 16.5: Lateral collateral ligament

Functions of LCL

- It resists varus stress across the knee.
- It limits lateral rotation of tibia in conjunction with postero-lateral capsule.
- It also resists combined lateral rotation with posterior displacement of tibia in conjunction with popliteal tendon.

Causes of LCL injury

- Abduction of tibia on femur.
- Hypextension varus force.
- Varus stress on knee.
- Overuse injury in sports activities like:
  - Cross country running.
  - Long distance skiing.

Nature of Injury

Chronic sprain of LCL are more common than acute sprain. Complete rupture of LCL are very rare and if occurs is at mid-substance or at fibular insertion (Fig. 16.6). In young individuals injury to the growth plate occurs prior to ligamentous injury. The ligament is usually avulsed from fibular head along with piece of bone.

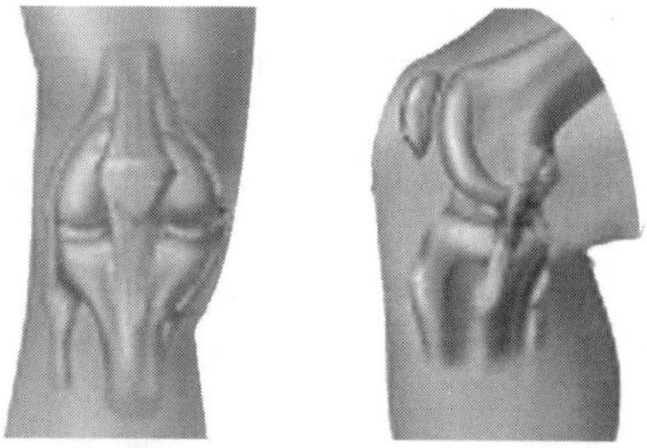

Fig. 16.6: Rupture of LCL

Associated Injury

- *Posterior cruciate ligament injury:* Excessive varus instability in knee extension as well as flexion indicates involvement of posterior cruciate ligament.
- Common peroneal nerve injury.
- Arcuate ligament injury.
- Biceps femoris injury.
- Popliteus tendon injury.

Clinical Features

In case of acute sprain of LCL, clinical features are similar to MCL injury but are localised to lateral side of the joint.

- *Pain:* The patient experiences light aching pain initially which goes off with rest. The intensity of pain decreases gradually and it takes longer time to settle. Pain is present on lateral side of knee towards fibular head.
- *Tenderness:* Marked tenderness is present over the ligament and fibular head but no tenderness is detected over the joint line.
- *LCL is taut in full extension:* The patient may experience lateral knee pain when the knee is over pressured into full extension.

Clinical Diagnostic Test

Varus Laxity Test (Fig. 16.7): The patient is positioned in supine with the knee first in full extension and then in 30° of flexion. The therapist stands on the side of the injured leg and applies varus stress in both extended and 30° flexed position (Fig. 16.8). The therapist compares the firmness of resistance and the amount of joint separation in both the knees.

The femur and tibia will be felt to separate with varus force and clink back together when the force is released, in case of LCL injury.

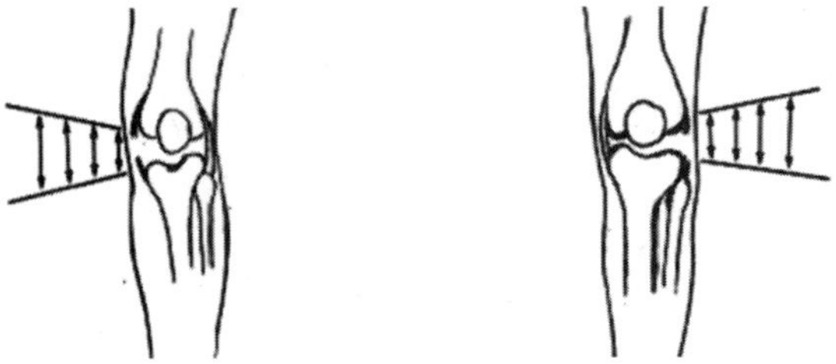

Fig. 16.7: Varus laxity test

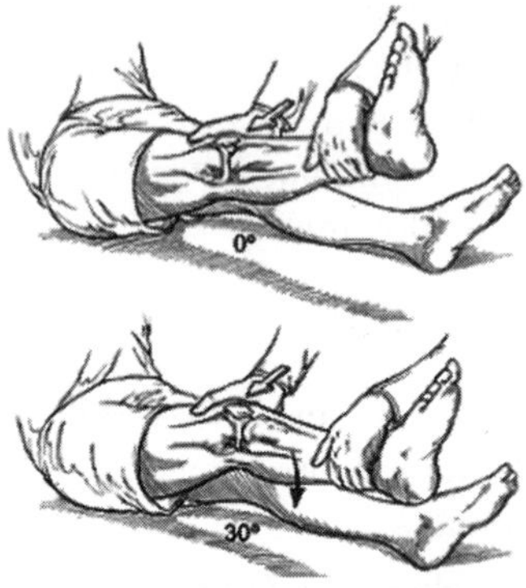

Fig. 16.8: Varus laxity test

Prognosis

The recovery of the LCL injury is always remarkable and full as there are many other stabilizing agents on lateral side of knee. Following are the stabilizing agents that aid in achieving full recovery after LCL injury:

- Iliotibial tract.
- Biceps femoris.
- Popliteus tendon.
- Arcuate ligament.

There is no significant long-term disability after LCL injury rehabilitation.

Physiotherapy Management

The physiotherapy management follows the same lines as for medial collateral ligament emphasizing upon lateral aspect of the knee joint.

MENISCAL INJURIES

Menisci are the semilunar cartilages mainly composed of collagen fibers with some elastic tissue present on the proximal surface of the tibial condyles (Fig. 16.9). The knee menisci are dependent on the synovial fluid for their nutrition as they lack blood vessels except at the outer margins where blood vessels are present.

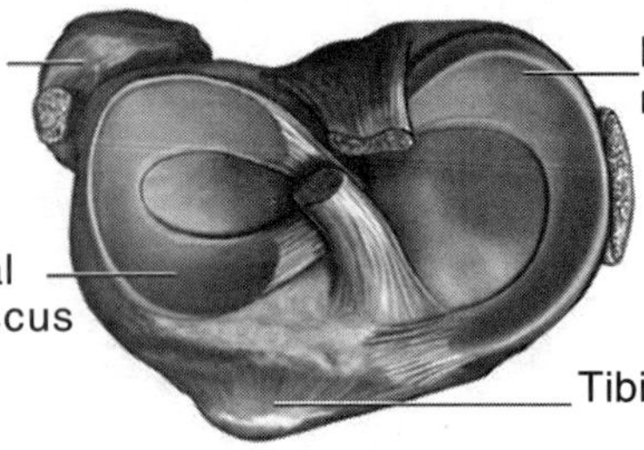

Fig. 15.9: Menisci of the knee

Function of Menisci

- Shock absorption.
- Deepening of articular surface of tibial condyles.
- Facilitation of knee rotation.

Aetiology

The medial meniscus is torn three times more often than the lateral, as it is non-mobile and firmly attached to medial collateral ligament.

Age: It is common in young adults of age group 18-45 years.

Gender: Males are affected more than females.

Occupation: Professional sports (football, rugger, gold, tennis), miners, labourers.

Mechanism of Injury

It is usually a twisting injury in which sudden rotation of knee in partial flexion during weight bearing causes the menisci to be trapped between joint surfaces.

Types of Meniscal Tear

All the meniscal tears begin as the longitudinal split in the substance of the menisci which on further exertion or injury develops one of the following three types of meniscal tears:
- Bucket handle tear
- Posterior horn tear
- Anterior horn tear

Bucket Handle Tear:

It is the most common type of meniscal tear in which longitudinal split extends throughout the length of the menisci with fragments remaining attached at both the ends (Fig. 16.10). The femoral condyle rolls upon the tibia through rent in the meniscus. The centrally displaced fragment blocks the normal play of femoral condyle during extreme range of extension causing locking of the joint.

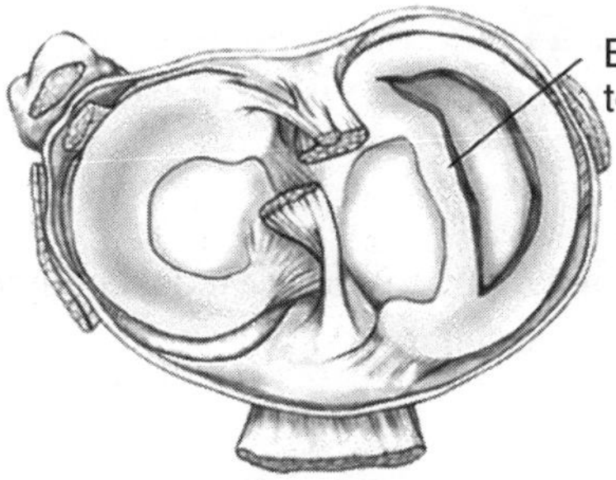

Fig. 16.10: Bucket handle meniscal tear

Posterior Horn Tear:

The tear starts at the concave border of the meniscus with the formation of a pedunculated tag which remains attached at the posterior horn of the meniscus.

Anterior Horn Tear:

In this case the pedunculated tag is formed at the anterior part of the concave border but remains attached to it.

Clinical Features

- *Pain:* There is acute pain in the knee joint. The patient complains of deep joint pain often around the medial joint margin.
- *Swelling:* Swelling is in the form of effusion of excess of synovial fluid in suprapatellar bursa and in between the joint surfaces.
- *Position of the joint:* The patient present with the affected knee in 20° of flexion.
- *Range of Motion:* The range of knee flexion is complete but the extension is limited. It is regarded as locking i.e. patient is not able to extend the knee due to trapped meniscal fragment.
- *Muscle Power:* Quadriceps gets atrophied especially the vastus medialis.
- *Tenderness:* There is sharp tenderness at the anteromedial aspect.
- *End Feel:* On passively extending the knee joint physiotherapist feels a springy elastic end feel.

Clinical Diagnostic Tests

Mc Murray Test (Fig. 16.11):

The patient lies in supine with knee completely flexed. The examiner medially rotates the tibia and extends the knee. If there is a loose fragment of lateral meniscus, this action causes a snap or click, accompanied by pain. The tibia is then laterally

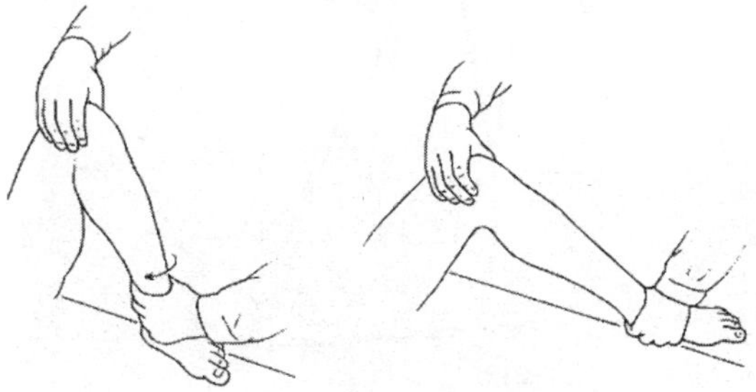

Fig. 16.11: Mc Murray test

rotated and process is repeated to test the medial meniscus.

Apley's Test:

The patient lies in prone with knee flexed to 90º. The patient's thigh is anchored to examination table. The examiner medially and laterally rotates the tibia combined with distraction (Fig. 16.12) while noting any restriction, excessive movement or discomfort. Then the process is repeated with compression (Fig. 16.13). If rotation along with distraction is more painful, then the injury is ligamentous but if rotation along with compression is more painful or shows decreased rotation relative to normal side, the lesion is meniscal injury.

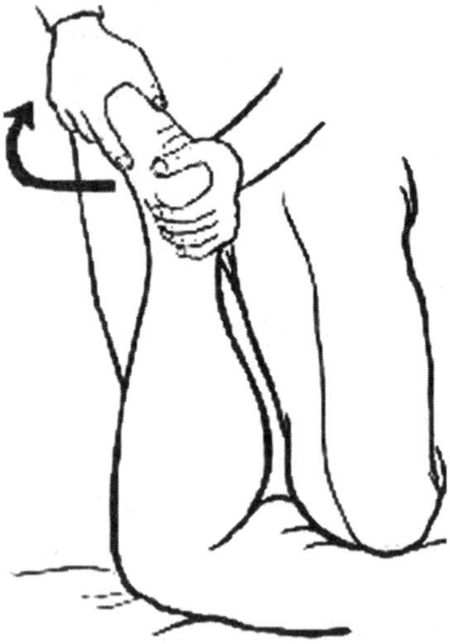

Fig. 16.12: Apley's distraction test

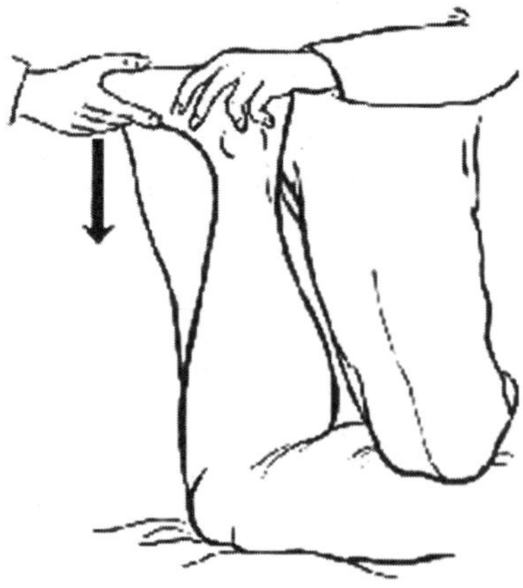

Fig. 16.13: Apley's compression test

Bounce Home Test:

The patient lies in supine and the heel of patient's foot is cupped in examiner's hand. The patient's knee is completely flexed and the knee is passively allowed to extend. If extension is not complete or has rubbery end feel i.e. springy block, the most likely cause of block is a torn meniscus.

Investigations

Radiographic Examination:

X-ray in cases of meniscal injuries do not reveal any changes and appears to be normal.

Magnetic Resonance Imaging:

MRI is a non-invasive method of detecting meniscal tears. It does reveal useful information.

Arthrography:

It is rarely used being an invasive technique. In this X-rays are taken after injecting radio-opaque dye into the knee. The dye outlines the menisci so that tear if present can be visualized.

Arthroscopy:

It is a technique in which thin endoscope about 4-5 mm in diameter is introduced into the joint through a stab wound, inside is visualized.

Treatment

The treatment of a meniscal tear will depend upon the chronicity of the injury.

Acute Cases

- *If the knee joint is locked:* If the knee joint is locked into flexion, it is manipulated under general anesthesia. No special maneuver is needed. As the knee relaxes the menisci falls into place and knee is unlocked. The knee is then immobilized into Robert-Jones compression bandage.

- *If the knee joint is not locked:* If locking of the joint is absent, the immobiliization with Robert-Jones bandage is sufficient.

Chronic Cases

In the chronic cases of meniscal tears, the treatment is always surgical.

- *Arthrotomy:* The displaced fragment of the menisci is excised either by opening the joint or by arthroscopically.
- *Menescorraphy:* It refers to meniscal repair through suturing of the torn menisci.

Physiotherapy Management after Meniscal Repair

The physiotherapeutic management after meniscal repair is divided into three phases:
Phase 1: Maximum protection.
Phase 2: Moderate protection.
Phase 3: Advanced phase.

Phase 1: Maximum Protection (Day 1-Week 6)

The phase of maximum protection extends till 6 weeks from the first post-operative day emphasizing upon pain relief, muscle strengthening and knee mobilization.

Stage 1: Day 1-Week 3

- To reduce inflammation: Ice, compression and elevation.
- Scar tissue mobilization.
- Passive ROM at the affected knee joint with maximum flexion of 90°. It should be progressed based on pain assessment scale.
- Patellar mobilization.
- Knee strengthening exercises.
- Electrical muscle stimulation to quadriceps and hamstrings.
- Isometrics to quadriceps and hamstrings.
- Weight bearing as tolerated with crutches and brace locked at 0°.
- Proprioceptive training.

Stage 2: Week 4 - Week 6

- Progressive resisted exercises, (PREs) for the knee musclature.
- Toe raises.
- Mini squats.
- Free cycling without any resistance.
- Flexibility exercises.

Phase 2: Moderate Protection (Week 6 - Week 10)

The physiotherapeutic regime after meniscal repair could be progressed to phase 2 of moderate protection when the following criteria is achieved:

- Knee ROM 0-90°
- No change in pain or effusion
- Good quadriceps control

Goals

- To normalize knee ROM.
- To increase strength, power and endurance.
- To prepare the patient for advance exercises.

Physiotherapeutic Intervention

- Knee strengthening with PRE.
- Flexibility exercises.
- Mini squats.
- Isokinetic exercises.
- Endurance training with swimming, cycling, pool running.
- Coordination program:
  - Balance board.
  - Pool sprinting.
  - Backward walking.
- Plyometric exercises.

Phase 3: Advanced Phase (Week 11 – Week 15)

Once the patient achieves the following criteria, the treatment regime could be progressed to the advanced phase:

- Full non-painful ROM
- No pain or tenderness
- Satisfactory isokinetic test and clinical examination

Goals

- Increase power and endurance.
- Emphasize return to skill activities.

Intervention

- Emphasize more on plyometric and pool exercises.

- Initiate running program.
- Continue the rest of the exercises.

In case of professional sports player, the athelete patient could return to activity once the clinical examination and isokinetic testing is satisfactory along with full and non-painful ROM.

OSTEOCHONDRITIS DISSECANS

Osteochondritis dissecans is the problem that affects the knee at the distal end of the femur. The lesion commonly affects the medial femoral condyle (Fig 16.14), which is under constant stress due to body weight.

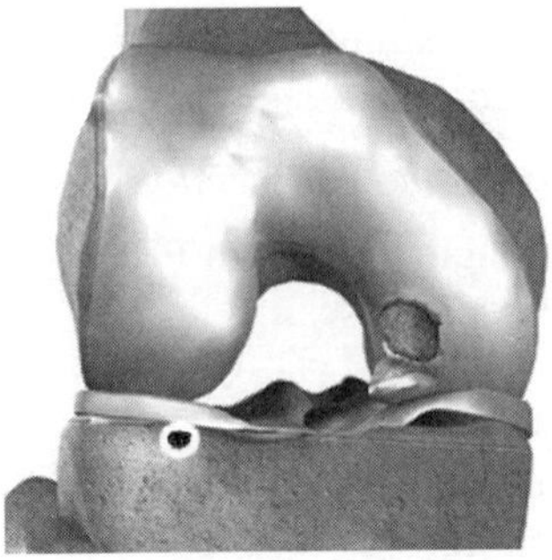

Fig. 16.14: Osteochondral lesion at medial femoral condyle

Cause

The disease is common in athletes involved in competitive sport due to repeated stress on bone.

Pathogenesis

The femoral condyles are covered with the articular cartilage, which allow bones of knee joint to slide smoothly against each other. The problem occurs where the cartilage of the knee attaches to bone underneath. The area of the bone just under the cartilage surface is injured leading to damage of blood vessels of bone. Without blood flow, area of the damaged bone actually dies. The area of the dead bone can be seen on a radiograph (Fig. 16.15).

As the condition worsens the area of bone affected may collapse causing a notch to form in smooth joint surface. The cartilage over this dead section of bone becomes damaged. There occurs the feeling of snapping or catching as the knee joint moves across the notched area. In some cases the dead bone becomes detached from rest of femur forming a loose body (Fig. 16.16).

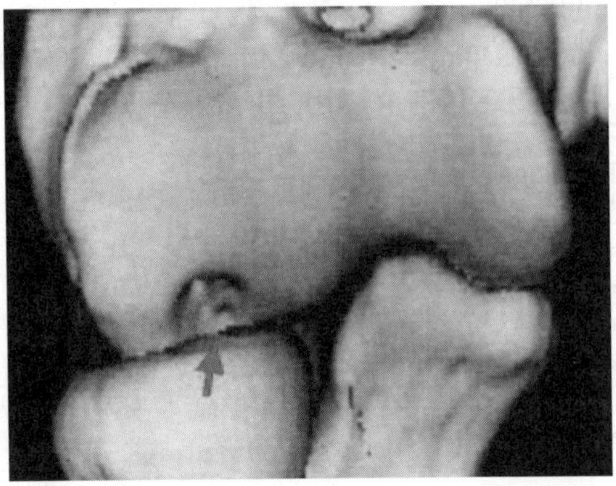

Fig. 16.15: Necrotic lesion on a radiograph

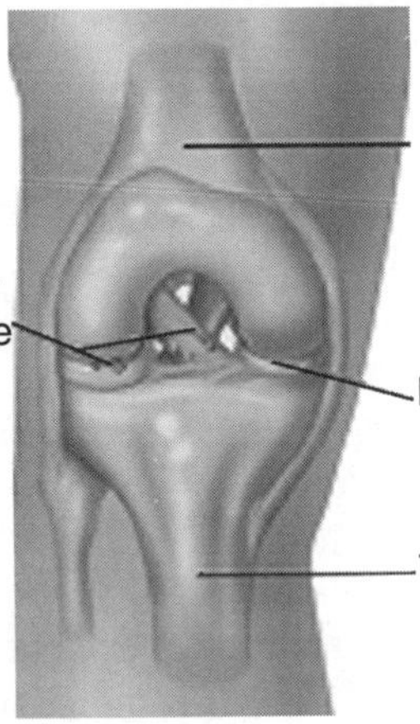

Fig. 16.16: Loose body

Clinical Features

The clinical features of the disease vary from mild to worse as the disease progresses. The patient presents with the following symptoms:

- Mild aching pain
- Painful knee movement
- Swelling
- Tenderness
- Inability to bear full weight on the affected knee.

- Locking of the knee joint due to presence of loose body.

Diagnosis

The diagnosis can be made by observing the clinical features of the disease. The confirmation can be made by:
- Radiographs.
- Bone scan.
- Magnetic Resonance Imaging (MRI).

Management

The joint surfaces damaged by osteochondritis dissecans does not heal naturally due to constant stress on the affected site.

Conservative Treatment

The conservative treatment involves the immobilization of the affected joint into a plaster cast so as to avoid the stress on the bone and to give it time to heal. The patient is allowed to do crutch walking without placing weight on the affected limb.

Surgical Treatment

The surgical treatment is only used when the joint cavity contains a loose body. The removal of loose body can be done either using arthroscopy or open method.
If a loose bone fragment is in a weight bearing area of a bone, fragment repair is necessary. The lesion is reattached using metal screws.
If the fragment of bone has to be removed from the weight bearing area of the bone, the lesion site has to be filled using:
- Osteochondral autograft.
- Allograft transplant.
- *Autologous chondrocyte implantation:* This is an experimental technique which involves use of chondrocytes (cartilage cells) to help regenerate the articular cartilage.

Non-Surgical Rehabilitation

Goal

The goal of non-surgical treatment is to prevent the injured area of the cartilage while improving the knee motion and strength.

Intervention

- The patient is asked to avoid heavy sports or work activities for at least 8 weeks.
- As the symptoms ceases range of motion and stretching exercises for the affected knee are initiated. In the initial stage those exercises should not be involved in which weight is placed through foot.
- The athletic patients are advised to use shock absorbing shoe insoles to reduce impact on knee.
- Strengthening exercises for the hip and knee musculature are initiated.

Post-Surgical Rehabilitation

- Post-surgically weight bearing is restricted on the affected knee joint for six weeks except in the arthroscopic procedures, as the bone needs time to heal. If transplantation at the lesion site is done the weight bearing is restricted for four months.
- The patient is advised to use walker/crutches to ambulate for the initial period of six weeks.
- Ensure safe weight bearing on the affected joint.
- *Continuous passive movement (CPM):* It is used for gaining range of motion at the knee joint and alleviate joint stiffness.
- The physiotherapeutic measures are used to control pain and swelling after surgery.
- Improvisation of strength and range of motion at knee: Various exercises are chosen to help improve the knee motion and to get muscles toned and active again. The emphasis is placed on exercising the knee in positions and movements that don't strain the healing part of cartilage.

ANTERIOR CRUCIATE LIGAMENT (ACL) INJURY

Rupture of anterior cruciate ligament has been the commonest among the ligamentous injuries of the knee, (Fig. 16.17) and has greatest potential to cause both short term and long term disability.

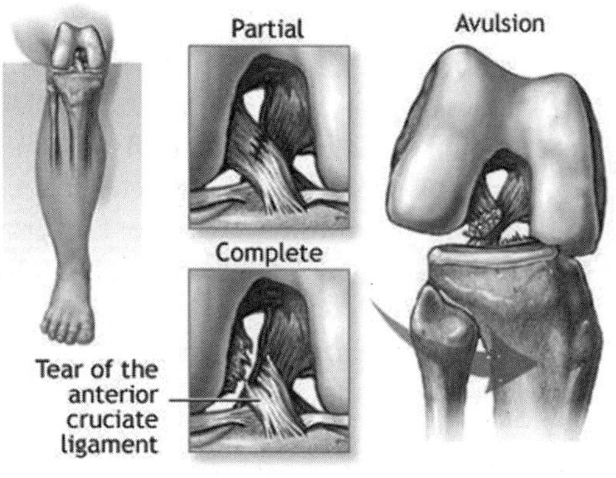

Fig. 16.17: Anterior cruciate ligament injury

Functional Anatomy

ACL is the broad ligament joining the anterior tibial plateu to the posterior femoral intercondylar notch (Fig. 16.18). The tibial attachment is to a facet, in front of and lateral to anterior tibial spine. The femoral attachment is high on the posterior aspect of the lateral wall of intercondylar notch.

The biomechanical function of ACL complex is that it provides both mechanical stability and proprioceptive feedback to the knee. In its stabilizing role it has four major functions:

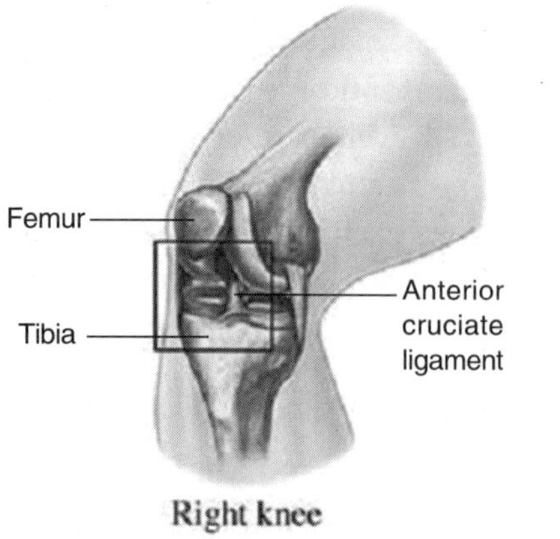

Fig. 16.18: Anterior cruciate ligament

- Restrains anterior translation of tibia.
- Prevents hyperextension of the knee.
- Acts as secondary stabilizer to valgus stress, reinforcing medial collateral ligament.
- Controls rotation of tibia on femur in femoral extension of 0–30°.

Causes of ACL Rupture (Fig. 16.19)

The most common cause of ACL rupture is a traumatic force being applied to the knee in a twisting moment. This can occur with either a direct or indirect force. Non-contact causes of ACL rupture are:

- Side stepping.
- Pivoting.
- Landing from a jump.
- On football field.
- On snow fields.
- Motor vehicle accidents.
- Skiing injuries usually occurring during a fall in inexperienced skier.

History

The classic history of a patient is cutting, side-stepping or landing from a jump and the knee giving way.

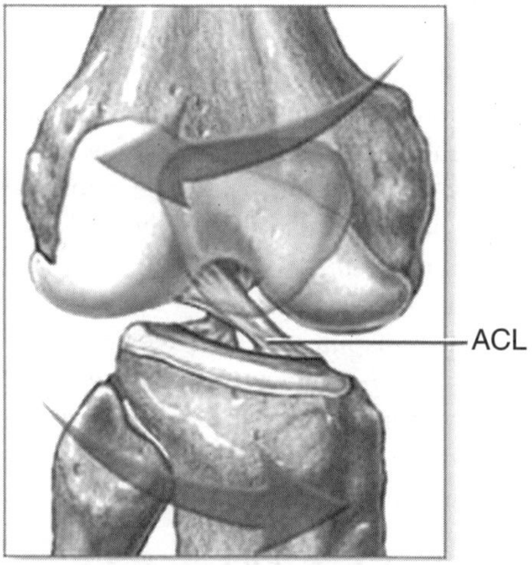

Fig. 16.19: ACL injuries occur when bones of the leg twist in opposite directions under full body weight

Clinical Features

At the time of an ACL injury, signs and symptoms may include:

- A loud 'pop' sound.
- Severe pain.
- Knee swelling within 4 to 12 hours.
- Feeling of instability with weight bearing.

The pain and swelling usually subsides after 2 to 4 weeks, but the knee remains unstable. It may give way during twisting or pivoting movements, or feel like it wants to slip backwards.

Rapid intra-articular swelling following injury is nearly always due to haemarthrosis due to bleeding from vessels within the torn ligament.

Clinical Diagnostic Tests

The diagnosis of ACL tear can be confirmed by following tests:

- Lachman test.
- Dynamic extension test
- Lateral pivot jerk test

Lachman Test (Fig. 16.20):

The patient lies supine with involved leg beside the examiner. The examiner holds the patient's knee between full extension and 30 degrees of flexion. The patient's femur is stabilized with one of the examiner's hand while the proximal aspect of tibia is moved forwards with other hand applying an anterior translation force. A positive sign is indicated by a mushy or soft end feel when the tibia is moved forwards on the femur and disappearance of the infrapatellar tendon slope.

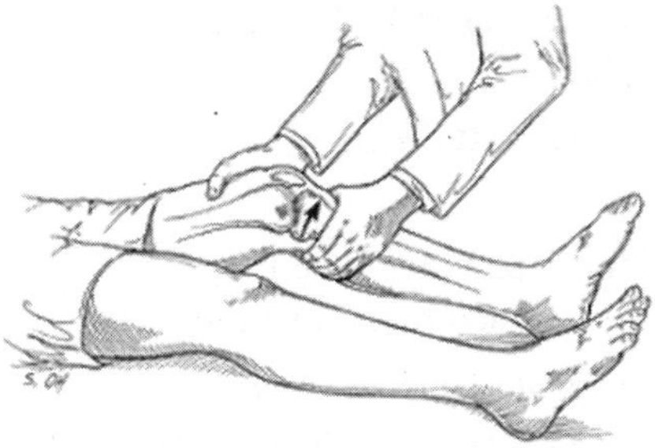

Fig. 16.20: Lachman test

Lateral Pivot Jerk Test:

The patient lies supine with the hip both flexed and abducted 30 degrees and relaxed in slight medial rotation. The examiner holds the patient's foot with one hand while the other hand is placed at the knee, holding the leg in slight medial rotation. This is done by placing the heel of the hand behind the fibula and over the lateral head of gastrocnemius muscle with the tibia rotated medially, causing the tibia to subluxate anteriorly as the knee is taken into extension. A giving way feel to the patient indicates a positive test.

The lachman and dynamic extension tests are helpful in making a diagnosis, particularly in acute injury, the lateral pivot jerk test is most important.

This test reproduces the rotator subluxation that occurs in ACL deficiency.

Differential Diagnosis

- Osteochondral fracture.
- Peripheral meniscal tear.
- Retinacular tear associated with patellar dislocation or subluxation.
- Posterior cruciate ligament tear.
- Bleeding disorders.

Rationale for Treatment

Rupture of ACL causes significant short term and long term disability. With each episode of ACL instability there is subluxation of tibia on the femur, causing stretching of the enveloping capsular ligaments and abnormal shear forces on the menisci and on the articular cartilage. Delay in diagnosis and treatment gives rise to increased intra-articular damage as well as stretching of the secondary stabilizing capsular structures.

The long term outlook of ACL deficient knee is development of significant osteoarthrosis. Thus it is important to make an early diagnosis of ACL rupture so that consequent meniscal injury and long term degenerative damage is to be minimized.

Treatment

Initial Treatment of an ACL Injury Aims to

- Reduce pain and swelling.
- Regain normal joint movement.
- Strengthen the muscles around the knee.

To Treat Acute Injury

- Use ice.
- Elevate the affected knee.
- Wrap an elastic bandage around the knee.
- Use a splint or advice walking with assistive devices.
- Range of motion and muscle strengthening exercises.

Surgical Treatment

Surgery is indicated if:

- Knee is unstable and gives way during daily activities or sports.
- The patient is very active and wants to resume heavy work, sports or other recreational activities.
- Other structures such as meniscus or other ligaments are also injured.
- To prevent any further injury to knee.

ACL reconstruction is the procedure of choice which is done by utilizing a graft, either autograft or allograft.

Non-Surgical Rehabilitation

A rehabilitation program without surgery includes physical therapy, activity modification and knee bracing.

Indications of non-surgical rehabilitation:

- Patient does not participate in sports that involve cutting, pivoting or jumping.
- The patient's knee is not painful or unstable during normal activities.
- Patient lead a fairly sedentary lifestyle.
- Patient's knee cartilage has not been damaged.

Rehabilitation

The major goals of rehabilitation following ACL surgery are:

- Restoration of joint anatomy.
- Provision of static and dynamic stability.
- Maintenance of the aerobic conditioning and psychological well being.
- Early return to work and support.

These have required the development of an intensive rehabilitation program in which the patient has to take an active involvement.

The graft undergoes physiological changes during its incorporation, as fibroblastic activity changes the biology of the graft to become more liamentous. The graft is weakest between 6 and 12 weeks post operatively, so programs must be designed to protect the graft during this period. On the other hand investigations into the ligamentous healing have shown that the progressive controlled loading provides a stimulus for healing which improves the quality of graft incorporation. Moreover early immobilization has advantages such as maintenance of articular cartilage nutrition and retention of bone mineralization.

Kinematic research has shown quadriceps contraction causes greatest strain on the anterior cruciate ligament graft between 10° and 45° of flexion. The ACL graft lacks the normal mechanoreceptors that provide biofeedback in the uninjured knee. All these factors must be taken into account when designing rehabilitation program.

The accelerated rehabilitation program is divided into four phases:

First Phase (1–2 Weeks):

Aims:

- To decrease pain and swelling.
- To increase knee range of motion.

Physiotherapeutic Intervention:

- A post-operative brace that maintains the knee into ranges between 30 to 90 degrees is used until there is adequate quadriceps control.
- CPM is used immediately after surgery.
- An emphasis is laid on static contraction of hamstrings and co-contraction of hamstrings and quadriceps.
- Crutch walking with partial weight bearing is allowed.

- Electrotherapeutic modalities are used to reduce pain and swelling.

Second Phase (2 – 6 Weeks):

Aims:
- To increase range of motion.
- To improve weight bearing.
- To gain hamstrings and quadriceps control.

Physiotherapeutic Intervention:
- The patient is usually out of brace by third to fourth week.
- Commencement of gait re-education and static proprioception exercises include balancing on affected leg and biofeedback techniques.
- Hydrotherapy can be utilized to maintain conditioning and range of motion.

Third phase (6 – 12 Weeks):

Aims:
- To improve muscular control.
- To improve proprioception.
- General muscular strengthening.

Physiotherapeutic Intervention:
- Proprioceptive work progresses from static to dynamic techniques including balance exercises on the wobble board and eventually jogging on a mini-tramp.
- The patient should have full range of motion during this stage and gentle resistance work should be added.
- By the end of this period patient should be able to cycle normally, swim with a straight leg kick and be able to jog freely on the mini-tramp.

Fourth Phase (12 Weeks – 6 Months):

Aims:
- Gradual re-introduction of sports specific exercises.
- To improve agility and reaction times.
- To increase total lower extremity strength.

Physiotherapeutic Intervention:
An elite athlete who has had an early reconstruction of ACL followed by an adequate and successful rehabilitation program, should be able to return to field of his chosen sport between six and nine months.

Prevention

To reduce the chances of an ACL injury, following should be taken care of:
- Training programs that have been shown to be effective in preventing ACL injuries include stretching and strengthening exercises, aerobic conditioning, plyometrics, or jumping exercises and risk awareness training. Exercises that improve balance also can help.
- Women athletes should take care to strengthen and stretch their hamstrings as well as quadriceps muscles.
- Conditioning exercises.
- Learn and use proper sporting techniques.

POSTERIOR CRUCIATE LIGAMENT INJURY

Posterior cruciate ligament injury (Fig. 16.21) happens far less than injury to ACL. In case of injury to PCL, patient may experience pain and swelling at the back of knee. Occasionally, this injury can cause a feeling of instability or looseness in the knee.

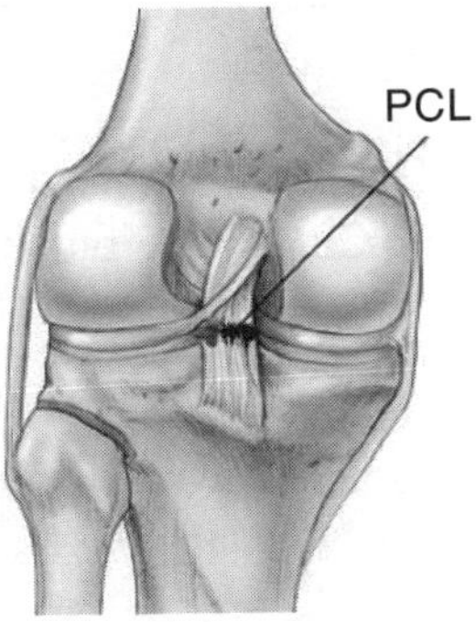

Fig. 16.21: Posterior cruciate ligament injury

Causes

The PCL can tear if tibia is hit hard or if the patient falls on a bent knee. These injuries are most common during:
- *Motor vehicle accidents:* Dash board injury occurs when the driver's or passenger's bent knees slams against the dashboard, pushing in shin bone just below the knee and causing the PCL to tear.

- *Contact sports:* Athletes in sports such as football or soccer may tear their PCL when they fall on a bent knee with their foot pointed down. The shin bone hits the ground first and it moves backwards. Being tackled with bent knee can also cause this injury.

Signs and Symptoms

- Mild to moderate pain at the back of the knee.
- Sudden knee swelling (within three hours of the injury) and tenderness.
- Pain while kneeling or squatting.
- A slight limp or difficulty walking.
- Feeling of instability or looseness in the knee or giving way of knee during activities.
- Pain while running, slowing down, or walking up or down stairs or ramps.

Diagnosis

- *History:* The therapist must ask about the accident or injury, duration of the symptoms.
- *Physical examination of the knee:* The therapist must evaluate the extent of swelling, tenderness, any injury marks, posture of the knee and any observable deformity.
- *Posterior Drawer test:* (Fig. 16.22).
- *X- Ray:* X-ray picture of the bones and tissues won't show a PCL injury, but it can show damage to bones and cartilage, a sagging shin bone or an avulsion fracture.
- *Magnetic Resonance Imaging:* An MRI scan can clearly show a PCL tear and can determine if other knee structures are also injured.
- Arthroscopy evaluation.

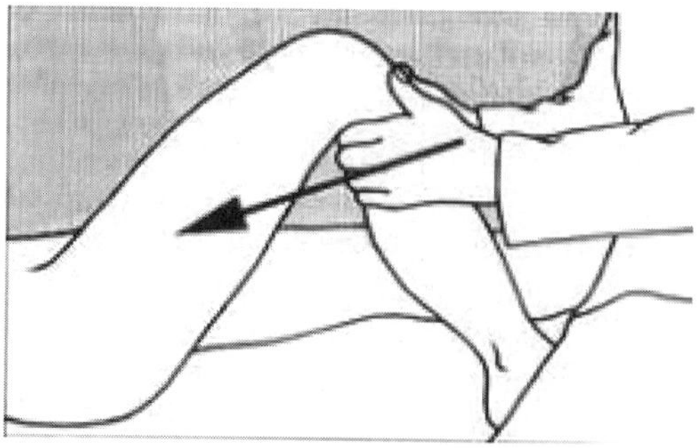

Fig. 16.22: Posterior drawer test

Treatment

The treatment option will depend upon the type and extent of the injury. For an isolated PCL tear, with no damage to other parts of the knee joint or tibia, the patient can be treated conservatively. Many patients with minor PCL injury can return to their previous level of activity after completing a rehabilitation program, which may take from 1 to 4 months.

If the patient has a bad PCL tear combined with other torn ligaments, cartilage damage or a broken bone, surgery is needed to reconstruct a joint. Surgery may also help if knee remains unstable after rehabilitation. After surgery the patient has to go through a rehabilitation program. Full recovery may take several months.

To treat acute injury:

- Rest.
- Apply ice packs for 20-30 minutes every three to four hours for two to three days or until the pain goes away.
- Wrap an elastic bandage around the knee.
- Use a splint or make the patient walk with an assistive device. The patient is required to avoid putting weight on the injured knee for several weeks. The patient must wear a knee brace to protect the knee during activity and keep it stable.

Prevention

- Strengthening exercises for quadriceps and hamstrings.
- Stretching exercises for lower extremity.
- Proper techniques while playing sports or exercising.

REHABILITATION PROTOCOL FOR POSTERIOR CRUCIATE LIGAMENT INJURIES

Non-Operative Rehabilitation Protocol

Phase 1 (Day 0 – Week 3):

Day 1 – Day 7:

- Electrical stimulation to quadriceps.

- Isometric quadriceps strengthening.
- Knee range of motion 0 – 60°.
- Hip abduction and adduction exercises.
- Weight bearing with crutches.

Week 2 – Week 3:

- Knee range of motion 0 – 60°.
- Stationary cycling for both range of motion and strengthening.
- Resistive exercises using weight cuffs.
- Leg press 0 – 60°.

Phase 2 (Week 3 – Week 6):

- Knee range of motion as tolerated by the patient.
- Stationary cycling and rowing.
- Progressive resistive exercises.
- Mini squats, leg press.
- Toe calf raises.
- Step ups.

Phase 3:

- Continue all strengthening exercises.
- Gradual return to sports.

Post-Operative Rehabilitation Protocol

Phase 1 (Day 0 – Week 4)

Aims:

- To protect the healing structures.
- To minimize the effects of immobilization.

Physiotherapy Intervention:

- For the initial one week post-operatively brace is locked at 0°. After a week brace is unlocked to perform passive range of motion exercises.
- The patient is allowed to bear weight with crutches and brace locked in extension.
- The stretching of calf and hamstrings are administered.
- The patient is asked to place a pillow under proximal posterior tibia to prevent posterior sagging.
- The patient must perform the following exercises:
  - Ankle pumps.
  - Isometric quadriceps sets.
  - SLR.
  - Hip abduction and adduction.
  - Prone passive flexion and extension.

Phase 2 (Week 4 – Week 12)

Aims:

- To increase flexion range of motion.
- To restore normal gait.
- To increase quadriceps strength.
- To gain flexibility in hamstrings.

Physiotherapy Intervention:

Week 4 – Week 8:

- In the period of 4–6 weeks the brace is unlocked for controlled gait training and after that it can be unlocked for all the activities.
- The patient uses crutches for weight bearing.
- Aquatic therapy for gait training: The patient is advised to practice normal heel toe gait pattern in the pool.
- The patient must practice the following exercises:
  - Wall slides.
  - Mini squats.
  - Leg press.
  - *Hip exercises with knee fully extended:* Flexion, extension, abduction and adduction.

Week 8 – Week 12:

- The brace is discontinued.
- The patient can discard the crutches if there is no quadriceps lag, knee flexion range is 90°–100° and normal gait pattern.
- The patient practice balance and proprioception activities.
- Use of stationary bike must be continued.
- The patient must practice:
  - Seated calf raises.
  - Leg press.

Phase 3 (3–6 months)

Aims:

- To restore any residual loss of motion.
- To improve functional strength and proprioception.
- To prevent patellofemoral irritation.

Physiotherapy Intervention:

- Progression of closed chain kinetic exercises.
- Treadmill walking.
- Swimming.

PRE-PATELLAR BURSITIS

Prepatellar bursitis is defined as the inflammation of the bursa lying in front of the lower half of the patella and upper part of patellar tendon which is prone to inflammation.

Other Name: The prepatellar bursitis is also known as housemaid's knee.

Causes

- Frequent kneeling: Occupational or handicapped patient.
- Infectious.

Types

- Irritative prepatellar bursitis.
- Suppurative prepatellar bursitis.

Irritative Prepatellar Bursitis

This type of prepatellar bursitis is caused by repeated friction as in case of frequent kneeling due to occupation such as of housemaid or the patient is stressing the bursa with his/her body weight while knee walking as in case of amputees. The wall of the bursa gets thickened and is distended with fluid.

Clinical Features

- Soft fluctuating swelling in the vicinity of bursa. The swelling is always extracapsular.
- Painful quadriceps activity.
- Tenderness over the bursa.

Treatment

- Aspiration of the inflammed bursa.
- Infiltration of hydrocortisone injection.
- Operative excision of bursa.

Suppurative Prepatellar Bursitis

This type of prepatellar bursitis is caused due to infection by pyogenic organism. This organism may reach the bursa directly through the open wound or through any infected lesion in the leg. The wall of the bursa is acutely inflammed and the sac is distended with pus.

Clinical Features

- Pyrexia.
- Signs of inflammation: Reddened and hot skin.
- Pain.
- Extracapsular swelling.
- Tenderness on palpation.
- Enlarged and tender inguinal lymph nodes.
- Limited knee flexion due to the unwillingness of the patient as tension over the inflammed bursa increases with flexion.

Treatment

- Antibiotic therapy.
- Incision and drainage of bursal abscess.

PHYSIOTHERAPY MANAGEMENT

Conservative Management

- Rest to the affected knee joint either with the use of:
  - Crepe bandage.
  - Pressure bandage.
  - Knee cap.
- The afflected limb should be kept in elevation so as to reduce swelling and improve the circulation.
- Electrical stimulation to the quadriceps in order to avoid the atrophy of the muscle.
- Isometeric quadriceps exercises.
- Assisted SLR.
- Knee movements in pain free range are initiated.

Post-Operative Treatment

- Elevation of the affected limb.
- Strong active movements of toes, ankle and hip.
- Isometeric quadriceps exercises.
- Self-assisted knee swinging exercises.
- Friction massage.
- Range of motion exercises initiated as passive movements progressed gradually to active-assisted, active and then to active-resisted exercises.
- Re-education of walking.

Precautions

- Avoid kneeling.
- Strong and jerky knee movements.
- Pressure positions of knee.

UNIT NINE

ANKLE AND FOOT CONDITIONS

17. ANKLE CONDITIONS

CHAPTER 17

ANKLE CONDITIONS

ANKLE SPRAIN

The term ankle sprain is used for the ligamentous injury either of medial or lateral ligament of the ankle. The ligaments of the ankle are more susceptible for sprain as the unstable ankle joint depends largely on its ligaments for its stability.

Deltoid (Medial) Ligament (Fig.17.1)

This is a strong triangular ligament present on medial side of ankle having a superficial and a deep part. Both the parts originate from apex and margins of the medial malleolus of tibia, with lower attachments as follows:

Superficial Part

- Anterior fibers (tibionavicular) are attached to the tuberosity of the navicular bone and to medial margin of spring ligament.

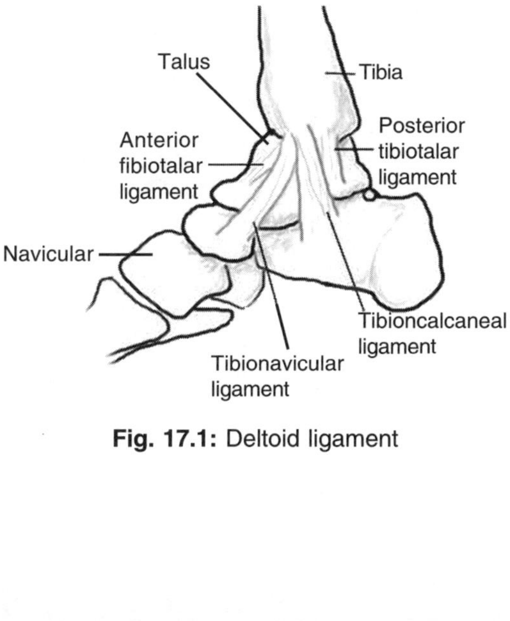

Fig. 17.1: Deltoid ligament

- The middle fibers (tibiocalcaneal) are attached to whole length of the sustentaculum tali.
- The posterior fibers (posterior tibiotalar) are attached to medial tubercle and to adjoining part of medial surface of talus.

Deep Part (Anterior tibiotalar)

It is attached to anterior part of medial surface of talus.

Lateral Ligament (Fig. 17.2)

- The anterior talofibular ligament is a flat band passing from anterior margin of lateral malleolus to neck of talus just in front of fibular facet.

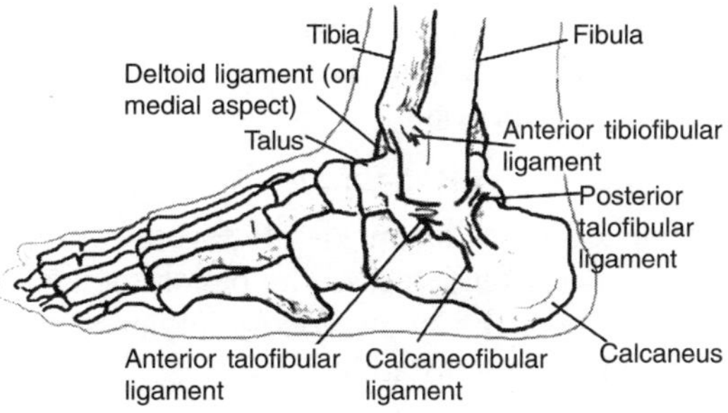

Fig. 17.2: Lateral ankle ligament

- The posterior talofibular ligament passes from lower part of malleolar fossa to the lateral tubercle of talus.
- The calcaneofibular ligament is a long rounded cord, which passes from notch on lower border of lateral malleolus to tubercle on lateral surface of calcaneum.

The lateral ligament of the ankle is sprained more commonly than the medial as the medial ligament is stronger and inversion injuries are more common than eversion injuries.

LATERAL LIGAMENT SPRAIN

The lateral ligament of the ankle is the commonly injured ligament amongst the two ligaments.

Mechanism of Injury

The lateral ligament of the ankle is sprained when the foot is forced into inversion and plantar flexion. It could be either during the sports activities or during walking or running on uneven surfaces. The common sports activities in which the ligament is injured are pole vaulting, cross-country running and hiking.

Grades of Injury

Grade 1–Mild Ankle Sprain

The ligament is stretched with no macroscopic tear. There is minimal swelling and tenderness. The joint is stable with no functional impairment.

Grade 2–Moderate Ankle Sprain

The ligament is partially torn with moderate swelling and tenderness. The joint is mildly unstable with some loss of function.

Grade 3 –Severe Ankle Sprain

Complete tear of the ligament with severe swelling, ecchymosis and tenderness. The patient is unable to bear weight on the involved extremity presenting as mechanical joint instability.

Clinical Features

- *History:* Patient gives a history of twisting injury to the ankle with tearing sensation or a pop felt by the patient over lateral ankle.
- *Pain:* The patient complains of pain just below and anterior to lateral malleolus which aggravates on passive stretching and weight bearing.
- *Swelling:* Swelling is evident from lateral border of tendoachillis over lateral malleolus along dorsum of foot.
- *Bruising:* This appears under lateral malleolus and over the dorsum of the foot.
- *Weight bearing:* Weight bearing on the affected extremity is extremely painful.
- *Gait:* The patient walks with short stance on affected foot.

Clinical Diagnostic Test

The injury to the lateral ankle ligament could be easily diagnosed by the following clinical tests:
- Stress test
- Anterior drawer test
- Talar tilt test

Stress Test

The patient experiences severe pain if the torn ligament is subjected to stress by following maneuvers:
- Inversion of plantar flexed foot for anterior talofibular ligament sprain.
- Inversion of foot in neutral position for complete sprain of the lateral ligament (Fig.17.3).

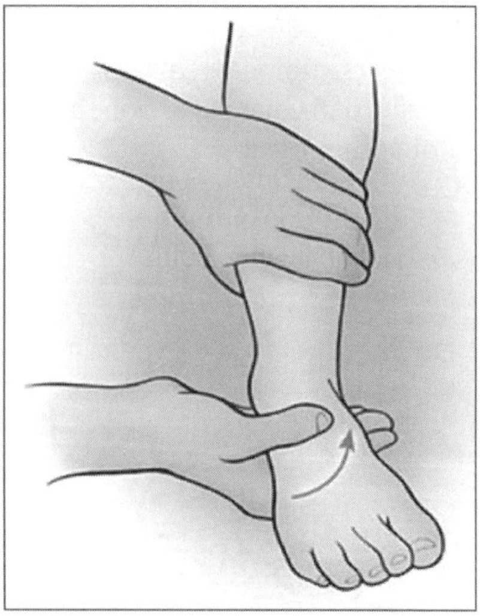

Fig. 17.3: Stress test

Anterior Drawer Test (Fig. 17.4)

The test is performed by stabilizing the tibia anteriorly with one hand and pulling the slightly plantar flexed foot forward with other hand behind the heel. A positive finding of more than 5 mm of anterior translation indicates a tear of anterior talofibular ligament.

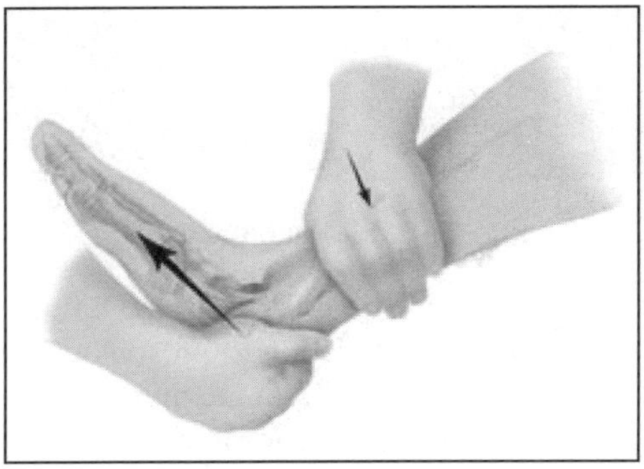

Fig. 17.4: Anterior drawer test

Talar Tilt Test (Fig.17.5)

The test is performed by stabilizing the distal tibia with one hand and inverting the talus and calcaneum as a unit with other hand. A positive finding of more than 5 mm translation with soft end feel indicates combined injury to anterior talofibular ligament and calcaneofibular ligament.

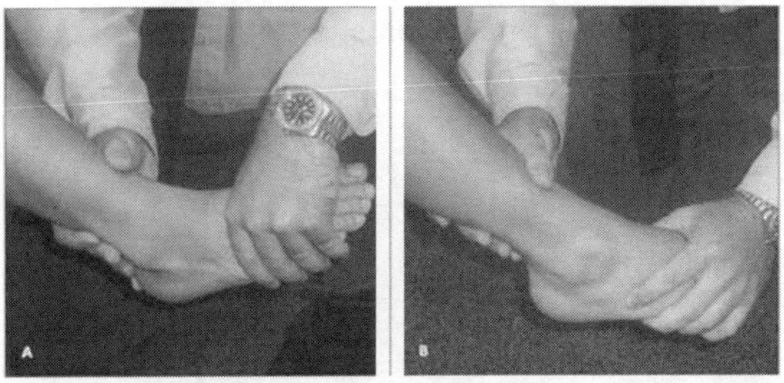

Fig. 17.5: Talar tilt test

Radiological Examination

X-rays of ankle both AP and lateral view are usually normal. Stress X-ray is done to judge the severity of the sprain.

Management

The treatment of the ankle sprain depends upon the severity of the injury. The affected ankle is usually immobilized in a plaster cast for a period of two weeks, four weeks and six weeks for grade 1, grade 2, and grade 3 injuries respectively. The immobilization is followed by mobilization. The grade 3 ligament injury is managed by operative repair for young athletic individual by some surgeons.

Physiotherapy Management

Phase 1: Acute Phase

The acute phase of the treatment varies according to the grade of injury. The acute phase for grade 1 is 1-3 days, grade 2 is 2-4 days and grade 3 is 3-7 days.

Goals of Treatment

- To reduce pain and swelling.
- To protect the patient from re-injury.
- To maintain appropriate weight bearing status.

Intervention

Physiotherapeutic intervention in acute stage of ligamentous injury follows the principle of "PRICE".

P - Prevention from further injury or protection

R - Rest

I - Ice

C - Compression

E - Elevation

- Prevention from further injury or protection of injured ankle can be done by the following methods in acute stage:
  - Taping.
  - Functional bracing (Fig. 17.6)
  - Removable cast boot (Fig. 17.7) for grade 2 and grade 3 sprains.
  - Crepe or elastic bandage (Fig. 17.8) for minor sprain.

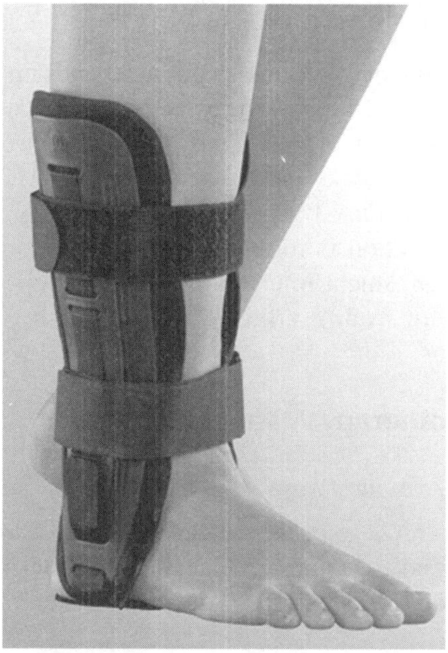

Fig. 17.6: Functional ankle brace

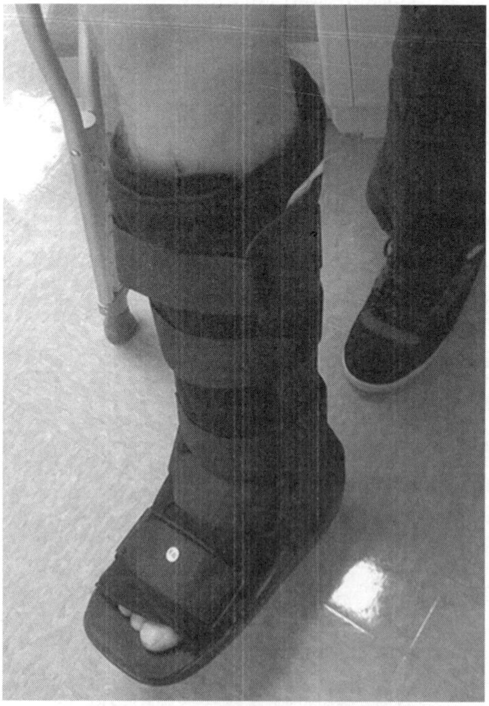

Fig. 17.7: Removable cast boot

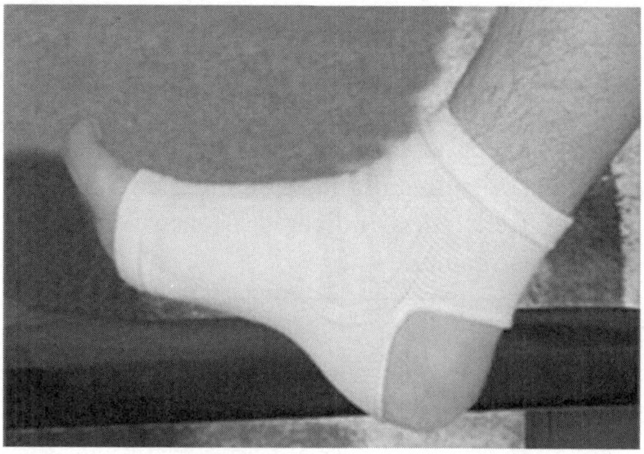

Fig. 17.8: Elastic bandage

- Rest to the injured limb is given in the form of crutches during ambulation to prevent any gait deviation along with weight bearing.
- Application of cold in the form of ice packs, ice massage or ice toweling is of importance in the acute stage of injury so as to reduce inflammation.
- Compression to the injured area can be provided with:
  - Crepe or elastic bandage.
  - Elastic wrap.
  - TED hose (Fig. 17.9).
  - Vasopneumatic pump.
- Elevation of the injured limb is important; the injured ankle should be lifted above the heart level. This should be in combination with ankle pumps.

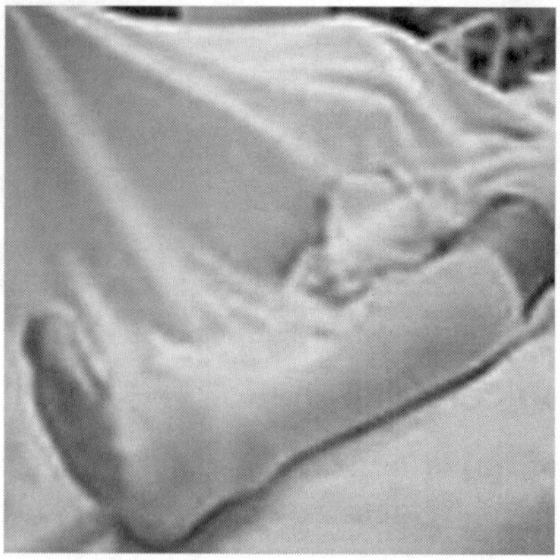

Fig. 17.9: TED hose

Phase 2: Subacute Phase

The subacute phase of treatment for grade 1 sprain is 2-4 days; grade 2 is 3-5 days; grade 3 is 4-8 days.

Goals of Treatment

- To reduce pain and swelling.
- To increase range of motion.
- To gain muscle strength.
- Proprioceptive training.

Intervention

To Reduce Pain and Swelling

- Ice or contrast bath.
- Electrical stimulation by high voltage galvanic or interferential current.
- Ultrasound should be applied over the site of injury to limit adhesion formation and to stimulate the repair of collagen.
- Massage in the form of kneading, effleurage and cross friction should be done as early as possible to prevent consolidation of fluid.

To Increase Range of Motion

- Active ROM exercises as dorsiflexion, plantar flexion, inversion, eversion, and foot circles.
- Passive ROM by the physiotherapist only plantar flexion and dorsiflexion.
- Stretching of tendoachilles should be done gently.
- Grade 1 or grade 2 mobilizations by the therapist for plantar flexion and dorsiflexion.

To Gain Muscle Strength

- Isometrics to the ankle in pain free range.
- Toe curls with towel.
- Picking up of objects with toes.

Proprioceptive Training

- Wobble board.
- Ankle disc.
- Weight bearing is permitted as the symptoms regresses. If there are no signs of antalgic gait weight bearing could be progressed from partial to full.

Phase 3: Rehabilitative Phase

The rehabilitative phase of treatment for grade 1 injury is of 1 week; grade 2 injury is of 2 weeks; grade 3 injury is of 3 weeks.

Goals of Treatment

- To gain pain free range of motion.
- Progression of strength.
- Propriceptive training.

Intervention

To Gain Pain Free Range of Motion

- Joint mobilization for the movement of dorsiflexion, plantar flexion and eversion. The joint mobilization of grade 3 is done.
- Stretching of gastrocnemius and soleus to be done with increased intensity.

Progression of Muscular Strength

- Weight bearing exercises to the affected ankle are started in form of:
  - Heel raises.
  - Toe raises.
  - Squats with gym ball (progressing from quarter to full).
  - Stepping up and down of a stair.
- Invertors, evertors, plantar flexors and dorsiflexors are strengthened using thera bands and weight cuffs.

Proprioceptive Training

It advances from non-weight bearing to controlled weight bearing to full weight bearing single leg balance activities.

The use of modalities for reducing pain and swelling should be continued after the exercises.

Taping Technique for Lateral Ligament Sprain:

In order to do the protective taping which provides support to the lateral aspect of ankle, the patient should be in high sitting position with lower leg supported.

Three anchors are applied to the lower leg starting distal to the belly of gastrocnemius. The lower anchor should slightly overlap the proximal one. The third anchor must be placed just proximal to malleoli. After the anchors are applied it must be checked that the motion is not restricted at the ankle joint.

Three supports are applied to the lateral malleolus. The first support starts proximal to lateral malleolus angled downwards towards posterior aspect of calcaneum and then pulled upwards to the level of first anchor covering the posterior part of lateral malleolus. The second support starts proximal to the first support directed downwards passing anterior to medial malleolus then continuing on top of first and then pulled upwards covering the anterior half of lateral malleolus extended till first anchor. The third support is placed in center of first two.

Three more anchors are re-inforced over the original anchors covering the supports.

HEEL PAIN–PLANTAR FASCITIS

Functions of Plantar Fascia

- Fixes the skin of the sole.
- Protects deeper structures.
- Helps in maintaining the longitudinal arches of the foot.
- It gives origin to muscles of first layer of foot/ sole.
- The main function of plantar fascia in regard to the condition is that it provides stability to foot by increasing the longitudinal arch during propulsion phase of gait by means of Windlass mechanism.

Prevalence

Plantar fascitis is the most common foot condition affecting as much as 10% of the population over the course of lifetime.

Pathoanatomical Features

The plantar aponeurosis or fascia consists of 3 bands: lateral, medial and central. It is the central band that originates from medial tubercle on the plantar surface of calcaneum and that travel towards the toes as a solid band of tissues dividing just prior to the metatarsals head into 5 slips (Fig. 17.10).

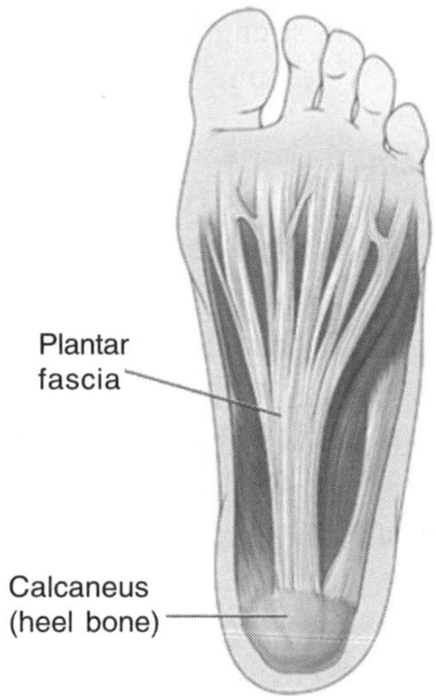

Fig. 17.10: Plantar fascia attachments

Each slip then divides in half to insert on the proximal phalanx of each toe. The central band only attaches to the calcaneum and the proximal phalanx of each toe. When the toes are extended, the plantar fascia is functionally shortened as it wraps around each metatarsal head. Hicks was the first to describe this functional shortening as 'windlass effect' of plantar fascia. The windlass effect can assist in supinating the foot during the later portion of the stance phase.

The most common site of abnormality in the individuals complaining of heel pain diagnosed as plantar fascitis is near the origin or enthesis of central band of plantar aponeurosis at the medial plantar tubercle of the calcaneum (Fig.17.11). On occasion, the individual will complain of pain and symptom in mid-portion of central band just prior to splitting into the five slips.

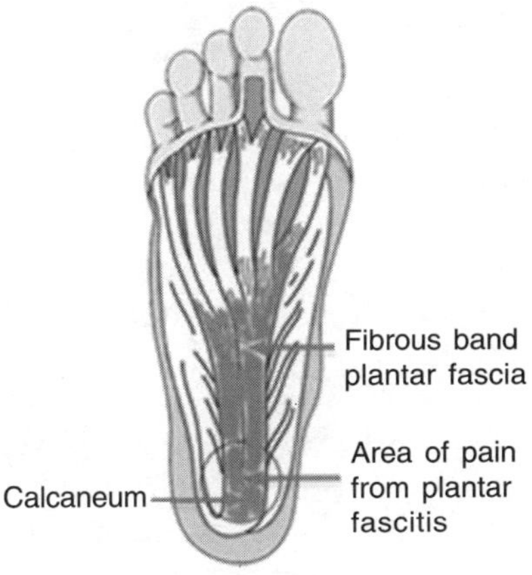

Fig. 17.11: Area of pain

Risk Factors

The specific cause of plantar fascitis is poorly understood and is multifactorial.

- Reduced ankle dorsiflexion.
- *Work related weight bearing:* Spending majority of workday on the feet.
- *Obesity:* Body mass index of greater than 30 kg/m^2.
- Decreased first metatarsophalangeal joint extension.

Diagnosis

The diagnosis of plantar fascitis is made with a reasonable level of certainty on the basis of clinical assessment alone:

- Patients report an insidious onset of pain under the plantar surface of the heel upon weight bearing after a prolonged period of non-weight bearing.
- The pain in plantar heel region is most noticeable in the morning with the first steps after waking or after a period of inactivity.
- In some cases, the pain is so severe that it results in an antalgic gait.
- The patient usually reports that heel pain will lessen with increasing levels of activity but tend to worsen towards the end of the day.
- The history usually indicates that there has been a recent change in activity level, such as increased distance with walking or running, or an employment change that required more time standing or walking.
- The patient will initially complain of sharp, localized pain under the anteromedial aspect of plantar surface of the heel.

Differential Diagnosis

The following differential diagnoses have been suggested for plantar heel pain:

- Calcaneal stress fracture.
- Bone bruise.
- Fat pad atrophy.
- Tarsal tunnel syndrome.
- Soft tissue, primary or metastatic bone tumors.
- Paget disease of bone.
- Sever's disease.
- Referred pain as a result of an S1 radiculopathy.

Examination

- *Active and Passive Ankle Dorsiflexion*
  The amount of active ankle dorsiflexion ROM is measured with knee extended. The patient is positioned in prone with feet over the edge of the treatment table. The examiner asks the patient to dorsiflex the ankle for an active measurement, or the examiner passively dorsiflexes the ankle, while ensuring that the foot does not evert or invert during the maneuver.
- *Windlass Test*
  Extension of the first metatarsophalangeal joint in both weight bearing and non-weight bearing causes windlass effect (Fig.17.12) of plantar fascia and is used to determine if the patient's heel pain is reproduced.
  - Non-weight bearing windlass test
    With the patient sitting, the examiner stabilizes the ankle joint in neutral with one hand placed just behind the first metatarsal head. The examiner then extends the first metatarso-

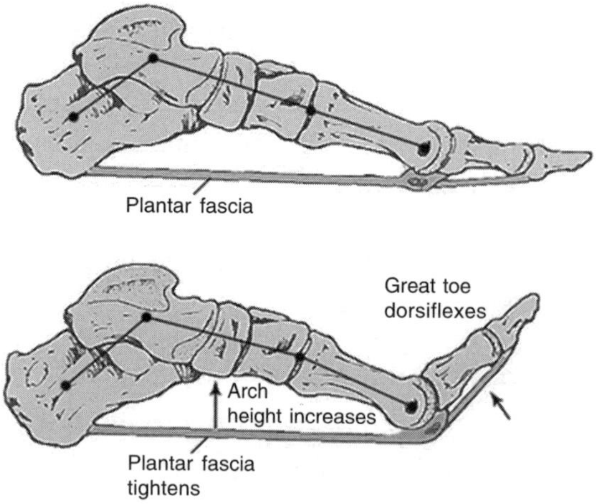

Fig. 17.12: Windlass effect

phalangeal joint (Fig.17.13), while allowing the interphalangeal joint to flex. Passive extension of the first MTP joint is continued to its end of range or until the patient's pain is reproduced.

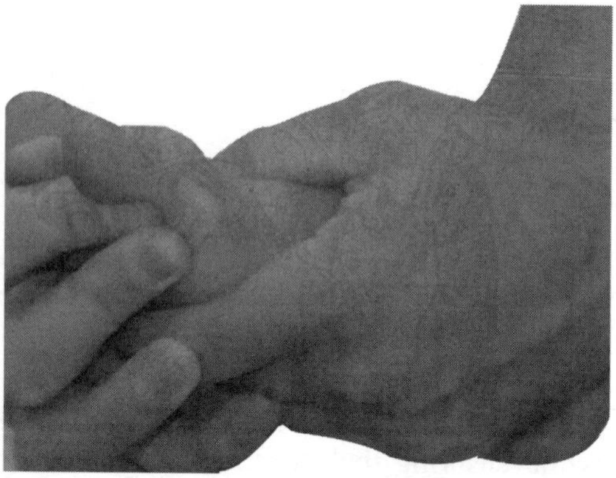

Fig.17.13: Non-weight bearing Windlass test

– Weight bearing windlass test
  The patient stands on a step stool and positions the metatarsal heads of the foot to be tested just over the edge of the step. The subject is instructed to place equal weight on both the feet. The examiner then passively extends the first MTP joint (Fig.17.14) allowing interphalangeal joint to flex. Passive extension of first MTP is continues to its end of range or until the patient's pain is reproduced.

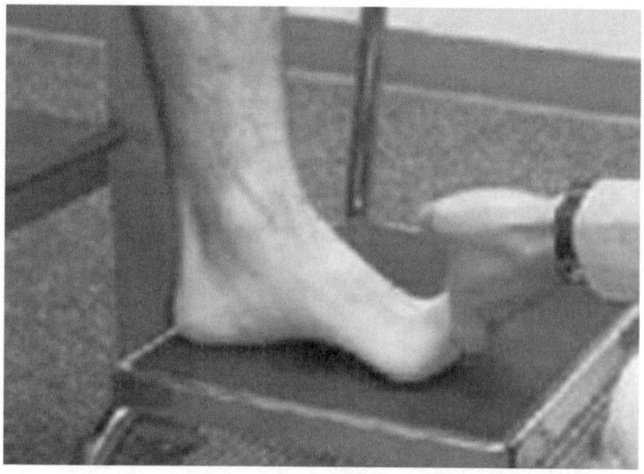

Fig. 17.14: Weight bearing windlass test

- *Longitudinal Arch Angle*
  The angle formed by a line projected from the medial malleolus to the navicular tuberosity in relation to second line projected from the most medial prominence of the first metatarsal head to the navicular tuberosity (Fig.17.15).

With the patient standing with equal weight on both feet, the midpoint of medial malleolus, the navicular tuberosity and the most medial prominence of the first metatarsal head are identified using palpation and marked with a pen. A goniometer is then used to measure the angle formed by the 3 points with navicular tuberosity acting as the axis point. The longitudinal arch angle provides a measure of foot structure and function that would be related to the development of plantar fascitis.

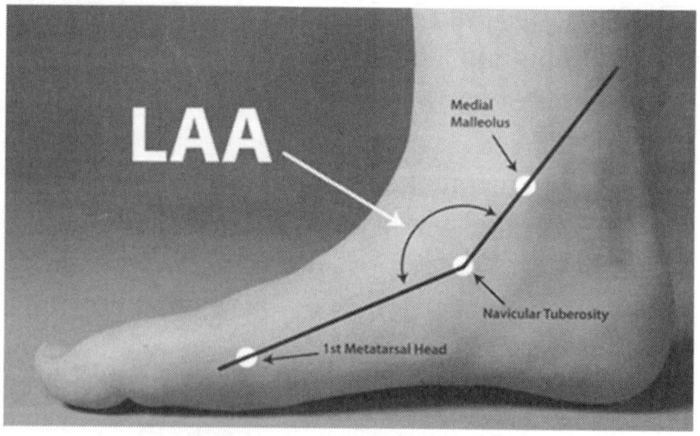

Fig.17.15: Longitudinal arch angle

Intervention

Numerous interventions have been described for the treatment of plantar fascitis, but few high qualities randomized controlled trials have been conducted to support these intervention therapies.

- *Medications:* Anti-inflammatory agents.
- *Modalities:* Iontophoresis using 0.4% dexamethasone sodium phosphate, 0.9% sodium chloride, 5% acetic acid provides short term (2 to 4 weeks) pain relief and improves function.
- *Manual Therapy:* There is minimal evidence to support the use of manual therapy and nerve mobilization procedures to provide short-term (1 to 3 months) pain relief and improved function. Suggested manual therapy procedures include:
  - Talocrural joint posterior glide.
  - Subtalar joint lateral glide.
  - Anterior and posterior glides of first metatarsophalangeal joint.
  - Subtalar joint distraction.
  - Subtalar joint mobilization.
  - Passive neural mobilization procedures.
- *Stretching*
  Calf muscle and/or plantar fascia specific stretching can be used to provide short-term (2 to 4 months) pain relief and improvement in flexibility. The dosage for stretching can be either 3 times or 2 times a day utilizing either a sustained (3 minutes) or intermittent (20 seconds) stretching time. The stretching could either be done passively by the therapist or actively by the patient himself. The method of active stretching should be taught to the patient and is as follows:
  - *Calf Muscle Stretching (Fig.17.16)*
    The continuity of connective tissue between the Achilles tendon and the plantar fascia as well as the fact that decreased ankle dorsiflexion is a risk factor in the development of plantar fascitis, provides justification for calf stretching. The calf stretch is performed in standing while leaning into the wall with the non-affected foot behind the leg being stretched.

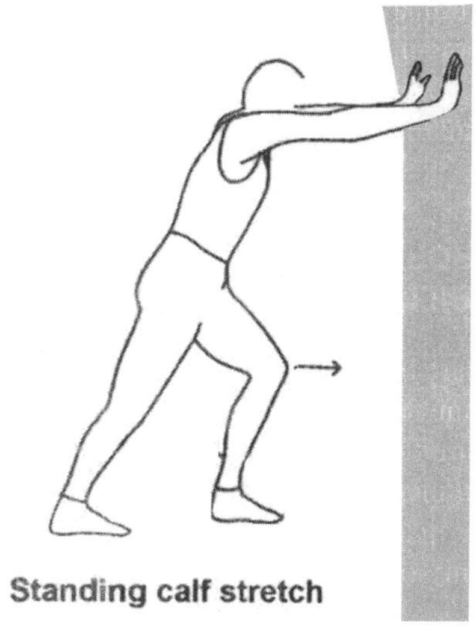

Fig.17.16: Calf Stretch

  - *Plantar Fascia Specific Stretch* (Fig. 17.17)
    The plantar fascia specific stretch is performed in sitting, with the patient placing the fingers of one hand across the toes of the involved foot, then pulling the toes back towards the shin until stretching is felt in arch

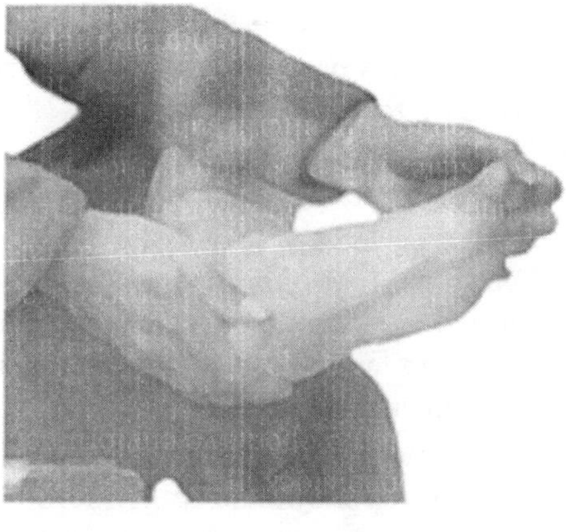

Fig.17.17: Plantar fascia stretch

- *Taping*
  Calcaneal or low dye taping (Fig.17.18) can be used to provide short-term (7 to 10 days) pain relief. Studies indicate that taping does cause improvement in function. The calcaneal taping procedure was designed to invert the calcaneus thus to improve biomechanical position.

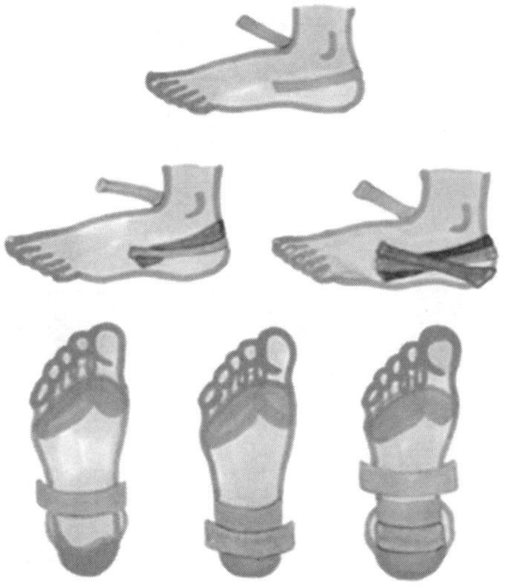

Fig. 17.18: Low dye taping

- *Orthotic Devices*
  Foot orthoses are frequently utilized as a component of the conservative management plan for plantar fascitis. The justification given for the use of foot orthoses is to decrease abnormal foot pronation that is thought to cause increased stress on the medial band of plantar fascia. Different orthoses used are:
  - Silicone heel pad (Fig. 17.19).
  - Felt arch insert (Fig. 17.20).
  - Rubber heel cup (Fig. 17.21).
  - Functional foot orthoses

Prefabricated or custom foot orthoses can be used to provide short term (3 months) reduction in pain and improvement in function.

- *Night Splints*
  Night splints should be considered as an intervention for patients with symptoms greater than 6 months in duration. The desired length of time for wearing the night splint is 1 to 3 months. The type of night splint used (posterior, anterior, sock-type) does not appear to affect the outcome.

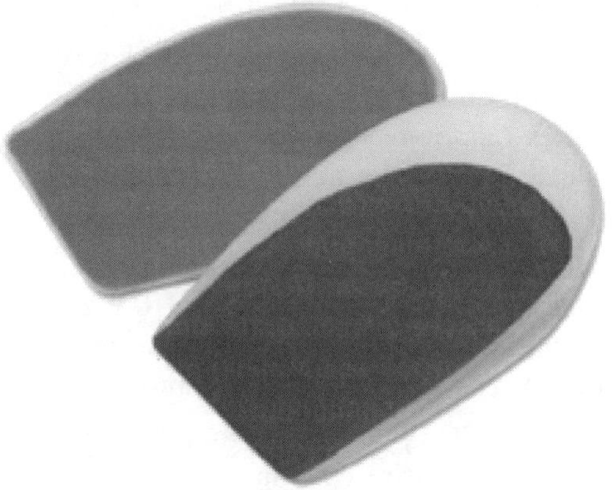

Fig. 17.19: Silicone heel pad

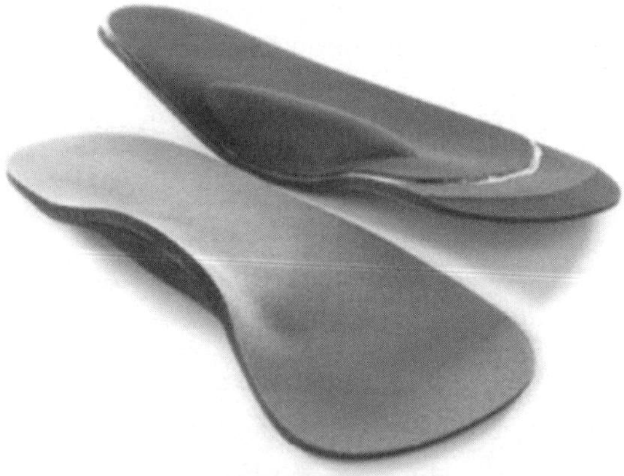

Fig. 17.20: Felt arch insert

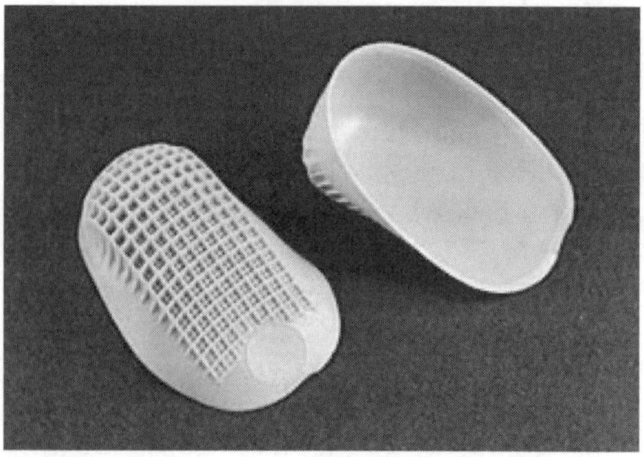

Fig. 17.21: Rubber heel cup

UNIT TEN

REPLACEMENT SURGERIES

CHAPTER 18

HIP REPLACEMENT

Hip replacement is a surgical procedure in which the hip joint is replaced by a prosthetic implant. Hip replacement surgery can be performed as a total replacement or a hemi replacement. A total hip replacement (total hip arthroplasty) consists of replacing both the components of hip joint i.e., acetabulum and the femoral head (Fig. 18.1) while hemiarthroplasty generally only replaces the femoral head with artificial component (prosthesis).

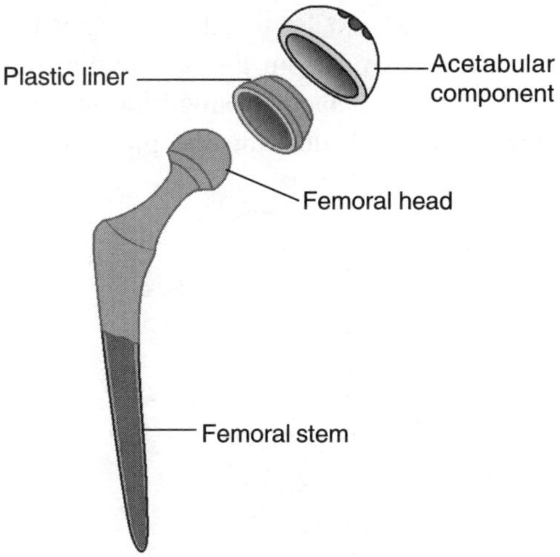

Fig. 18.1: Prosthetic components

INDICATIONS

- Incapacitating arthritis of hip either:
  - Osteoarthritis
  - Rheumatoid Arthritis
  - Traumatic Arthritis
  - Juvenile Rheumatoid Arthritis
- Avascular Necrosis
- Protrusio Acetabuli
- Certain Hip Fractures
- Benign And Malignant Bone Tumors
- Arthritis Associated with Paget's Disease
- Ankylosing Spondylitis

CONTRAINDICATIONS

- Overt or latent sepsis.

Types of Hip Replacement

Cemented Hip Replacement

In cemented hip replacement the prosthetic joint components i.e., acetabulum and/or femoral head is fixed with the help of bone cement, methyl methacrylate. It is usually indicated in elderly patients.

Uncemented Hip Replacement

No bone cement is required in this type of replacement surgery. It is usually indicated in younger patients.

Basic Surgical Approaches Used in Hip Replacement

There are several different incisions, defined by their relation to the gluteus medius. The approaches are:

- Posterior (Moore).
- Lateral (Hardinge or Liverpool).
- Antero-lateral (Watson-Jones).

- Anterior (Smith-Petersen).
- Greater trochanter osteotomy.

Posterior Approach

The posterior (Moore or southern) approach accesses the joint and capsule through the back, taking piriformis muscle and the short external rotators off the femur. This approach gives excellent access to the acetabulum and femur and preserves the hip abductors (gluteus medius) thus minimising the risk of abductor dysfunction post-operatively and facilitating early rehabilitation. It has the advantage of becoming a more extensile approach if needed. Immediate full weight bearing is allowed after the surgery. The movements of hip flexion, abduction and medial rotation should be strictly avoided for a period of six weeks post-operatively. The only disadvantage of posterior approach is that it is most vulnerable to dislocation.

Lateral Approach

The approach requires elevation of the hip abductors (gluteus medius and gluteus minimus) in order to access the joint. The abductors may be lifted up by osteotomy of the greater trochanter and reapplying it afterwards using wires (as per Charnley), or may be divided at their tendinous portion, or through the functional tendon (as per Hardinge) and repaired using sutures.

Antero-lateral Approach

The anterolateral approach develops the interval between the tensor fascia lata and the gluteus medius. It has an advantage of lower incidence of post-operative dislocation. Patient is allowed restricted weight bearing for six weeks. The movements of extension, adduction and lateral rotation should be restricted.

Anterior Approach

The anterior approach utilises an interval between the sartorius muscle and tensor fascia lata.

Minimally Invasive Approach

The double incision surgery and minimally invasive surgery seeks to reduce soft tissue damage through reducing the size of the incision. However, component positioning, accuracy and visualization of the bone structures is significantly impaired. This can result in unintended fractures and soft tissue injury. Surgeons using these approaches use intraoperative x-ray, fluoroscopy or computer guidance systems.

PROSTHESIS

Consideration About The Prosthesis Used

- Implant must be durable.
- It must permit slippery movement at the articulation.
- It must be firmly fixed to skeleton.
- It must be inert and do not provoke any unwanted reaction in the tissues.

Acetabular Cup

The acetabular cup (Fig. 18.2) is the component which is placed into the acetabulum . Cartilage and bone are removed from the acetabulum and the acetabular cup is attached using friction or cement. Some acetabular cups are one piece, others are modular.

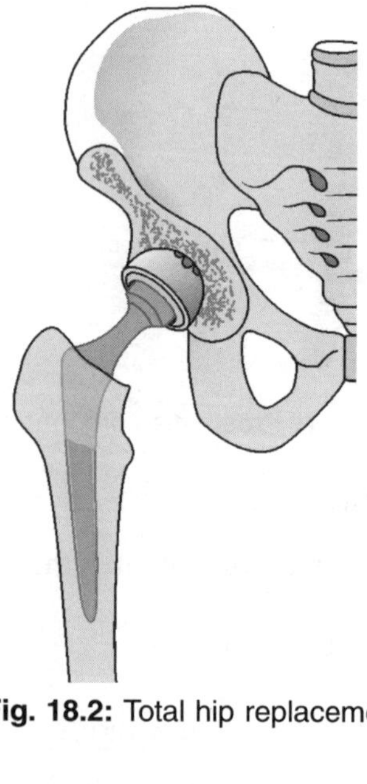

Fig. 18.2: Total hip replacement

One piece (monobloc) shells are either polyethylene or metal, they have their articular surface machined on the inside surface of the cup and do not rely on a locking mechanism to hold a liner in place. A monobloc polyethylene cup is cemented in place while a metal cup is held in place by a metal coating on the outside of the cup.

Modular cups consist of two pieces, a shell and liner. The shell is made of metal, the outside has a porous coating while the inside contains a locking mechanism designed to accept a liner. Two types of porous coating used to form a friction fit are sintered beads or a foam metal design to mimic the trabeculi of cancellous bone. Additional fixation is achieved as bone grows onto or into the porous coating. Screws can be used to lag the shell to the bone providing even more fixation. Polyethylene liners are placed into the shell and connected by a rim locking mechanism, ceramic and metal liners are attached with a morse taper.

Femoral Component

The femoral component is the component that fits in the femur. Bone is removed and the femur is shaped to accept the femoral stem with attached prosthetic femoral head (Fig. 18.2). There are two types of fixation: cemented and uncemented. Cemented stems use acrylic bone cement to form a mantle between the stem and to the bone. Uncemented stems use friction, shape and surface coatings to stimulate bone to remodel and bond to the implant. Stems are made of multiple materials (titanium, cobalt chromium and stainless steel) and they can be monolithic or modular.

Modular components consist of different head dimensions and/or modular neck orientations; these attach via a taper similar to a morse taper. These options allow for variability in leg length, offset and version.

Femoral heads are made of metal or ceramic material. Metal heads, made of cobalt chromium for hardness, are machined to size and then polished to reduce wear of the socket liner. Ceramic heads are more smooth than polished metal heads, have a lower coefficient of friction than a cobalt chrome head, and in theory will wear down the socket liner more slowly. Common sizes of femoral heads are 28 mm, 32 mm and 36 mm. While a 22.25 mm was common in the first modern prostheses, now even larger sizes are available 38–54+. Larger diameter heads lead to increased stability and range of motion whilst lowering the risk of dislocation. At the same time they also are subject to higher stresses such as friction and inertia.

Articular Interface

The articular interface is not actually part of the either implant, rather it is the area between the acetabular cup and femoral component. The articular interface of the hip is a simple ball and socket joint. Size, material properties and machining tolerances at the articular interface can be selected based on patient demand to optimise implant function and longevity whilst mitigating associated risks. The interface size is measured by the outside diameter of the head or the inside diameter of the socket.

Complications

- Deep vein thrombosis
- Dislocation
- Fracture
- Loosening
- Impingement
- Infection
- Osteolysis
- Metal sensitivity
- Nerve palsy
- Vascular injury
- Chronic pain
- Leg length inequality
- Death

Factors contributing to above mentioned complications:

- Previous hip surgery
- Severe deformity

- Lack of pre-operative training
- Inadequate bone stock
- Insufficient sterile operative enviornment

HEMIARTHROPLASTY

Hemiarthroplasty is a surgical procedure which replaces one half of the joint with an artificial surface and leaves the other part in its natural (pre-operative) state. This procedure is most commonly performed on the hip after a subcapital fracture of the femur. The procedure is performed by removing the head of the femur and replacing it with a metal or composite prosthesis. The most commonly used prosthesis designs are the Austin Moore prosthesis and the Thompson prosthesis. The bipolar prosthesis has not been shown to have any advantage over monopolar designs. The procedure is recommended only for elderly and frail patients.

HIP RESURFACING

Hip resurfacing is an alternative to hip replacement surgery. It is a bone conserving procedure that places a metal cap on the femoral head instead of amputating it. There is no long stem placed down the femur so it is more like a natural hip and may allow patients a return to many activities.

REHABILITATION AFTER TOTAL HIP ARTHROPLASTY

Goals

- To guard against dislocation of the implant.
- To prevent bedrest hazards.
- To obtain pain free range of motion within pain free limits.
- To strengthen hip and knee musculature.
- To teach independent transfers and ambulation.

Weight Bearing Status

Cemented Prosthesis

Weight bearing as tolerated by patient with walker for an initial period of 6 weeks, then use a cane in contralateral hand for 4-6 months.

Cementless Prosthesis

Toe touch weight bearing with walker for 6-8 weeks, then use a cane.

PHYSIOTHERAPY MANAGEMENT

The physiotherapy management of the patient undergoing total hip replacement is necessary not only post-operatively but it begins as soon as the patient is admitted in the hospital for surgery. Pre–operatively, it is important to discuss with the patient the post–operative regime to obtain a pain–free, mobile, stable and functionally acceptable hip joint.

Goals of physiotherapy management:

- To prevent post-operative complications.
- To gain pain free range of motion within permissible limit.
- To gain strength in hip and knee musculature.
- To teach independent transfers and ambulation.
- To gain functional strength.

Pre–operative Regime

The pre-operative regime includes evaluation of pre-operative status of the patient and education to the patient about the post-surgical complications, their prevention and the exercise regime to be followed during initial period.

Evaluation Includes

- Assessment of range of motion at hip joint and all the other lower extremity joints.
- Status of the muscles at involved hip: any atrophy if present.
- Evaluation of muscles strength.
- Detailed assessment of ambulation and gait.

Pre-Operative Education Includes

- Isometric exercise must be practiced for glutei, quadriceps and hamstrings to improve the strength and endurance which will help in post-operative period.

- Ankle pumps on the involved side to increase circulation and prevent post–operative complications.
- Deep breathing exercise and coughing are practised to avoid post–operative chest complications and improve vital capacity of lungs.
- Appropriate transfer techniques are taught to the patient pre–operatively so that patient can use it wisely.
- Range of motion and strengthening exercise which are required post operatively are taught on the sound limb.
- To facilitate early ambulation with walking aids, weight bearing muscles of the upper limb must be strengthened.
- Various precautionary measures that are needed to be followed by the patient post–operatively must be taught to the patient.

Precautions to be followed after Total Hip Replacement (Fig. 18.3)

- Avoid cross leg sitting.
- Do not use lower chair or toilet seat.
- While sitting on the chair, knees must be comfortably apart.

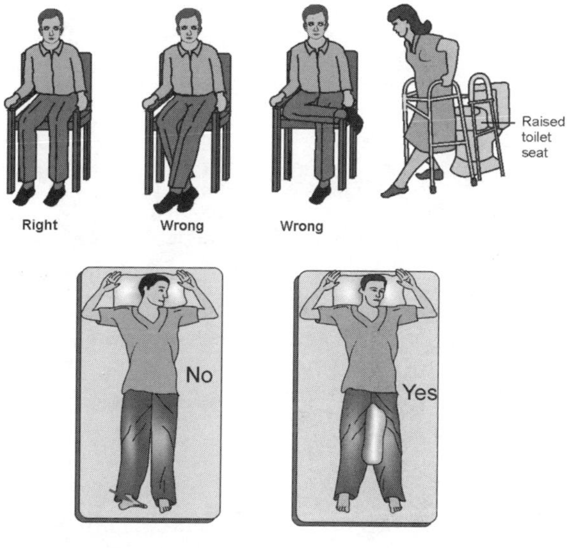

Fig. 18.3: Precautions after THR

- Never stand with toes turned in.
- While lying on your side, always place a pillow between your legs.
- Avoid flexion more than 80° at operated hip, so avoid touching your feet, pulling up pants, picking up something off the floor. Use of 'reaches" or 'grabbers' should be insisted.
- Supine lying must be a scheduled activity so as to avoid stiffness in the hip flexors.
- The patient must change the position quickly.
- Reclining sitting position must be taught to the patient.

Post-operative Regimen

Weight Bearing Status

Cemented Prosthesis: Patient is instructed to bear weight as tolerated on the operated extremity using walker for at least 6 weeks, followed by use of cane in the contralateral hand for 4 to 6 months.

Cementless Prosthesis: Patient is instructed for only touch down weight bearing with walker for initial 6 to 8 weeks, followed by use of cane in contralateral hand for 4 to 6 months.

Isometric Exercises

- Ankle pumps.
- Quadriceps isometric exercise sets.
- Gluteal isometric exercise sets.
- Isometrics to hip abductors in supine lying.

Stretching Exercises

- Initiate Thomas stretch 1 or 2 days post-operatively to stretch the anterior hip joint capsule and avoid flexion contracture of the operated hip.

Range of Motion Exercises

- Static bicycle with a raised seat can be used by the patient 4-7 days post-operatively. The seat may be progressively lowered within the safe parameters to enhance hip flexion.
- Hip abduction range of motion exercise in supine can be initiated 1-week post-operatively.

- Hip abduction range of motion exercise in side lying or standing can be initiated 5-6 weeks post-operatively.
- Prone lying hip extension should be practised.
- Hip flexion in the form of straight leg raising within the permissible limits should be performed with the contralateral hip and knee flexed.

Strengthening Exercises

- Continue with the isometric set of exercises.
- Hip abductors strengthening using therabands in supine lying and weight cuffs in side lying or standing must be practised.
- Gluteal strengthening in prone position with knee in flexion to isolate gluteus maximus and with knee extension for strengthening of both hamstrings and gluteus maximus must be practised.

Gait Rehabilitation

Gait rehabilitation is important at every phase, with assistive devices or during independent ambulation.Observation of faults or substitution while walking is important for correct gait re-education. Proper heel-toe pattern should be taught to the patient and made to practice. Hip abductor strengthening plays a very important role to avoid limp during walking.

Ascending and descending stairs should be taught to the patient initially with the use of assistive devices and railing followed by independent practice.

CHAPTER 19

KNEE REPLACEMENT

Knee replacement, or knee arthroplasty, is a surgical procedure to replace the weight-bearing surfaces of the knee joint to relieve the pain and disability.

Knee replacement surgery can be performed as a partial or a total knee replacement. In general, the surgery consists of replacing the diseased or damaged joint surfaces of the knee with metal and plastic components shaped to allow continued motion of the knee.

The operation involves substantial postoperative pain, and includes vigorous physical rehabilitation. The recovery period may be 6 weeks or longer and may involve the use of mobility aids (e.g. walking frames, canes, crutches).

TECHNIQUE

The surgery involves exposure of the front of the knee, with detachment of vastus medialis from the patella. The patella is displaced to one side of the joint allowing exposure of the distal end of the femur and the proximal end of the tibia. The ends of these bones are then accurately cut to shape using cutting guides oriented to the long axis of the bones. The cartilages and the anterior cruciate ligament are removed; the posterior cruciate ligament may also be removed but the tibial and fibular collateral ligaments are preserved. Metal components are then impacted onto the bone or fixed using polymethyl-methacrylate (PMMA) cement. Alternative techniques exist that affix the implant without cement. These cementless techniques may involve osseointegration, including porous metal prostheses.

A round ended implant is used for the femur, mimicking the natural shape of the bone. On the tibia the component is flat, although it often has a stem which goes down inside the bone for further stability. A flattened or slightly dished high density polyethylene surface is then inserted onto the tibial component so that the weight is transferred from metal to plastic not metal to metal (Fig 19.1). During the operation any deformities must be corrected, and the ligaments balanced so that the knee has a good range of movement and is stable. In some cases the articular surface of the patella is also removed and replaced by a polyethylene button cemented to the posterior surface of the patella. In other cases, the patella is replaced unaltered.

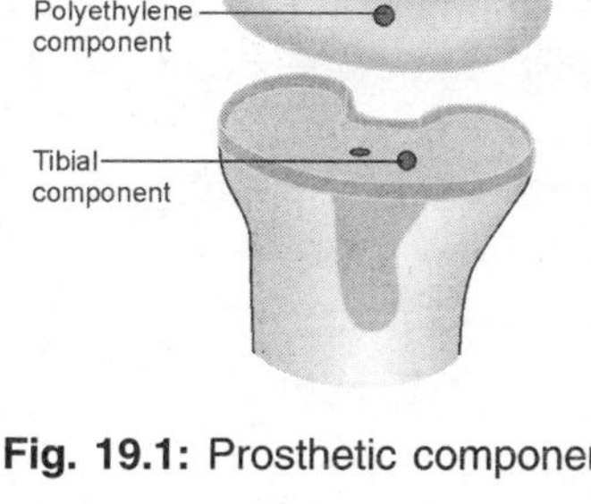

Fig. 19.1: Prosthetic components

Partial Knee Replacement

Unicompartmental arthroplasty, also called partial knee replacement is an option for some patients. The knee is generally divided into three "compartments": medial, lateral, and patellofemoral. Most patients with arthritis severe enough to consider knee replacement have significant wear in two or more of the above compartments and are best treated with total knee replacement. A minority of patients have wear confined primarily to one compartment, usually the medial, and may be candidates for unicompartmental knee replacement. Advantages include smaller incision, easier post-operative rehabilitation, better post-operative ROM, shorter hospital stay, less blood loss, lower risk of infection, stiffness, and blood clots, and easier revision if necessary.

Risks and Complications

Risks and complications in knee replacement are similar to those associated with all joint replacements. The most serious complication is infection of the joint, which occurs in <1% of patients. Deep vein thrombosis occurs in up to 15% of patients, and is symptomatic in 2-3%. Nerve injuries occur in 1-2% of patients. Persistent pain or stiffness occurs in 8-23% of patients. Prosthesis failure occurs in approximately 2% of patients at 5 years.

Deep Vein Thrombosis

According to the American Academy of Orthopedic Surgeons (AAOS), deep vein thrombosis is the most common complication of knee replacement surgery. Deep vein thrombosis occurs in up to 15% of patients, and is symptomatic in 2-3%. Physiotherapist can outline a prevention program, which may include periodic elevation of legs, lower leg exercises to increase circulation and support stockings.

Fractures

Periprosthetic fractures are becoming more frequent with the aging patient population and can occur intraoperatively or postoperatively.

Loss of Motion

The knee at times may not recover its normal range of motion (0 - 135 degrees) after total knee replacement. Much of this is dependent on pre-operative function. Most patients can achieve 0 - 110 degrees, but stiffness of the joint can occur. In some situations, manipulation of the knee under anaesthesia is used to improve post operative stiffness. There are also many implants from manufacturers that are designed to be "high-flex" knees, offering a greater range of motion.

Instability

In some patients, the patella is unstable post-surgically and dislocates laterally. This is painful and usually needs to be treated by surgery to realign the kneecap. However this is quite rare.

Implant Loosening

In the past, there was a considerable risk of the implant components loosening over time as a result of wear. As medical technology has improved however, this risk has fallen considerably. Knee replacement implants can now last up to 20 years.

Infection

The most serious complication is infection of the joint, which occurs in <1% of patients. While it is relatively rare, periprosthetic infection remains one of the most challenging complications of joint arthroplasty. A detailed clinical history and physical examination remains the most reliable tool to recognize a potential periprosthetic infection. In some cases the classic signs of fever, chills, painful joint, and a draining sinus may be present, and diagnostic studies are simply done to confirm the diagnosis. In reality though, most patients do not present with those clinical signs, and in fact the clinical presentation may overlap with other complications such as aseptic loosening. In those cases diagnostic tests can be useful in confirming or excluding infection.

Rehabilitation after Total Knee Replacement

Weight Bearing Status

The weight bearing status of the patient postoperatively depends upon the type of prosthesis used i.e. cemented or non-cemented.

- In case of cemented prosthesis, patient is allowed to bear comfortable weight on the affected foot but walking aid must be used to share the weight.
- In case of non-cemented prosthesis, patient is allowed to do only toe touch weight bearing on the affected limb for a period of 4-6 weeks.

Physical Therapy Evaluation

The therapist must evaluate the affected limb for the following both pre and post-operatively. This evaluation will affect the treatment protocol of the patient. Following need to be evaluated:

- *Posture:* The patient is assisted for the alignment of low back, pelvis, knee and ankle as all of these in combination will affect the status of the knee.
- *Swelling:* Careful observation must be made to assess the swelling around the knee and the ipsilateral ankle and foot.
- *Atrophy:* The patient is assured for the atrophy or wasting of the affected quadriceps muscles by comparing it to the contralateral limb.
- *Range of Motion:* The affected knee joint is examined for the range of motion both flexion and extension. Patellar mobility must also be examined.
- *Gait Analysis*
- *Muscle Strength:* The strength of the muscles around the knee especially quadriceps and hamstrings must be assessed pre and post-operatively. The muscles around the hip and ankle must also be assessed.
- *Girth Measurement:* It is important, as the girth is an indication of swelling or atrophy when compared to the contralateral limb. The girth measurement is done around thigh, knee and the calf area.

Physiotherapeutic Intervention

The following physiotherapy interventions should be used post-operatively.

- *To Ease Pain:* It is important to take rest immediately after the surgery. The patient is advised to avoid all the movements and the activities that increase pain. Use of walker must be advocated during ambulation. The patient must put the right amount of weight through affected limb as directed.Immediately post-operatively ice can be used as an important adjunct to control pain and inflammation. Ice could be used either as ice packs or ice massage for a period of 10-15 min.
- *To control Swelling:* Following are the modalities that are used to control swelling:
  - Massage
  - Cold whirlpool treatment
  - Compression therapy
  - Electrical stimulation

  The most beneficial combination to reduce swelling is cold compression and elevation.
- *To improve Range of Motion:* Following are the techniques that are used to improve range of motion at the operated knee joint.
  - Graded joint mobilization
  - Patellar mobilization
  - Continuous Passive Motion (CPM)
  - Manual Stretching
- *Gait Training:* Gait training is important post-operatively for the patient either using the assistive devices or bearing full weight on the operative leg to prevent antalgic gait.

Aquatic Therapy

While the patient is in water, it is easier to begin walking with less stress on knee. The properties of buoyancy and warmth will ease the movement and could give resistance to some exercise. The warmth of the water relaxes the muscles, improves circulation and eases soreness.

Muscle Strengthening Exercises

Post-operatively the affected muscles may respond in the following manner:

- *Muscle weakness:* Especially the quadriceps muscle is weakened.
- *Muscle imbalance:* The muscles lengthened become weak and the muscles that are stronger become shortened. The following intervention could be used to strengthen the weakened muscles:
- *Biofeedback:* Muscle control is the basis of strength so biofeedback is used to gain control of quadriceps muscle. If could also set to alert the patient if other muscles are overpowering the weak muscles and to know if the patient is actually working the right muscle.
- *Functional Electrical Stimulation:* By functional electrical stimulation the muscles are artificially stimulated and the patient is asked to contract the muscles when the current is on. It is specially used for deconditioned muscle.
- *Progressive Resistive Exercises (PRE):* In PRE graded resistance is applied to the muscle group to gain endurance and strength. These exercises typically start with lighter weight-more repetitions progressing to more amount of weight with lesser repetitions. Following techniques are used.
  - Pulley system
  - Rubber tubing
  - Free weights
  - Manual resistance
  - Computerized exercises device
- Balance Training

REHABILITATION PROTOCOL AFTER TOTAL KNEE ARTHROPLASTY

Day 1–Day 10

Goals of Treatment

- Control of swelling and inflammation
- Active quadriceps muscle contraction
- Improving knee flexion upto 90° and knee extension to 0°
- Development of isometric control
- Independent ambulation

Physiotherapy Intervention

Day 1-Day 2

- Cryotherapy to control inflammation
- Adequate chest physiotherapy
- Prophylactic measures must be taken to prevent deep vein thrombosis
- Knee flexion to 40°
- The patient must use assistive device during ambulation
- Ankle pumps with leg elevated
- Passive knee extension exercises: 90° -30° of knee extension
- Isometric quadriceps exercises

Day 4–Day 10

- Continue the use of cryotherapy to control inflammation
- Weight bearing as tolerated by the patient
- Patient is allowed to do safe ambulation and must be instructed while doing transfers.
- Continuous passive motion (CPM) must permit knee flexion to 90°
- Practice the following exercises
  - Ankle pumps with legs elevated
  - Quadriceps isometric exercises
  - Straight leg raises
  - Hip abduction-adduction
  - Passive knee extension strength: 90°-0° of knee extension
  - Active-assistive knee flexion

Week 2–Week 6

Goals of Treatment

- To reduce swelling and inflammation
- To improve range of motion
- To develop muscular strength and endurance
- To enhance dynamic joint stability
- To establish patient's return to functional activities

Outline of Rehbilitation of Total Knee Replacement

Pre-operative	• Education on surgical process and outcomes • Instructions of post operative exercise program • Assessment of home environment
• Post-op Day 1	• Bed side exercise: ankle pumps, quadriceps sets, gluteal sets • Review weight bearing status • Bed mobility and transfer training
• Post-op Day 2	• Exercises for active assistive and active range of motion • Terminal knee extension exercises • Patellar mobilization • Strengthening exercises: ankle pumps quadriceps sets, gluteal sets, isometric hip adduction, heal slides • Gait training with assistive with device and functional transfer training
• Post-op Day 3-5	• Progression of range of motion and strengthening exercises to patient's tolerance • Progression of ambulation on level surfaces with least assistive devices • Progression of ADL training
• Post-op Day 5-4 weeks	• Strengthening exercises: Seated leg extension, knee bends, short arc quadriceps • Stretching of quadriceps and hamstrings • Progression of ambulation distance • Progression of independence in ADL

Physiotherapy Intervention

Week 2–Week 4

- If inflammation still persists cryotherapy can be used.
- Patient is allowed to ambulate with assistive devices.
- Patient is allowed to do stationary bicycle to improve knee range of motion.
- The knee extension must be practiced from 90°-0° with stress on terminal knee extension 45°-0°
- Hip movements of flexion-extension and abduction-adduction must be practiced.
- Hamstring curls are initiated.
- Isometric quadriceps exercises.
- Stretching to hamstrings, gastrocsoleus and quadriceps.
- Squats (mini) are initiated.

Week 4–Week 6

Same program as for week 2-Week 4 must be continued, with following additions.

- Aquatic therapy must be started.
- Front lunges are initiated.

Week 7–Week 12

Goals of Treatment

- To increase knee range of motion from 110° to above.
- To improve strength and endurance
- To enhance functional activity of the patient.

Physiotherapy Intervention

- Emphasize upon eccentric concentric control of the knee.
- The patient must be encouraged to do progressive walking.
- Lunges, squats and step-ups to a greater height can be initiated.

CHAPTER 20

SHOULDER REPLACEMENT

TOTAL SHOULDER ARTHROPLASTY

Total shoulder replacement or arthroplasty involves replacement of both the components (humeral head and glenoid cavity) of shoulder joint by prosthetic material. It is considered to improve overall functions regardless of pain levels experienced by the patient.

Indications

- Severe pain
- Loss of motion
- Stiffness
- Arthritis
- Degenerative joint disease

Goals

- The primary goal of the procedure is pain relief to the patient.
- The secondary goals of the procedure are to restore motion, strength and function of the affected shoulder joint.

Contraindications

- Active infection.
- Loss or paralysis of both rotator cuff and deltoid muscles.
- Disease of the nervous system affecting the shoulder joint.

Anaesthesia

Patient can be operated either under the regional anaesthesia with interscalene block or general anaesthesia depending upon the discretion of the surgeon. The patient is in a breech chair position during surgery.

Implant Materials (Fig 20.1)

Affected humeral head is replaced with a metal (cobalt chrome) ball component with a stem (titanium metal) that extends down into the humerus distal to the head component. The stem component is cemented only if the fitting is not exact. In most of the cases stem is uncemented that promotes natural bone growth (ingrowth) into the material.

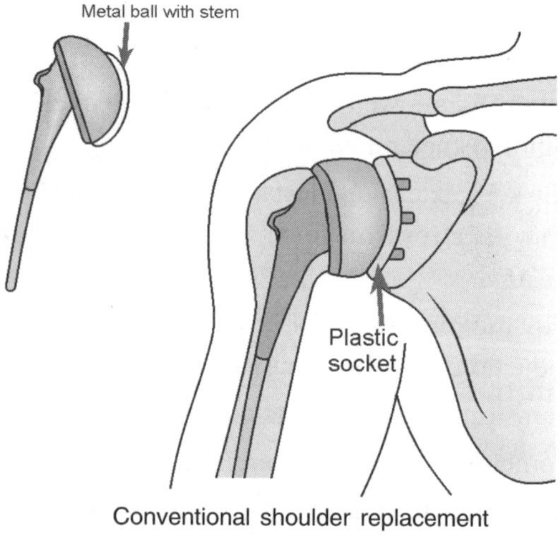

Fig. 20.1: Implants used in total shoulder arthroplasty

Procedure

The patient is either under general or regional anaesthesia. The surgeon adopts an anterior approach to the shoulder joint from a nerve free area to minimize the nerve damage. Incision is given in the rotator cuff muscles along with separation of the deltoid and pectorals. This is followed by the removal of the damaged parts and replacing them with prosthetic components.

Post surgically the extremity is immobilized in a sling with arm by the side. Immediate X-rays are taken to document the position of implants.

Rehabilitation

Shoulder is the most unstable joint in the body and therefore rehabilitation plan has to prevent shoulder dislocation and stress on the repaired tendons. The pre-surgical condition of the shoulder muscles and tendons plays an important role in patient's outcome. If tendons and muscles are in good shape, rehabilitation will be minimal.

Phase I: Immediate post-surgical (0-3 weeks)

Goals

- To reduce pain and inflammation.
- To allow healing of soft tissues.
- To maintain joint integrity.
- To prevent muscular inhibition.
- To restore active range of motion of elbow, wrist and hand of the involved extremity.
- To increase passive range of motion of the shoulder.
- To restore independence in activities of daily living with modification.

Precautions

- Keep the incision dry and clean.
- Full time sling wearing is necessary for first week post operatively and then gradual weaning off.
- In supine lying place a small cushion or towel roll behind the elbow to avoid scapular hyperextension and stretch to anterior capsule or subscapularis.
- Do not support body weight on the involved extremity.

Interventions

Day 1

- Education to the patient regarding proper joint positioning and protection techniques.
- Frequent cryotherapy sessions to reduce pain and inflammation.
- Pendular exercises to the involved shoulder.
- Active exercises to the elbow, wrist and hand of the involved extremity.
- Passive shoulder exercises in supine lying:
  - Passive forward flexion as tolerated.
  - External rotation in scapular plane upto 30º.
  - Passive internal rotation to chest.

Day 2–Day 10

- Continue cryotherapy.
- Continue above mentioned exercises.
- Initiate active assisted elbow range of motion.
- Assisted shoulder exercises:
  - Assisted flexion and abduction in shoulder plane.
  - Assisted external rotation.
  - Pulley exercises for flexion and abduction.
- Initiate isometrics for scapular musculature.
- Initiate sub-maximal pain free shoulder isometrics in neutral position.

Day 10–Day 21

- Continue previous exercises.
- Restore active elbow range of motion.
- Strengthening of the distal musculature of the involved extremity.
- Progression to active-assisted motion in pain free ranges.
- Progress passive range of motion as the motion allows.

Phase II: Weeks 3–6

Criteria for Progression to Phase II

- Tolerance to passive range of motion program.
- Patient must atleast have the following passive range of motion at the operated joint:
  - 90^0 of flexion and abduction.
  - 45° of external rotation and 70° of internal rotation in plane of scapula.
- Ability of the patient to isometrically activate the shoulder and scapular musculature.

Goals

- To control pain and inflammation.
- To allow healing of soft tissues.
- To restore and progress active and passive range of motion.
- To re-establish dynamic shoulder stability.

Intervention

Week 3
- Continue use of cryotherapy.
- Continue exercises for active-assisted and passive range of motion.
- Continue exercises for shoulder and scapular musculature.
- Initiate assisted horizontal adduction.
- Initiate gentle joint mobilization.
- Initiate rhythmic stabilization.

Week 4–6
- Wean off the sling completely.
- Initiate active forward flexion, internal rotation, external rotation and abduction in pain free ranges in supine lying.
- Initiate isometrics for rotator cuff and peri-scapular muscles.
- Progression of scapular strengthening exercises.

Phase III: Week 6-12

Criteria for Progression to Phase III

- Tolerance of active assisted and passive range of motion.
- Tolerance to isometric exercises.
- Patient must atleast have following passive range of motion at the operated shoulder joint:
  - 140° of flexion and 120° of abduction.
  - 60° of external rotation and 70° of internal rotation in scapular plane.

Goals

- Gradual restoration of strength, power and endurance of shoulder muscles.
- Optimize neuromuscular control.
- Gradual return to functional activities with involved upper extremity.

Intervention

Week 6–8
- Increase anti-gravity forward flexion and abduction.
- Active internal rotation and external rotation in scapular plane.
- Advance passive range of motion as tolerated.
- Initiate light stretching exercises at the operated joint as tolerated.
- Initiate internal rotation behind the back.
- Initiate light functional activities.

Week 8-10
- Initiate anterior deltoid strengthening (progressive supine active elevation) with light weights.

Week 10-12
- Progress strengthening of internal and external rotators.
- Progress internal rotation behind back from active assisted to active range of motion.
- Initiate resisted flexion, abduction and external rotation with thera bands/sports cords.

Phase IV: Beyond 12 weeks

Criteria for Progression to Phase IV

- Patient must atleast have following active range of motion at affected shoulder:
  - 140° of flexion and 120° of abduction in supine.
  - 60° of external rotation and 70° of internal rotation in scapular plane.

Goals

- Maintain full non-painful active range of motion.
- Improve muscular strength, power and endurance.
- Gradual return to more advanced functional activities.
- Progression to closed chain exercises.

Intervention

- Gradual progression of strengthening program.
- Gradual return to moderately challenging functional activities.
- Return to recreational activities.

REVERSE SHOULDER ARTHROPLASTY

This is indicated in deficient rotator cuff shoulder in which traditional shoulder arthroplasty has been less than optimal due to loss of force coupling of supraspinatus-deltoid complex resulting in a rocking horse phenomenon (proximal subluxation of humeral head on glenoid rim), contributing to loosening of glenoid component and at times prosthetic failure.

In reverse shoulder arthroplasty, a ball like convex surface replaces the glenoid cavity and the humeral head is replaced by glenoid like concave surface (Fig. 20.2). This provides stability and creates increase moment arm of deltoid and prevent superior migration of humeral head.

Indications

- Severe osteoarthritis or rheumatoid arthritis with massive irrepairable rotator cuff tear.
- Comminuted proximal humeral fracture with tuberosity malposition and non-union.
- Failure of traditional arthroplasty.
- Failed rotator cuff surgery with antero-superior shoulder instability and superior migration of humeral head.
- Following surgery of proximal humerus tumors with associated rotator cuff resection.

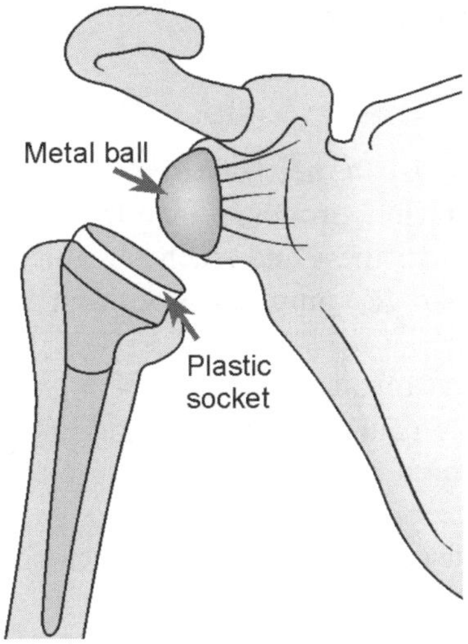

Reverse total shoulder replacement

Fig. 20.2: Implants used in reverse shoulder arthroplasty

Goals

- Improvement in range of motion (active lateral rotation may be limited long term without an intact teres minor).
- Improvement in function below shoulder height (scapular substitution may be necessary for functions above shoulder height).
- Improvement in functions for lighter activities above shoulder height).

Physiotherapy Intervention

Education to the patient

Patient has to be educated about long term joint protection measures in order to prevent instability or prosthetic failure. Patient has to avoid contact sports and high demand leisure activities.

Physiotherapy intervention depends upon

- Level of pain
- Stage of post-operative recovery
- Associated soft tissue repairs
- Associated medical conditions

Phase I: Weeks 2–4

Goals

- To emphasize the need of active participation in rehabilitation processs in oder to prevent excessive stiffness and reach functional goals.
- To encourage compliance without immobilization.
- To protect repair.
- To reduce pain and oedema.
- To promote normal elbow, wrist and hand motion.
- To initiate gentle pain free shoulder passive range of motion.
- To educate the patient regarding transfers.

Precautions

- No active range of motion.
- No strengthening and resistive exercises.

Intervention

- Address postural impairments of scapula and thoracic spine.
- Pendular exercises within 24 to 48 hours.
- Initiate active assisted range of motion in supine to assume good scapular stabilization using the uninvolved arm for guidance and support and progress to passive range of motion.
- Limit external rotation to less than 30^0 , flexion $<120^0$, abduction $< 45^0$ as there is no rotator cuff integrity.
- Address limitation of periscapular muscle length and trunk immobility.
- Address limitation of range of motion in distal upper extremity.

Phase II: Weeks 4-6

Goals

- Continue joint protection education.
- Initiate glenohumeral joint mobility primarily in elevation.
- Improve passive range of motion into full external rotation in neutral, elevation $< 140^0$, internal rotation as tolerated.

Precautions

- No strengthening or resistive exercises.
- No forceful stretching or passive range of motion.

Intervention

- Continue joint protection education.
- Encourage natural arm swing.
- Encourage the functional use of affected arm for activities of daily living (ADL) and instructional ADLs.
- Initiate anti-gravity active range of motion exercises in elevation, external rotation, internal rotation and adduction.

Phase III: Weeks 8-12

Goals

- Increase glenohumeral joint mobility primarily in elevation and external rotation.
- Progressive strengthening of shoulder girdle musculature particularly deltoid.

Precautions

- No weight lifting above shoulder height.
- Avoid overloading to teres minor while performing strengthening exercises.

Intervention

- Strengthening exercises for improving deltoid muscle balance and functional strength using:
  - Low resistance thera-bands
  - Light weights
  - Pool exercise program
- Progression from sub-maximal isometrics to limited range to full range isotonics.
- Encourage resisted exercises below shoulder height.

INDEX

T

W